Forensic Toxicology

A Comparative Approach

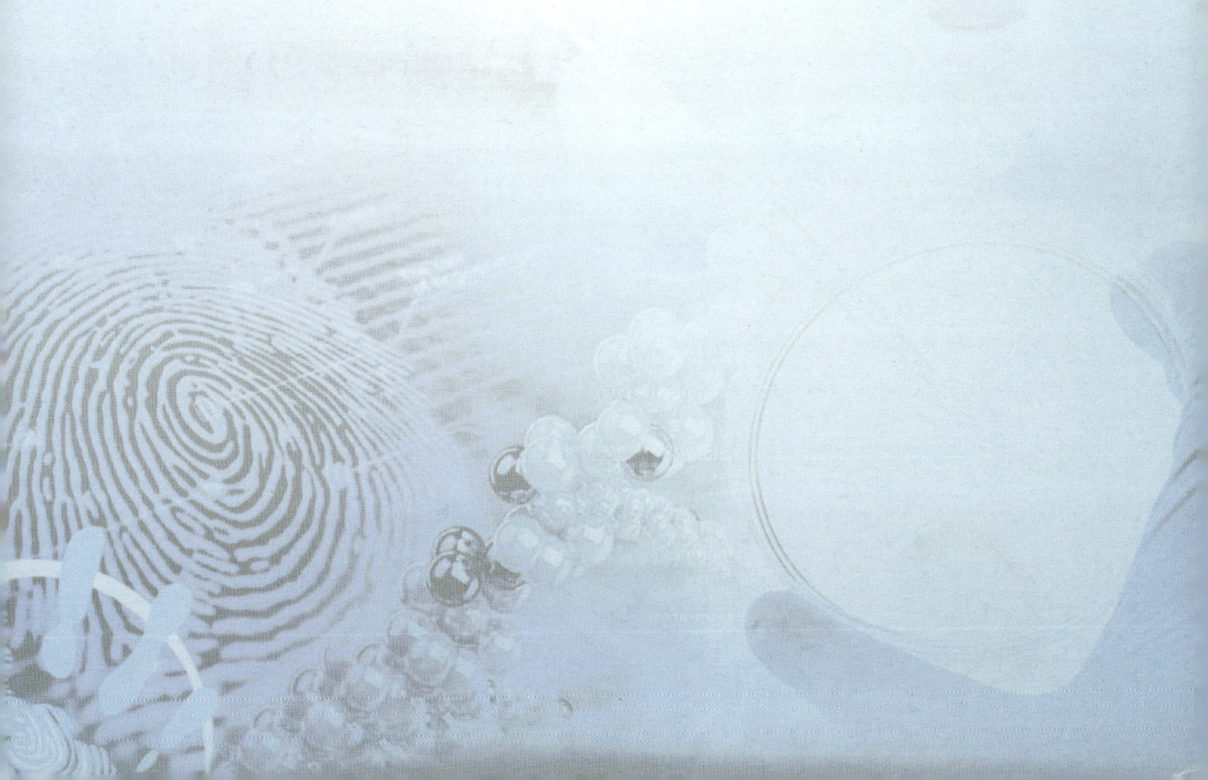

Forensic Toxicology

A Comparative Approach

Vipul Ambade MBBS, MD, LLB
Associate Professor
Department of Forensic Medicine
Government Medical College
Nagpur, Maharashtra

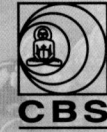

CBS

CBS Publishers & Distributors Pvt Ltd

New Delhi • Bengaluru • Chennai • Kochi • Kolkata • Mumbai
Hyderabad • Nagpur • Patna • Pune • Vijayawada

Forensic Toxicology
A Comparative Approach

ISBN: 978-81-239-2932-3

First Edition: 2016

Published by Satish Kumar Jain and produced by Varun Jain for
CBS Publishers & Distributors Pvt Ltd
4819/XI Prahlad Street, 24 Ansari Road, Daryaganj, New Delhi 110 002, India.
Ph: 23289259, 23266861, 23266867   Website: www.cbspd.com
Fax: 011-23243014   e-mail: delhi@cbspd.com; cbspubs@airtelmail.in.
Corporate Office: 204 FIE, Industrial Area, Patparganj, Delhi 110 092
Ph: 4934 4934   Fax: 4934 4935   e-mail: publishing@cbspd.com; publicity@cbspd.com

Branches

- **Bengaluru:** Seema House 2975, 17th Cross, K.R. Road, Banasankari 2nd Stage, Bengaluru 560 070, Karnataka
  Ph: +91-80-26771678/79   Fax: +91-80-26771680   e-mail: bangalore@cbspd.com

- **Chennai:** 7, Subbaraya Street, Shenoy Nagar, Chennai 600 030, Tamil Nadu
  Ph: +91-44-26680620, 26681266   Fax: +91-44-42032115   e-mail: chennai@cbspd.com

- **Kochi:** Ashana House, No. 39/1904, AM Thomas Road, Valanjambalam, Ernakulam 682 018, Kochi, Kerala
  Ph: +91-484-4059061-65   Fax: +91-484-4059065   e-mail: kochi@cbspd.com

- **Kolkata:** 6/B, Ground Floor, Rameswar Shaw Road, Kolkata-700 014, West Bengal
  Ph: +91-33-22891126, 22891127, 22891128   e-mail: kolkata@cbspd.com

- **Mumbai:** 83-C, Dr E Moses Road, Worli, Mumbai-400 018, Maharashtra
  Ph: +91-22-24902340/41   Fax: +91-22-24902342   e-mail: mumbai@cbspd.com

Representatives

- **Hyderabad** 0-9885175004   • **Nagpur** 0-9021734563   • **Patna** 0-9334159340
- **Pune**   0-9623451994   • **Vijayawada** 0-9000660880

Printed at Rashtriya Printers, Delhi-110095

to

---

my parent
Late Shri Namdeorao Ambade
and
Smt Chandraprabha Ambade

Preface

It is a great pleasure that I am presenting the book *Forensic Toxicology: A Comparative Approach*. Taking into the consideration that toxicology is very vast and difficult to remember, this book is presented in a simple and lucid language. The most important distinguishing feature of this book is that the different poisons of a group are discussed in a comparative point-wise manner in a tabular form for better understanding, learning and easy comparison. Apart from the numerous tabular charts, more than 180 photographs and figures related to poison/autopsy findings are included in this book. A separate chapter on preservation of viscera and other materials containing guidelines for collection, preservation and dispatch; and a new chapter on biological and chemical warfare are also included. Latest trends in the management of poisoning cases have been tried to cover in the book.

While preparing this book, I have gone through various textbooks and journals, and I am indebted to these authors. This book is primarily designed for undergraduate students and I hope it will make toxicology easier for students to learn and study. It will surely help the postgraduate students in preparing for examination and prove useful to the medical officers/practitioners while dealing the case of poisoning. I would definitely welcome the valuable suggestion and healthy criticism, which will be of immense help for future improvement of this book.

Vipul Ambade

vipulambade@rediffmail.com

Acknowledgments

I began my career in forensic medicine about 20 years back under the guidance of my teacher Dr AC Mohanty, a man with great vision and tremendous knowledge. While working with him, he not only made me realize the importance of the subject but also changed my outlook towards the dead victim. I gratefully acknowledge him for his guidance and influence which made me to persist my career in forensic.

It is with a great pleasure and deep sense of gratitude that I acknowledge my debt to my respected teacher Dr AP Dongre (Ex-Dean, Government Medical College, Yeotmal) for his affectionate guidance and constant support.

I am indebted to my revered teacher Dr AN Keoliya (Dean, Government Medical College, Gondia) for fostering me while learning and exploring my potential for different administrative and non-administrative work.

I am obliged to Dr Abhimanyu Niswade (Dean, Government Medical College, Nagpur) for allowing to embrace this work in the institution.

I am very grateful to my senior colleagues during postgraduation, Dr Ashesh Wankhede (Professor and Head, Forensic Medicine, Government Medical College, Jagdalpur, Chhattisgarh), Dr Anil Batra (Professor and Head, Forensic Medicine, Government Medical College, Akola) and Dr Kailash Zine (Professor and Head, Forensic Medicine, Government Medical College, Aurangabad) for being the first teachers who taught me medicolegal work.

I am also thankful to my classmates Dr Prakash Mohite (Professor and Head, Forensic Medicine, Medical College, Sawangi) and Dr Manish Shrigiriwar (OSD, Super-speciality Hospital, Nagpur) for their constant encouragement and unremitting help.

I respectfully thanks to Dr PG Dixit, Professor and Head, Forensic Medicine, Government Medical College, Nagpur, for permitting to carry out this work in the department.

I am respectfully thankful to Dr LK Bade, Dr HT Katade, Dr SS Gupta, Dr RK Singh (Raipur), Dr BH Tirpude (Sevagram), Dr SD Nanandkar, Dr SC Mohite, Dr Harish Pathak (Mumbai), Dr VR Agrawal (Pune), Dr HV Godbole, Dr RN Kagne (Pondicherry) for their guidance and blessing.

I am grateful to my friend Dr Linesh Khobragade (Consultant Pharmacologist, Sarjah), Dr Satin Meshram and Dr Nilesh Tumram (Department of Forensic Medicine, Government Medical College, Nagpur) without whom this endeavor would not have been possible.

I am thankful to Vinia Ambade (BE, Pune), Dr Raj Bhagwatkar (BDS, Nagpur), Dr Avinash Turankar (Department of Pharmacology, Nagpur) and Dr Pravin Shingade (Department of Medicine, Nagpur) for their help while preparing and editing the manuscript.

I am also thankful to Dr Hemant Kukde (Mumbai), Dr Nitin Barmate (Raipur), Shri Pramod Mandekar, Mr Sudesh Rathod (Yeotmal), Shri Gurudyal Pathak, Shri Ghodmare (Nagpur), Mr Arun Gujar (Pune), Mr Shantnu Sarkar and Mr Rajesh Shrivas (Nagpur) for their kind help.

Finally, I express my sincere gratitude and acknowledgment to my wife Dr Hemlata and lovely daughters Vidhi and Aarohi in accomplishing the task.

Vipul Ambade

Contents

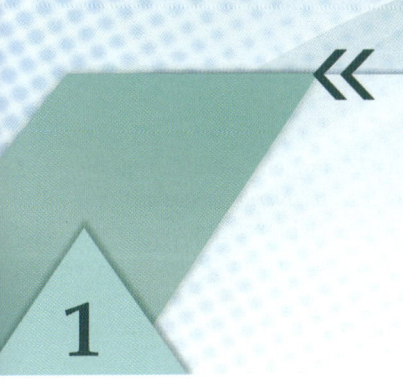

General Toxicology

Toxicology is defined as the branch of science which deals with the poisons in all its aspect. Thus, it is the study of poison deals with source, properties, absorption, fate, action, fatal dose and fatal period, signs and symptoms, laboratory investigation, diagnosis, treatment, postmortem findings and medicolegal aspect of different poisoning cases.

Forensic toxicology	*Clinical toxicology*
It deals with medicolegal aspects of poisoning, including causes and circumstances of death.	It deals with mechanism of action, clinical manifestations, laboratory investigation, diagnosis and treatment of a poison.
Poison	*Drugs*
Poison is defined as a substance which when ingested, injected, inhaled, applied or administered causes disease, ill health or death of a person. It is used to curtail the life or to minimise the life or to get rid of life.	Whereas, drug is any substance used in the diagnosis, treatment, investigation, and prevention and modification of disease. It is used to sustain or to prolong life or to get relief.

Difference between poison and drug
All drugs are poison when taken in **excess dose** and with **intention** to cause harm. But all poisons are not drugs even when taken in low dose.

Legal difference
There is no legal definition of poison. Legally the poison and drug are differentiated on the **basis of the intention** with which the substance is given.

When the substance is given with the **intention of causing harm** or death, it is considered as **poison.**	When a substance is given with the **intention of sustaining life,** it is considered as a **drug**, irrespective of the dose given.

Medical difference
The difference between the poison and the drug is of **dose with which that substance is given**. Since a drug in therapeutic dose or lesser dose produces desirable or beneficial effect but the same drug when given in higher dose produces deleterious effect and acts as a poison, e.g. digitalis, barbiturates, analgesics, tranquilizers, etc.

CLASSIFICATION OF POISONS

Poisons can be classified according to the

1. Action of poison
2. Nature of poison
3. Source of poison

ACCORDING TO MODE OF ACTION OF POISON

Poisons are classified into 2 groups as shown in Table 1.1.

1. Local
2. Systemic

Table 1.1: Classification of poison on the basis of action

Local	Systemic

1. Corrosives
  a. Acids:
    i. Inorganic: Sulfuric acid, hydrochloric acid, nitric acid
    ii. Organic: Acetic acid, oxalic acid, carbolic acid
  b. Alkalies:
    i. Hydroxide of sodium, potassium and ammonium
    ii. Carbonates of sodium, potassium and ammonium
  c. Metallic: Mercuric chlorides
	1. Cardiac poisons: Cyanogen, aconite, digitalis, tobacco, *Cerbera thevetia*, *Nerium odorum*
	2. Respiratory poisons (asphyxiant gases), e.g. CO, CO_2, SO_2, H_2S, NH_3, phosphine (PH_3), war gases and sewer gases
	3. Hepatotoxic poisons: Phosphorus, chloroform, trichloroethane, carbon tetrachloride.
	4. Nephrotoxic poisons: Mercury, carbolic, oxalic, snake poison
	5. Miscellaneous: Food poison, drug abuse

2. Irritants
  a. Mechanical:
    i. Glass pieces or powder
    ii. Hairs and fibers
    iii. Metallic chips, nails, pins
    iv. Diamond dust or powder
  b. Chemicl:
    i. Inorganic
    Non metals: Phosphorus, iodine, fluorine, chlorine, bromine
    Metals: Arsenic, lead, mercury, copper, iron, zinc, thallium
    ii. Organic: Agricultural poisoning
    Insecticidal: Organophosphorus, organochlorine, carbamate, pyrethroids:
    Rodenticidal
    Fungicidal
    Herbicidal
  c. Vegetables: *Abrus precatorius*, *Ricinus communis*, *Croton tiglium*, *Semicarpus anacardium*, Calotropis, *Plumbago rosea*, Capsicum
  d. Animals: Snakes, scorpions, bees, wasps, spiders, cantharides, and poisonous fish
	6. Neurotics
	  a. Cerebral:
	    i. Somniferous: Opium and its alkaloids like morphine, codeine, thebaine, papaverine, noscapine, and narcine
	    ii. Inebriants:
	    Alcohols
	    Anaesthetic agents: Ether, chloroform, nitrous oxide.
	    Coal tar derivatives, e.g. naphthalene
	    iii. Deliriants: Datura, cannabis, cocaine
	    iv. Depressant (sedatives and hypnotics): Barbiturates, benzodiazepam, chloral hydrate, paraldehyde
	    v. Stimulants: Amphetamines, camphor, caffeine, cocaine
	    vi. Hallucinogens: LSD (lysergic acid diethylamide), mescaline (peyote)
	  b. Spinal:
	    i. Excitants: *Strychnos nux-vomica*
	    ii. Depressants: *Lathyrus sativus* (khesari daal), gelsemium (jasmine).
	  c. Peripheral: Conium, curare

Nature of poison: For the medicolegal purpose, poisons are classified as:

1. Homicidal Poisoning

There is no ideal homicidal poison.

The near ideal homicidal poisons are: Thallium and fluoride (is present in some of rodenticides).

The commonly used poisons: Arsenic, aconite, lead, strychnine, snake venom, opium. Rarely bacterial culture is used.

2. Suicidal Poisoning

There is no ideal suicidal poison.

The near ideal suicidal poisons are: Opium and barbiturates.

Poisons which are commonly used for suicidal purpose in India are: Insecticides, cyanides, carbolic acid (phenol), barbiturates, opium, celphos.

Table 1.2: Characteristics of an ideal homicidal and suicidal poison

Ideal homicidal poison	Ideal suicidal poison
1. Cheap	Cheap
2. Easily available	Easily available
3. Highly toxic	Highly toxic
4. Odorless, colorless, tasteless	Tasteless, odorless, colorless/pleasant
5. Capable of being easily given with food or drinks	Capable of being easily taken with food or drinks
6. Produces features that resembles natural disease to avoid suspicion	Should lead to painless death
7. There should be no antidote available	Not necessary
8. Should be completely metabolised so that it is not detected on CA/PM examination	Not necessary

3. Accidental Poisoning

It occurs due to:

a. Mistaken with other material

b. Carelessness in storing poisons

c. Quack remedies

d. While working or exposure in industry, in agricultural fields or in laboratory

e. Bites by snakes, scorpions or insects

f. Leakage of gas from industries

g. Accidental consumption of poison by children

h. Food poisoning

i. Drug overdose or misuse or addiction

Accidental poisoning can occur due to any poison but commonly occurs due to insecticides, snake bite, and gas leakage from industries.

4. Other Types of Poisoning (Table 1.3)

Table 1.3: Classification of poison on the basis of its nature

Nature of poison	Description	Examples
1. **Homicidal:**	These are the poisons used for killing other	Arsenic, lead, strychnine, etc.
2. **Suicidal:**	These are the poisons used to commit suicide	Insecticides, cyanides, carbolic, barbiturates, etc.
3. **Accidental:**	These are the poisons which causes poisoning due to accidental circumstances	Insecticides, snakes bites, food poisoning, gas leakage, etc.
4. **Abortifacients:**	These are the poisons which are used for inducing criminal abortion	Arsenic, lead, ergot, quinine, Calotropis, Plumbago, Nerium, *Cerbera thevetia*, aconite, strychnine, etc.
5. **Aphrodisiac agents:**	These are the poisons which increases the sexual desire	Alcohol, Datura, cocaine, Cannabis preparations
6. **Arrow poisons:**	These are the poisons which are commonly applied on the arrow head	Strychnine, Curare, aconite, Abrus, Calotropis, Plumbago and snake venom
7. **Cattle poisons:**	These are the poisons used for killing cattle	Strychnine, Curare, aconite, Abrus, Calotropis, Plumbago, Nerium, *Cerbera thevetia*
8. **Stupefying poisons:**	These are the poisons which alter the consciousness of the person and are commonly given for purpose of rape, robbery, dacoity and theft	Datura, cocaine, Cannabis preparations, alcohol
9. **Malingering purpose:**	These are the poisons used for malingering purpose to avoid duty or to make false charges against enemy	*Semicarpus anacardium*—branding; Abrus—conjunctivitis
10. **Vitriolage:**	Agents used to cause bodily injury	Corrosives

Source of poison: Depending upon the source, poisons are classified as (Table 1.4).

Table 1.4: Source of poison with its examples

Source	Examples
1. Domestic/household	Detergents, disinfectants, phenols, kerosene, etc.
2. Agricultural	Organophosphorus, organochlorine, carbamates
3. Vegetables	All vegetable irritants, Datura, Cannabis, etc.
4. Animals	Snakes venoms, insect bite
5. Medicinal source	Wrong medication, over medication and abuse Barbiturate, diazepam, opium, etc.
6. Industrial source	Factories where poisons are produced as by-products, e.g. carbide, methyl isocyanate, phosphine, carbon monoxide, cyanides, etc.
7. Commercial source	From storehouse, selling shops, etc. e.g. alcohols, opium, cocaine, etc.
8. Food and drink	Preservatives of food grains, additives like coloring and odoring agents, and food poisoning itself
9. Miscellaneous	Sewer gases

PROPERTIES

Color, odor, taste, solubility, form, etc. in relation to particular poison is described in particular chapter.

ABSORPTION: May be direct or indirect through mucous membrane or skin.

Direct: Through parenteral routes.

Mucous membranes: Sublingual, inhalation, oral and other orifices.

Skin: Example phosphorus, phenol, insecticidal poison.

Routes of Administration

1. Oral
2. Parenteral/injection—SC, IM, IV, intra-dermal, intra-arterial, etc.
3. Inhalation
4. Sublingual
5. Other natural orifices (e.g. nasal, rectal, vaginal and urethral, etc.).
6. Contact poisoning, i.e. through skin or wounds, or ulcers
7. Through pellets (chemical or bacterial poison pellets fired with air gun).

Injured or ulcerated skin absorbs poison quicker than intact skin. When taken by mouth various factors influence the absorption of poison.

FATE OF POISON

1. Eliminated as such by defecation or vomitus.
2. Neutralized or inactivated in GIT.
3. Metabolized or detoxified in the body.
4. Eliminated after absorption by urine, breath, bile, milk, sweat, saliva, tear, etc.
5. Gets deposited in some organs or tissue. Heavy metals and radioactive substances stored in epidermis, hair, nails and bones and organophosphorus compounds in fat.

ACTION OF POISON

The action of a poison may be:

1. Local
2. Systemic/remote: Specific and non-specific
3. Both: Local as well as remote
4. General action

1. **Local action:** The action of the poison occurs at the local site of contact, e.g. corrosion with corrosives (mineral acids), GIT irritation with irritants, dilatation of pupil with atropine, tingling and numbness with aconite and local anesthesia with cocaine.

2. **Systemic action:** The poison has purely systemic action after absorption of the poison. The remote action could be:

   a. Specific: A particular specific part of the body is involved, e.g. barbiturates act on cerebrum, digitalis on heart, strychnine on spinal cord, curare on peripheral nerves.

b. Non-specific: No particular organ is involved but there is a non-specific remote action. For example shock with corrosives.

3. **Combined local and remote action:** The poison has local action at the site of contact and also evokes a remote action after its absorption, e.g. snake venom, organic corrosives, phosphorus.

   i. Snake venom—a local action at the site of bite and remote action depending upon type of snake.

   ii. Oxalic acid and carbolic acid have a local corrosive action and a remote action leading to CNS toxicity and nephrotoxicity.

   iii. Phosphorus has local action on GIT and remote action on liver and CNS.

4. **General action:** The response due to poisoning is not restricted to some organs and there is a generalized involvement of the whole body, e.g. arsenic, mercury, lead, DDT, etc.

FACTORS INFLUENCING THE ACTION OF POISONS

1. **Dose:** Normally, the action of the poison is directly proportional to the dose. Higher the dose more will be the fatality and lesser the dose less will be the fatality with the following exceptions:

   a. Idiosyncrasy: It is the abnormal response of a drug or hypersensitivity due to inborn peculiarities. This is the inherent hypersensitivity to a particular drug or agent so that even a small dose may cause death, e.g. morphine, quinine, aspirin, cocaine, etc.

   b. Allergy: It is the hypersensitivity acquired as a result of previous exposure due to the formation of antibodies, e.g. penicillin, other protective sera.

   c. Tolerance: It is the capacity of the body to sustain the action of certain drugs or agents without any immediate harm. e.g. alcohol, opium, tobacco, Cannabis, etc. The repeated and chronic use of these agents results in addiction and drug dependence.

d. Synergism: The final response due to combination of substances is more than the sum of their individual action, e.g. alcohol with cocaine or barbiturates or with antidepressants, anticonvulsants, tranquilizers and antihistaminic.

e. Cumulative poisons: Some poisons are not readily excreted from the body and are retained or tend to accumulate in the body and may not cause any toxic effect when ingested/enter the body in a low dose, e.g. lead, arsenic, digitalis, carbon monoxide (CO), strychnine, and barbiturates.

2. **Form of poison**

   a. Physical form: The poison in gaseous/vapor form is more poisonous than liquids, and liquids are more toxic than solids. The solid poison which is in fine powder form is more poisonous than coarse form.

   [Gases/vapors > liquid > solid (fine > coarse)]

   b. Chemical form: Pure arsenic and mercury are not poisonous while their compounds are highly poisonous.

   Similarly, some compound of an individual metal is not toxic and other compound of the same metal is deadly toxic, e.g. barium sulfate is non-toxic and used in barium meal in radiological investigation; whereas barium sulfide is highly toxic.

   c. Concentrated form: Normally more the concentration more will be the absorption and more its toxicity. But the dilute solution of oxalic acid is more rapidly absorbed and is much more fatal.

3. **Condition of stomach:** It delays or facilitates the absorption of poison and it depends on:

   a. Empty stomach—absorbs poison rapidly.

   b. Food contents in stomach:
   - Presence of food stuff in the stomach acts as diluents.
   - Fatty food delays the absorption process of poisoning except phosphorus.

c. Abnormal conditions of the stomach also lead to delay in the absorption of poison.
- Pyloric stenosis which delays the emptying of food.
- Gastrojejunostomy causes repeated backward flow of gastric contents.

d. Achlorhydric subjects—the salts of cyanides is ineffective due to lack of hydrochloric acid (HCl) in the stomach which is required for their conversion to hydrogen cyanide before absorption.

4. Routes of administration of poison

a. Route: Rate of absorption depends upon the route of administration. Through some routes, poisons are absorbed very rapidly and exert their action promptly. Poisoning through inhalation is more effective than intravenous; than intramuscular; than other parenteral; than oral; than direct contact with skin. Poisoning through mouth is more effective than rectal poisoning.

b. Different route: The action of poison is different when they are introduced through different routes, e.g.
- Snake venom is effective only when injected and harmless when taken orally.
- Cocaine: On ingestion acts as deliriants, on injection it acts as local anesthetic.
- Curare: On ingestion is inert, on injection it is highly toxic.

5. General condition of the body

a. Age: Some poisons are better tolerated in some ages and badly in other ages. Opium is better tolerated by elderly and atropine is better tolerated by children.

b. State of body and health: Well built person with good physique and health will tolerate poison better than weak and lean subject.

c. Presence of any disease: Usually, in disease conditions the effect of poison is more.
- In liver pathology, morphine is more poisonous.
- In renal damage, mercury is more poisonous.
- In head injury or raised ICP, morphine is more dangerous/lethal.
- However, some poisons are well-tolerated during disease conditions, sedatives and tranquilizers in manic and deliriant patients:
  - Digitalis in heart failure.
  - Strychnine in paralysis.
  - Cyanide in achlorhydria.

d. Sleep: Absorption is less during sleep due to slow metabolism and hence has slow action but depressant drugs may cause more harm during sleep.

e. Exercise: Action of alcohol on CNS is slowed during exercise because more blood is drawn to the muscles during exercise.

DIAGNOSIS OF POISONING

The diagnosis of poisoning is not always possible due to various reasons.

1. Usually patient is not in a position to narrate the story or to give the history.
2. Sometimes in spite of knowing the nature of poisoning consumed by the patient, the relatives do not come forward due to fear of being involved in police investigation.
3. Also due to ignorance of the importance of giving proper history of poisoning to the doctor, the physician's task becomes more difficult as none is willing to give correct history to avoid police investigation.

In Living Subject

1. History of the case as stated by patient, relatives or friends:
   It includes time of onset, symptoms, progress, in relation to food/drink and condition of others who took the same, possible source of poison, any past history of poisoning, history of depression and about the properties of the poisonous material like smell, taste, color, consistency, etc.
2. Signs and symptoms
3. Detailed physical examination

4. Laboratory investigation of vomitus, excreta, blood, etc. or any material brought by the relatives. The chemical analysis of gastric lavage fluid, blood, urine, stools and vomitus confirms the nature of the poison.

The detection of the poison in suspected food, fluid or utensils help as corroborative evidence.

In Dead Subject

1. History as provided by police or relatives should be taken in the same line as in case of living victims. In addition, history should also contain:
   i. Period of survival after poisoning and their symptoms.
   ii. Details of treatment if given.
2. Postmortem examination of a body
   a. External examination
      i. Stain of vomitus on the clothes.
      ii. Smell of poison from the body.
      iii. Presence of froth at the nose and mouth, e.g. in cyanides, opium, barbiturates, organophosphorus and strychnine.
      iv. Color of PM lividity, e.g. cherry-red in carbon monoxide, bluish-green in hydrogen sulfide, pink with cyanides, almost black in opium.
      v. Color and condition of the skin, e.g. jaundiced with phosphorus, cyanosed in asphyxiants and yellow in acute copper poisoning.
      vi. Condition of gums and teeth.
      vii. Marks of injection on the body.
      viii. Condition of natural orifices.
   b. Internal examination: Examination should be done of all the organs/viscera, the most important is examination of stomach and its contents for color, smell, softening, congestion and per-forations. (In poisoning changes are more marked at the cardiac end and at the greater curvature of stomach.)
3. Preservation of viscera and other materials for laboratory investigation like CA.

4. Moral and circumstantial evidence.
   i. Evidence of purchase of poison.
   ii. Evidence of ingestion of poison.
   iii. Suicide note.
   iv. History of quarrel.
   v. Presence of poison container near the dead body.
   vi. Eagerness on the part of relatives to dispose the dead body.

TREATMENT OF POISONING

If the specific nature of the poison is not known then it should be treated on the lines of general principles of treatment of poisoning which are as follows:

1. Removal of patient from the source
2. Removal of unabsorbed poison
3. Diluting the poison and delaying its absorption
4. Elimination of absorbed poison
5. Use of specific antidote
6. Symptomatic treatment

Aims

1. Removal of unabsorbed poison.
2. Removal of absorbed poison.

1. **Removal of patient from the source of exposure:** In gaseous/volatile poison-remove patient from the source or environment.
   In insecticidal poison—removal of clothes
   In corrosives poison—removal of soiled clothes

2. **Removal of unabsorbed poison:** It depends upon the route of administration of poison.
   a. In case of **contact poisoning** to skin/injuries: Removal of clothes.
      • Wash the area with lukewarm water or soap.
      • Application of local anaesthetic agents.
   b. In case of **intra-vaginal or other natural orifices:** Vaginal douching or irrigation with plain water.
   c. **Inhaled poison:** Removal of patient from source.
      • Ensure clear airway and respiration.

d. **Injected poison** (e.g. snake bite, arrow poison): Ligature/tourniquette application proximal to the site of bite.
  - Application of ice packs.
  - Antidote infiltration after washing of the site of bite.

e. **Ingested poison:** It is removed by:
  - Emesis/induction of vomiting.
  - Gastric lavage/stomach wash.
  - Purgatives and colonic lavage by means of sodium/magnesium sulfate or dulcolax, etc.

Emesis: At very early stage of poisoning within 4–6 hours, emesis is better than stomach wash.

Methods of emesis: Vomiting can be induced by:

a. Mechanical irritation of throat	Finger—stimulating the posterior wall of pharynx
b. Plain lukewarm water	Good amount of water
c. Common salt	1 TSF in one glass of water
d. Mustard powder	1 TSF in one glass of water
e. Copper sulfate	Weak solution
f. Ipecacuanha (contains emetine)	1–2 gm with one glass of water
g. Zinc sulfate	1–2 gm in one glass of water
h. Ammonium carbonate	1–2 gm in one glass of water
i. Apomorphine hydrochloride	1–2 ml IM, is centrally acting potent emetic agent. (contraindicated in coma and respiratory depression)

Household emetics : These are the emetics available in the house. Top four methods are the examples of household emetics.

Contraindications of emesis (5CVP)

a. Corrosives	Except carbolic acid (chances of perforation of the stomach)
b. Convulsions	(Chances of precipitating convulsions)
c. Coma	(Chances of aspiration)
d. Children	(Chances of aspiration)
e. Volatile poison	(Chances of inhalation of fumes)
f. Cardiorespiratory diseases	(Chances of heart failure)
g. Pregnancy	(Chances of abortion)

Gastric lavage: It is done by means of following tubes:
  - In adults—stomach tube (Boa/Ewald).
  - In children—male urinary rubber catheter.
  - In infants—Ryle's tube.

Indications of Stomach Wash

1. Any **ingested poison** within 4–6 hrs.
2. Even if the poison has been ingested more than 6 hrs earlier, gastric lavage may be useful since in case of depression, unconsciousness, the gastric emptying time is increased.
3. In **injected morphine poisoning** due to its property of re-secretion in the stomach.

Contraindications of Gastric Lavage

a. Corrosives	Except carbolic acid. Absolute contraindication
b. Convulsions	Anesthetize or sedate the patient first
c. Coma/petroleum	Do cuffed intubation in such cases
d. Children	Use Ryle's tube or rubber catheter
e. Esophageal varices	Lead to massive hemorrhage

Stomach Tube (Boa's or Ewald's Tube)

It is 1–1.5 meter long, 12.7 mm broad, rubber tube, thick enough to pass without bending and has the following parts:

1. **Funnel end:** to pour in fluid and to take out fluid after lavage.

2. **Suction bulb (sometimes absent)**
   a. To force open the perforations, if blocked by food material.
   b. To take out fluid, if siphon action fails.

3. **Mouth gag:** It is a wooden to avoid damage to the teeth and has a central large hole for the passage of rubber tube, one end pointed to help force open the clenched teeth, 2 side holes to enable to tie a thread to the head of the patient, in case the patient is violent.

4. **Rubber tubing:** Marked at 40 cm, 50 cm and 60 cm.

5. Lower rounded perforated end: Rounded to avoid damage to the GIT during its passage.

Procedure

After positioning the patient (semiprone or prone to the left side with head lower), the teeth are opened and the mouth gag is placed in them. The lower end of the tube is lubricated with water, liquid paraffin or castor oil and is passed through the opening of the mouth gag, till the 50 cm mark, ensuring that the tube has reached the stomach (Fig. 1.1).

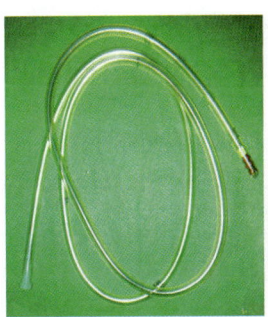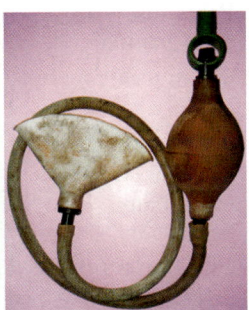

Fig. 1.1: Ryle's tube and stomach tube

In case it enters respiratory passages
  a. Cough reflex starts
  b. Hissing sounds heard at funnel end
  c. Air bubbles seen on dipping the funnel end in water.

To confirm the tube to be in stomach, air is blown from funnel end and it is auscultated at the area of stomach.

The first washing is done with fresh lukewarm water or normal saline since that sample is to be sent for chemical analysis. Small amount only is used (100–200 ml) to avoid pushing forward of the poison into intestines. Later, lavage is done with plain warm water or KMnO$_4$ solution (1 : 1000), i.e. 1 gm/1 liter or specific antidote. Each time about 300 ml of fluid is passed into the funnel held at a level higher than the body. The fluid enters by gravity. After 15–30 seconds the funnel end is taken lower than the level of the body then fluid from the stomach will come out due to siphon action. The process is repeated till the color and nature of ingoing and outgoing fluid is same. Pinch the tube before

removing it to avoid aspiration to respiratory tract.

Volume of Each Wash

For adult:	300–350 ml
For child:	150–200 ml
For infant:	<100 ml

For whole procedure, about 10 liters of the fluid is required (about 20 washings).

To take care of poison that may be re-secreted in stomach (e.g. morphine) or remains sticking to stomach walls, one of the following can be left in the stomach:
  a. KMnO$_4$ solution
  b. Demulcents
  c. Sodium/magnesium sulfate as purgatives
  d. Sodium bicarbonate (in case of acidity)
  e. Activated charcoal (as adsorbent)

3. Diluting the poison and delaying its absorption: it is done by giving:
  a Water to drink that helps in two ways:
    • It reduces the local damaging action
    • It delays the rate of absorption
  b. Bulky bland food, e.g. banana, boiled potato, mashed rice.
  c. Demulcents/fats: It delays the process of absorption and also protects the stomach wall. This method is of **no use in oxalic acid poisoning** (where dilution is contraindicated), and **phosphorus poisoning** (where fats are contraindicated).

4. Elimination of absorbed poison: It is done by:
  a. Diuresis (increased urination/forced diuresis) by using fluids and drugs like frusemide or mannitol infusion.
  b. Diaphoresis (increased sweating/perspiration) by applying hot packs and neostigmine or pilocarpine injection.
  c. Dialysis: In case kidney is not functioning (peritoneal or hemodialysis).
  d. Chelating agents
  e. Exchange transfusion

5. Specific antidote: Antidote is the substance which counteracts the deleterious effects of the poison without itself being harmful to the body. It is indicated when poison is absorbed from the GIT or shows clinical systemic manifestation of poison.

Types and Uses of Antidotes

I. Physical (mechanical) antidotes: These are the antidotes which **prevent the action of poison mechanically** without destroying or neutralizing the poison.

a. Demulcents: Oil, ghee, butter, milk, egg albumin (egg white), starch, barley water, etc.

- These substances have soothing action and **form a protective layer on the mucous membrane of stomach,** so that absorption of poison does not occur. It is not used in phosphorus poisoning.

b. Bulky foods: Example banana, mashed potato, boiled rice, vegetables, etc.

- These substances **engulf the poison and make it unavailable** for causing effects and for its absorption.

c. Adsorbent, e.g. activated charcoal.

It adsorbs the alkaloid poison in their pores so that poison is not available for absorption in stomach.

d. Diluents, e.g. water, milk, drinks, etc.

- It dilutes the poison, thereby delaying the absorption of poison.

Physical antidote	Uses
Demulcent	Corrosive/irritant, except phosphorus
Bulky foods	Mechanical irritant
Adsorbent	Irritant poison
Diluents	Corrosive/irritant, except Oxalic

II. Chemical antidotes: These are the substances which **chemically react with the poison** and thereby disintegrate or inactivate it.

Examples are:

Chemical antidote	For action/forms
a. Weak non-carbonated alkali (CaO, MgO)	Acid poison (neutralizing the acids)
b. Weak vegetables acid (citric, acetic)	Alkali poison (neutralizing alkali)
c. Copper sulfate	Phosphorus (forms copper phosphide)
d. Egg albumin	Mercury chloride (forms mercuric albuminate)
e. Fresh ferric oxide	Arsenic (forms ferric arsenate)
f. Potassium ferrocyanide	Copper
g. Calcium carbonate	Oxalic acid (forms calcium oxalate)
h. $KMnO_4$	Opium/morphine
i. Sodium thiosulfate	Iodine/cyanide

III. Pharmacological or physiological antidotes: These are the substances which have a pharmacologically opposite action as compared to the poison. Examples are:

Pharmacological antidote	Used
Naloxone	Opium/morphine
Physostigmine/neostigmine	Datura
Barbiturate	Strychnine
Atropine	Organophosphorus

IV. Universal antidote: It is so-called because it can be used in all cases of poisoning, especially when the nature of poison is not known. It is the combination of physical and chemical antidote. Dose is 15–30 gm orally. It can be repeated 12–24 hourly.

Universal antidote is prepared as follows

Contents	Obtained from	Parts	Action
Charcoal	Burnt bread/toast	2	Adsorbs poison
MgO	Milk of magnesia	1	Neutralizes acid
Tannin	Strong tea	1	Precipitates metal, alkaloids, and glucosides

V. Chelating agents: These are the substances which act on the absorbed metallic poison and form a non-ionized complex with the metal ion freely available in the blood circulation, so that the metal ion is not available for absorption and thereby cannot affect the enzyme system of the body.

Examples of chelating agents

a. Dimercaprol or BAL (British antilewisite): is chemically dimercaprol or 2 : 3 dimercapto-propanol). It has two SH radicles which binds with metal ion.

   Contraindications and complications Liver damage, hypertension and tachycardia.

b. EDTA (ethylenediaminetetra-acetic acid): Other forms are calcium disodium edetate (CaNa$_2$EDTA) and disodium edetate. As EDTA depletes serum calcium, CaNa$_2$EDTA is better. Trientine (cuprid) is a newer chelating agent.

   Contraindications and complications: Renal damage.

c. Penicillamine or cuprimine: It is a degradation product of penicillin. It has stable SH-radicle.

   Uses: It is also effective in Wilson's disease, i.e. hepatolenticular degeneration.

   Complications: Almost non-toxic but prolonged use may cause thrombocytopenia, agranulocytosis, skin rashes and nephrotic syndrome.

d. Desferrioxamine:

   Complications: Its adverse effects are allergic reactions, abdominal pain, loose motions, cramps and fever.

   Uses: It is also used in hemochromatosis and thalassemia.

Chelating agents	Dose	Uses
BAL (dimercaprol)	*Dose:* **3–4 mg/kg body wt, given deep IM in** the gluteus region, 4 hourly for the first two days, followed for by 12 hourly (1 BD) next 10 days. It cannot be given	Arsenic, mercury, copper.
	intravenously for danger of causing embolism due to arachis oil	
EDTA	*Dose:* **1 gm in 5% glucose by slow IV drip,** BD for 5 days. It is also given as: a. Orally: 1 gm BD for 5 days b. IV: 5 ml of 50% solution BD for 5 days	Lead, mercury, copper
Penicillamine	*Dose:* **30 mg/kg body weight, orally** in 4 divided doses for 5–10 days. OR 1–3 gm in slow normal saline drip for 2–4 days	Copper, mercury, lead
Desferrioxamine	*Dose:* **10 gm/day orally** for unabsorbed iron. OR 2 gm/day in 50% laevulose solution IV for absorbed iron	Iron poisoning

VI. Serological/biological antidotes: These are the substance prepared by injecting the antigen (like snake venom) in the animal blood, so that the sensitized animal serum can be used as an antidote, e.g. antivenom serum.

Household antidotes: These are the substances which are available usually in the house and can be used as antidotes in case of poisoning.

Household antidotes	Uses/used as
1. Common salt, mustard powder, plain warm water	Emetic agent
2. Charcoal from burnt toast	Adsorbent
3. Flour suspension	Engulf or even adsorb
4. Banana, potato, boiled rice	Physical antidote
5. Oil, ghee, butter, milk, egg albumin	Demulcent
6. Starch solution	Iodine poisoning
7. Milk of magnesia, tooth paste, wall scrapping	Acid poisoning
8. Vinegar, lemon/orange juice	Alkali poisoning
9. Milk	All ingested poison

6. Symptomatic treatment

A. Safeguarding respiration
1. Clearing the airways
2. Endotracheal intubation
3. Tracheostomy
4. Oxygen inhalation—6 liters/min
5. Artificial respiration
B. Maintenance of circulation
1. Vasoconstriction
2. Stimulants
3. Blood transfusion
4. Noradrenaline drip for peripheral circulatory failure
C. Electrolyte imbalance correction
1. IV fluids for dehydration/shock
2. Sodium/potassium for electrolyte imbalance
3. Other fluids
D. Other supportive treatments like
1. Atropine for abdominal pain
2. Diazepam for convulsions/restlessness
3. Adrenaline, antihistaminic and steroids in anaphylactic reactions
4. Morphine, pethidine for pain
5. Glucose for hypoglycaemia
E. Maintenance of general condition of the patient
1. Warm and comfortable condition
2. Good nursing care
3. Prophylactic antibiotics
4. Physiotherapy for rehabilitation
5. Psychotherapy in an attempted suicide

POSTMORTEM FINDINGS IN SUSPECTED POISONING

The postmortem (PM) findings are different in individual poisoning are dealt in respective chapter. However, the characteristic findings in different poisoning are as follows:

External postmortem findings

1. Postmortem lividity:	Typical lividity in different cases
Deep blue	Asphyxiant/aniline
Cherry-red	CO poisoning
Bright red	Cyanide
Brown	Phosphorus
Black	Opium
Green	Hydrogen sulfide
2. Froth from mouth and nose	Opium, barbiturate, OP (blood tinged)

3. Detectable smell	Insecticidal poison, volatile poison, opium, cyanide, kerosene, phenol
4. Deep cyanosis	Opium, CO_2, sewer gas,
5. Early rigor mortis	Strychnine, HCN
6. Resist decomposition	Arsenic, datura, formalin
7. Stain near mouth and on hands	Nitric acid, copper sulfate, paints
8. Ulceration on lips and mouth	Corrosives
9. Hemorrhage spots under skin/mucosa	Phosphorus
10. Staining, erosion, ulceration near external genital	Abortifacient agents, corrosives
11. Alopecia, hyperpigmentation, hyperkeratosis	Arsenic
12. Injection marks	Opium/cocaine abuser
13. Punctures marks	Bite marks of snakes, scorpion and insect
14. Constriction of pupil	Morphine, phenol, organophosphorus,
15. Dilatation of pupil	Datura, alcohol

Internal postmortem findings

1. Corrosion, ulceration and desquamation of lips, mouth, tongue	Corrosive
2. Soft, swollen, bleached tongue/mouth	Alkali
3. Chalky white teeth	Sulfuric acid
4. Blue lining on gums/teeth	Lead, mercury (chronic poisoning)
5. Corrosion, des-quamation, ulceration of GIT mucosa	Corrosives, irritant
6. MM of upper GIT Hard/white	Phenol
Yellow	Nitric acid
Bluish green	Copper sulfate
Green	Ferrous sulfate
Black	Sulfuric acid
Grey/slate color	Mercury chloride
Red velvety	Arsenic
Discolor/staining	Colored salts of arsenic, lead, copper

7. Stomach wall

Thickened and soft	Corrosive, irritant
Hard wall	Formaldehyde
Hard and leather-like	Carbolic acid
Hemorrhage/ ulcerated	Irritant
Ulceration and sloughing	Corrosive

8. Stomach contents

Blood	Corrosive, irritant
Bluish	Copper sulfate
Luminous in dark	Phosphorus
Powder/tablets	Drug tab, arsenic, oxalic
Detectable smell	Kerosene, alcohol, insecticides, cyanide, formaldehyde, etc.

7. **Small intestine:** It may show irritation, sometimes may show presence of poisonous remains.

8. **Large intestine:** May show ulcerations, as in case of HgCl₃, similar in appearance of ulcers of bacillary dysentery. It particularly involves the ascending and transverse colons.

9. **Brain and spinal cord:** Congestion and edema of brain and spinal cord in cases of cerebral and spinal poison (e.g. strychnine), respectively. Brain—may be congested, edematous with occasional hemorrhagic points at places in cases of asphyxiant poisons.

10. **Larynx and trachea:** Froth in case of opium and organophosphorus poisoning. Hyperemic and inflamed in case of inhalation of irritating gases, leaking of corrosive agents while ingestion or vomiting.

11. **Chest cavity:** Smell of volatile poisons, cyanide, opium, etc. can be detected.

12. **Lungs:** Voluminous, congested, presence of Tardieu's spots—in case of asphyxiant and inhaled poisons. Cut section gives blood stained frothy fluid in case of opium and other asphyxiant.

13. **Heart:** Presence of subendocardial hemorrhagic spots in case of arsenic, phosphorus, mercuric chloride, etc.

14. **Liver:** Different degenerative changes occur in cases of poisoning with phosphorus, carbon tetrachloride, chloroform, tetrachloroethylene and many other poisons. The type and extent of the degenerative changes occur depending on the type of the poison, dose, duration of the exposure and the physical condition of the patient.

15. **Kidneys:** Swollen, reddish, soft, sometimes greasy in touch with hemorrhage in the calyces and other degenerative changes in cases of poisoning with mercury, oxalic acid, carbolic acid, phosphorus, cantherides, viper snake venom and many others. In case of oxalic acid poisoning, white powder of oxalate crystals are present in the tubules and the calyces.

16. **Urinary bladder:** Hemorrhage in cases of *Abrus precatorius*, viper snake bite and cantheride poisoning.

17. **Uterus and vagina:** Staining, congestion, hemorrhage, ulceration in cases of attempted abortion by use of local abortifacient agents.

DUTIES OF DOCTOR IN CASES OF POISONING

1. **Treatment:** The foremost duty of doctor is to treat the patient. When the nature of poison is not known, then the treatment should be given on general principle of treatment of poisoning.
   If brought dead, inform police and send body for postmortem.

2. **Maintenance of records:** Detailed record should be maintained of complaints, examination, condition, progress, prognosis and treatment. All the preliminary data including name, age, sex, address, brought by/from, time, date and place of examination, consent of the patient or guardian (if minor or unconscious), marks of identification should be recorded.

3. **History:** The details of nature of the poison, time of consumption, time of onset of manifestations, nature of manifestations, nature of vomitus, any typical smell, treatment received, history of drug

hypersensitivity and motive of poisoning should be recorded. Judge whether poisoning is suicidal, homicidal or accidental.

4. Informed to authorities

a. The doctor must inform all cases of poisoning to police irrespective of whether it is suicidal or homicidal or accidental poisoning.

b. If the patient is about to die, then arrange for dying deposition or dying declaration.

c. If the patient dies, death certificate should not be issued, but police must be informed and the body should be sent for postmortem examination.

d. In case of accidental poisoning due to food/water, public health authorities should also be informed, so that precautions can be taken for public health safety.

5. Preservation of material for chemical analysis:
A doctor must preserve all possible evidence of suspected poisoning. He should preserve stomach wash, vomitus, urine, blood and also other suspicious articles and utensils used for preparing the poison.

POISONING AND LAW

1. Under Section 39 of CrPC, a doctor is bound to inform the legal authorities if his patient is suffering from homicidal poisoning. Noncompliance is punishable under Section 176 IPC.

2. A doctor in Government or Public Hospital, must inform all cases of poisoning to police. However, it is not obligatory for a doctor in private hospitals to inform to police in case of suicidal poisoning.

3. A doctor must preserve all possible evidence of suspected poisoning. Purposeful omission to do so with the intention of screening the offender is punishable under Section 201 IPC. Also releasing the dead body without inquest is punishable under Section 201 IPC.

4. Under Section 175 of CrPC a doctor is bound to supply all information in relation to the patient, when summoned by the investigating officer. Noncompliance or concealing any information is punishable under Section 202 IPC. Giving false information is punishable under Section 193 IPC.

5. For causing death or injury by administration of poison, a person may be tried under Sections 299, 304A, 324, 326 and 328 of IPC.

6. Indian penal code also describes the punishment specifically related to the poisoning and adulteration to deal offences related to drugs and poison.

a. Sec. 272 IPC: Punishment for adulterating food or drink intended for sale, so as to make the same noxious, may extend up to 6 months imprisonment of either term and/or fine of up to one thousand rupees.

b. Sec. 273 IPC: Punishment for selling noxious food or drink may be imprisonment of either description for a period of 6 months and/or fine of up to one thousand rupees.

c. Sec. 274 IPC: Punishment for adulteration of drugs in any form with any change in its effect knowing that it will be sold and used as unadulterated drug, may be imprisonment of either description for a period of 6 months and/or fine.

d. Sec. 275 IPC: Punishment for knowingly selling adulterated drugs with fewer efficacies or altered action serving it for use as unadulterated may be imprisonment of either description for 6 months and/or fine.

e. Sec. 276 IPC: Punishment for selling a drug as a different drug or preparation may be imprisonment of either description, which may extend up to 6 months and/or fine.

Note: In the State of West Bengal, the punishment for these offences described under Sections 272 to 276 may be up to imprisonment for life with or without fine.

f. Sec. 277 IPC: Punishment for fouling water of public spring or reservoir may be imprisonment of either description, which may extend up to a period of 3 months and/or fine.

g. Sec. 278 IPC: Punishment for voluntarily making atmosphere noxious to health is fine which may extend up to five hundred rupees.

h. Sec. 284 IPC: Punishment for negligent conduct with respect to poisonous substance may be imprisonment of either description, which may extend up to 6 months and/ or fine, which may extend up to one thousand rupees.

i. Sec. 328 IPC: Punishment for causing hurt by means of poison or any stupefying, intoxicating or unwhole some drug or any other thing with the intent to commit an offence shall be imprisonment of either description for a term which may extend to ten years with or without fine.

ACTS RELATED TO THE USE OF DRUGS AND POISON

In India, dealing of poisons and drugs are governed by Acts which are as follows:

The Opium Act, 1857

The Opium Act ,1878

The Poisons Act, 1919

The Dangerous Drugs Act, 1930

The Drugs Act, 1940

The Drugs and Cosmetics Act, 1940

The Drugs and Cosmetics Rules, 1945

The Pharmacy Act, 1948

The Drugs Control Act, 1950

The Drugs and Magic Remedies Act, 1954

Medicinal and Toilet Preparation Act, 1955

Drugs (Amendment) Act, 1964

Narcotic Drugs and Psychotropic Substances Act, 1985

1. **The Opium Act, 1857:** This Act empowers only the Central Government to cultivate poppy plants and manufacture opium with the help of farms authorized by the Government. It is amended in 1878.

2. **The Opium Act, 1878:** This Act prohibits import, export, transportation, possession and sale of opium. This Act was further amended in 1957.

3. **The Poisons Act, 1919:** This Act provides for the regulation of import of poisons and grant of license for dealing poisons. This Act also provides the central or the State Governments power for control on the possession and sale of poisons.

4. **The Dangerous Drugs Act, 1930:** This act regulates the import, export, cultivation, manufacture, possession, sale and use of dangerous drugs (drugs of abuse) e.g. opium, Cannabis and cocaine or drugs derived from these agents. This Act was further amended in 1933 and 1938.

5. **The Drugs Act, 1940:** This Act regulates the import, manufacture, distribution and sale of drugs in India. This Act was amended in 1962 to include cosmetics under the purview of the Act and is now known as "Drugs and Cosmetics Act of 1940".

6. **The Drugs and Cosmetics Act, 1940:** This Act empowered the Central Government to form a Drugs Technical Advisory Board, and to establish a Central Drugs Laboratory, to help and advice both the Central and the State Governments for enforcing uniformity in the implementation of the different provisions of the Act, all over the country. The Central Drug Laboratory analyses imported and manufactured drugs to know their constituents, purity and potency. This Act also provides that the formula of a patent or proprietary drug must be shown on a label on the container of the medicine. This Act was further amended to include Ayurvedic and Unani drugs under its purview in 1964.

7. **The Drugs and Cosmetics Rules, 1945:** The rules were framed under the provisions of the Drugs and Cosmetics Act of 1940 (former Drugs Act of 1940), which came into effect in 1945, known as Drugs and Cosmetics Rules of 1945, to regulate the function and procedure of Central Drugs Laboratory. This rule also regulates the import, manufacture, distribution and sale of drugs.

Under this rules, drugs are classified in certain schedules (and regulations are laid down for their storage, display, sale, dispensing, labelling, prescription, etc.) as follows:

Schedule C: Biological and special products;

Schedule E: List of poisons,

Schedule F: Vaccines and sera,

Schedule G: Hormone preparation,

Schedule H: Poisonous drugs which can not be sold without a prescription,

Schedule J: List of drugs used to cure disease which should not be advertised, and

Schedule L: Antibiotics, antihistaminics and other chemotherapeutic agents.

[Schedule H and L drugs cannot be sold without the prescription.]

This rule also dictates the procedure of sale of medicine by the retailer. The retailer should maintain a register, which should contain the name and address of patient and prescribing doctor, name and ingredients of drug, the serial number and date of the sale should be recorded along with the name of manufacturer, batch number of the product and the expiry date of the potency of the drug.

8. **The Pharmacy Act, 1948:** It regulates the Central and State Councils of Pharmacy and allow only the registered pharmacist to compound, prepare, mix or dispense any medicine on the prescription of doctor

9. **The Drugs Control Act, 1950:** It controls the sale, supply and distribution of any drug. It also gives power to Central Government to fix maximum price of a drug and the maximum quantity of retail sale of a drug.

10. **The Drugs and Magic Remedies Act, 1954:** It bans the advertisement of magic remedies in relation to: (i) abortion, (ii) prevention of conception, (iii) increase sexual potency/pleasure, (iv) treatment for menstrual disorders, (v) treatment and cure of venereal diseases, (vi) false or misleading information about a drug as to its nature and function.

11. **Medicinal and Toilet Preparation Act, 1955:** This Act provides for payment of levy and excise duty for medicinal and toilet preparations containing alcohol, Cannabis, opium and other similar drugs.

12. **Narcotic Drugs and Psychotropic Substances Act, 1985:** It repeals three Acts, namely The Opium Act, 1857 and 1878; and Dangerous Drugs Act, 1930. This Acts

    i. Consolidates and amends the existing laws relating to narcotic.
    ii. Strengthens existing control over drug of abuse.
    iii Makes stringent provision for the purpose of preventing, combating trafficking, and abuse of narcotic drugs and psychotropic substances.

To enforce the Act, Government of India had framed ND and PS Rules, 1985. Likewise, State Government have also formed their own rules to enforce this Act within their jurisdiction.

A narcotic drug is one that produces narcosis or sleep. A **narcotic drug** includes Cannabis, cocaine, opium, and their derivatives.

Psychotropic drugs are one that alters mental function by its action. "**Psychotropic substances**" means any substance or preparation of such substance that are included in the list of 77 psychotropic substances, e.g. hallucinogens—LSD, stimulants—amphetamines, hypnotic—barbiturate, tranquilizer diazepam, meprobamate.

Sec. 15–32 provides punishment of imprisonment for those dealing in these drugs and substance, for 10 years which may extend to 20 years with fine of ₹ 1 lakh extend to 2 lakhs.

Under Section 27, addict who is found to be in possession of a small quantity of any drugs or substance for his personal use or who consume any material under this Act is punishable for a period of one year with fine or both. By **small quantity means** such quantity as may be prescribed by Government and includes cocaine = 125 mg, heroine, smack, brown sugar = 200 mg, opium = 500 mg, ganja = 500 gm.

Preservation of Viscera and Other Materials

2

In poisoning deaths, viscera or blood is routinely preserved for chemical analysis to know the type of poison. In some medicolegal deaths, the cause of death is not clear at autopsy and the viscera and blood is preserved for chemical analysis to give a final opinion. Even in antemortem cases, the sample (like blood or gastric aspirate) is preserved to estimate the level of intoxicant. **Apart from such routine cases, the viscera and other materials like skin, hair, tissue, bones, urine, blood, etc. are preserved in different cases for various reasons.**

The viscera and other material from the human body may be preserved for the following reasons/purposes:

a. Chemical analysis (CA)—in poisoning, alcoholic intoxication, drug overdose.
   • Detection of toxin—in food poisoning
b. Blood grouping—in homicidal cases, sexual offences.
c. Biological/immunological study—in snakebites.
d. Detection of petroleum products—in burns.
e. Detection of residual and other material—in cases of firearm.
f. DNA fingerprinting—in disputed paternity and other cases.
g. Fingerprinting—in unknown persons for identification.
h. Diatoms detection—in drowning.
i. Biochemical estimation of certain elements and enzymes in poisoning (OP compounds), pathological condition and for time since death.
j. Microbiological examination: culture and sensitivity—in septicaemia,
   Virus detection—in dog bite cases, bacterial/protozoa detection in gastroenteritis and cholera.
k. Histopathological examination.
l. Histochemical examination.
m. Bone examination.

Apart from the above purpose, sometimes the organs or its part is preserved for museum purpose.

PRESERVATION FOR CHEMICAL ANALYSIS

1. In antemortem cases, usually the gastric aspirate/stomach wash for chemical analysis (in poisoning), blood for grouping (in sexual offences, assault cases), blood for chemical analysis (in alcoholic or intoxicating cases), and blood for DNA fingerprinting are preserved for further analysis.

2. However in postmortem cases, commonly the viscera is preserved for chemical analysis (in poisoning), followed by blood for chemical analysis (in alcoholic or intoxicating cases) and for grouping (in homicidal cases).

3. In cases of poisoning or where opinion is not possible on the autopsy findings alone or where death occurred in suspicious circumstances all of a sudden, viscera and body fluids/materials are to be preserved for chemical analysis.

4. Sometimes urine, feces, vomitus and other material are also preserved for chemical analysis.

5. In food poisoning, only the stomach contents are preserved without any preservative and sent to chemical analyser for the detection of toxins.
6. These materials are sent to regional forensic science laboratory (FSL) by the autopsy/treating doctor through the concerned police along with the related prescribed forms duly filled, signed and sealed.

INDICATION FOR VISCERA PRESERVATION FOR CHEMICAL ANALYSIS (CA)

1. The doctor conducting the autopsy suspects poisoning.
2. The investigating officer request for the same.
3. The cause of death is not known at autopsy—to exclude poisoning.
4. The cause of death is established but there is also suspicion of poisoning.
5. In traffic accidents especially of the driver when suspicion of alcohol consumption (blood for CA).
6. In homicidal deaths, to rule out any intoxication.

Routine viscera to be preserved: Since in majority of the cases, the poison is ingested and absorbs through stomach and intestines, is metabolized in liver and spleen and is excreted by kidneys in urine, the following viscera is routinely preserved (Table 2.1 and Fig. 2.1).

V1: Bottle No. 1: Stomach and intestinal loop and their contents.

V2: Bottle No. 2: Pieces of liver, ½ of spleen and ½ of both kidneys.

V3: Bottle No. 3: Blood 10–100 ml.

Gallbladder should be preserved along with liver since majority of the drugs can be

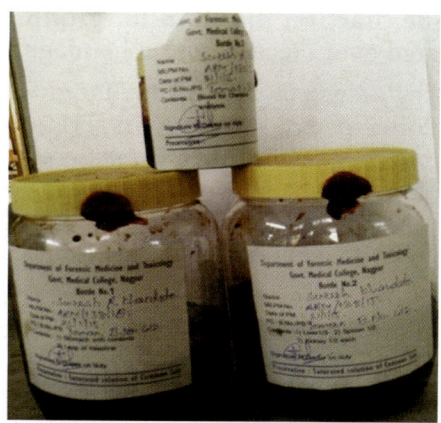

Fig. 2.1: Routine viscera for CA

Table 2.1: Guidelines for preservation of routine viscera in poisoning for CA

Viscera	Quantity	Preservatives
1. V1: Stomach with its contents + intestinal loop with its contents	Whole stomach with 300 ml **or** whole, if less is available 1 meter (2 meters in children, whole in infants) 100 ml **or** whole if less is available	Saturated solution of **common salt (not used in acid poisoning)** or rectified spirit (but not used in alcohol, phosphorus, acetic acid, phenol, paraldehyde, formalin, chloroform, chloral hydrate, anesthetic agents, etc.)
2. V2: Liver + gall bladder, spleen, and kidney	500 gm or 1/3rd of liver (whole in infants) 1/2 of the spleen (whole in infants) 1/2 of each kidney (whole in infants)	Saturated solution of **common salt (not used in acid poisoning)** or rectified spirit (but not used in alcohol, phosphorus, acetic acid, phenol, paraldehyde, formalin, chloroform, chloral hydrate, anesthetic agents, etc.)
3. V3: Blood	100 ml (postmortem) 10 ml (antemortem)	30 mg of potassium oxalate + 10 mg of sodium fluoride/10 ml of blood
4. Urine	100 ml (postmortem) 30–50 ml (antemortem)	3 ml of concentration HCl or 2–3 ml chloroform/100 ml of urine or 100 mg of **sodium fluoride** per 10 ml of urine
5. Gastric aspirate	500 ml or whole, if less is available	No preservatives

In food poisoning cases, stomach contents should be sent for detection of toxins to FSL, Mumbai

detected in it. Half of each kidney has to be preserved, as one kidney may be non-functional.

Blood for grouping: 2 ml blood from cubital vein in AM cases and from heart in PM cases in equal volume of 5% sodium citrate solution. However, it is preferred to prepare two blood stains of 5 cm diameter on sterile starch free cotton cloth and send in an envelope after complete air drying. Starch from the clothed is removed by successive washing the cloth with plain water and then drying. **But in routine practice, the stain for grouping is prepared over piece of cotton bandage.**

Dried blood stain over body for grouping: It is collected by taking stain scrapping if possible or transfer the dried stain onto the clean cotton cloth piece moistened with normal saline or distilled water, by gentle rubbing and send in an envelope after complete air drying.

Additional viscera/material to be preserved: Depending upon the specific site of action or affinity/storage of a poison for/in a particular organ, these organs are preserved as additional viscera, whenever indicated. Any additional viscera or material is preserved in a separate bottle (Table 2.2).

a. In injection deaths: The skin and muscles from around the site of injection are preserved **for detection of suspected drugs.** A similar part from opposite side is collected as control.

b. In burn cases: Skin, hair and clothes are preserved for the detection of **petroleum product** in cases where required. In presence of clothes, skin and hair is not required to send for preservation. If clothes are present then skin is not required for CA in such cases as it does not add any advantage.

c. In snakebite: Skin from bite site along with blood is preserved for detection of venom.

d. In electrocution cases: A part of skin from the site of electrocution injury is preserved for the detection of **metallic residues**; and part of skin for histopathology.

e. In cases of criminal abortion: The uterus, cervix, bladder and rectum are preserved.

f. In alcohol poisoning: Blood
g. In cerebral poisons: Brain
h. In strychnine poisoning: Spinal cord and brain
i. In cardiac poisons: Heart
j. In inhaled poisons: Lungs and brain
k. In heavy metal poisoning: Bone, bone marrow, nails and hair.

MATERIALS TO BE PRESERVED IN SEXUAL OFFENCES

In case of victims, following samples/articles are preserved for Forensic Science Laboratory (FSL):

a. Blood for grouping
b. Blood for CA
c. Urine for CA
d. Seminal stain for grouping and identification
e. Nail scrapping for detection of epithelium of assailant
f. Pubic hair: Plucked/loose
g. Foreign material: Hair/cloth fibers/skin fragment
h. Vaginal swabs for detection of seminal fluid (acid phosphatase, etc.)
i. Anal/buccal swabs: For detection of semen.
j. Clothes—usually the undergarments for seminal stains.

In case of accused, following articles are preserved for FSL:

a. Blood for grouping
b. Blood for CA
c. Urine for CA
d. Nail scrapping for detection of epithelium of suspect
e. Pubic Hair: Plucked/loose
f. Foreign material: Hair/cloth fibers/skin fragment
g. Anal/buccal swabs
h. Clothes

Apart from the above materials, the blood is preserved for culture; vaginal swab/smears for detection of sperms; penis/urethral swab/

Table 2.2: Additional viscera/materials and body fluids to be preserved in other specific cases apart from routine viscera

Specimen	Indication	Quantity	Preservative
1. Blood	Grouping	2 ml (from cubital vein in AM cases) 2 ml (from heart in PM cases) **or** cotton bandage soaked in blood and dried* **or** two blood stains of 5 cm diameter on sterile cotton cloth* **or** plucked hair* **or** muscle (in saturated saline) **or** molar teeth* **or** bones* as such *No preservative, it is sent in an envelope after completely dried	2 ml of 5% sodium citrate solution prepared as (5 gm sodium citrate + 0.25 ml of 40% formalin + distilled water to make it 100 ml).
	CA—for alcohol, poisoning cases	5–10 ml (from cubital vein in AM cases) 100 ml (from heart in PM cases)	1 mg of sodium fluoride + 3 mg potassium oxalate/ml
	Snakebite	5–10 ml of blood	5% sodium citrate (i.e. 5 gm in distilled water)
	Volatile poisons or irrespirable gases (CO)	2–5 ml (from heart in PM cases)	A layer of liquid paraffin added to top of blood to avoid losses
2. CSF	Alcohol	As much as possible	10 ml of Na fluoride/ml CSF
3. Brain	a. Dog bite i. For HP ii. For Negri bodies b. Alcohol, CO, HCN, anesthetic drugs, opiates, strychnine, barbiturate	Piece of brain from hippocampus cerebral cortex, medulla and cerebellum 300 gm of brain tissue	Formalin 50% glycerine in isotonic saline for Negri bodies Saturated solution of common salt
4. Spinal cord	Strychnine, gelsemium	Entire length	Rectified spirit
5. Lungs	Inhaled/volatile poison	One	Saturated solution of common salt
6. Skin with underlying tissue	a. Corrosive or injection death (insulin, cocaine morphine, heroin) b. Snakebite (skin from bite site + control) + venous blood c. Electrocution d. Burns	5–10 gm of tissue around site **or** 2 × 2 × 4 cm area with muscle + control skin from opposite side 5–10 gm of tissue around bite site + control skin 5–10 ml blood From the site of electrocution injury for detection of metallic residues Burnt site for detection of petroleum products	Common salt or rectified spirit Common salt 5% sodium citrate Common salt –
7. Heart	Cardiac poison	Complete	Saturated solution of common salt
8. Uterus its with appendages	Abortifacient agents in criminal abortion	Complete	Saturated solution of common salt

(Contd.)

Table 2.2: Additional viscera/materials and body fluids to be preserved in other specific cases apart from routine viscera *(Contd.)*

Specimen	Indication	Quantity	Preservative
9. Long bones	Heavy metal poisoning	15 cm of length or 200–300 gm, **or** bone marrow from sternum/femur	–
10. Scalp hair	Heavy metal	15–20 bands (20 gm) for detection of metals	–
	Burns	15–20 bands (20 gm) for detection of petroleum products	–
11. Pubic hair	Suspected sex violence	Plucking or combing in sterile envelope after drying	Immediately dried in desiccator
12. Vaginal or anal swab/ fluid and foreign body	Suspected sex violence	In test tube/slide immediately dried in desiccation and kept separated in TT	Sent in an envelope
13. Vomitus	Poisoning cases	500 ml or whole, if less	–
14. Stomach wash	Poisoning cases	Wash with distilled water— 500 ml or less	Saturated solution of common salt
15. Nail scraping	• Suspected sex assault • Homicidal/assault	Of all fingers, clipped without damaging underlying tissue to match with accused	–
16. Saliva	Grouping	Few drops in sterile test tube, **or** Two dried stains of 5 cm diameter on cloth	– Sent in envelope after drying
17. Soil	Exhumation articles	20 gm soil as much as possible	–
18. Clothes	Grouping—Homicidal Sexual offence Poisoning cases Burns	Blood stained cloth Undergarment or any stained cloth Soiled cloths For detection of petroleum products	Sent in envelope after complete air drying

smears for detection of vaginal epithelium. **These materials are not sent to FSL for examination.** Rather, it should be sent to department of microbiology/pathology or examined by oneself, if facilities are available.

MATERIALS PRESERVED IN FIREARM CASE

In every firearm case, the body is subjected to radiological examination prior to the autopsy for localization of projectiles (bullet/pellets) and for the track of firearm injuries.

Following materials are preserved in firearm cases and sent to FSL for further analysis (Table 2.3).

1. Skin from the site of entry and exit.
2. Projectile or related material.
3. Wash sample: Swab moistened with distilled water.
4. Clothes.

MATERIALS TO BE PRESERVED FOR DNA FINGERPRINTING (Table 2.4)

In living person
1. Usually 1.5 ml of blood in 2 plastic tubes containing EDTA.
2. One drop of blood on FTA paper.

In dead person
1. Blood if available from heart.
2. Autopsy tissue usually spleen—2 gm.
3. Bone, usually femur/manubrium.

IN UNKNOWN PERSONS FOR IDENTIFICATION

Identification is the main concern of investigation in unknown bodies. It can be known

Table 2.3: Materials to be preserved in firearm cases

Specimen	Quantity	Preservation technique
1. Skin	5–10 cm diameter around site or bearing shot holes	Keep in two plain white papers stapled to a thick cardboard and tied to another cardboard. Do not put in bottle or in any preservative
2. Pellets/fragments of bullet + other projectile like wad, etc.	As many as possible	Dried in air and put in bottle without any preservative
3. Bullet	Remove with finger or rubber tipped forceps	Dried and wrapped in cotton and put in a suitable container after putting identification mark on the base
4. Swabs a. Moist with distilled water b. Wet with 5% HNO_3 c. Control samples of cotton, HNO_3 and distilled water	From web and fingers of both hands separately in case of alleged firer	Dried in air and put in suitable container
5. Clothes	All or bearing shot holes	Dried in air and put in suitable container

Note: X-ray of the body is to be taken prior to the postmortem examination. Injury should be properly described, photograph with a scale attached or sketched and sent along with the articles to FSL for comparison purpose.

Table 2.4: Materials/tissue preserved for DNA profile

Specimen	Quantity	Preservative	Container	Freezing
Blood liquid	1.5 ml in 2 tubes—AM 2–5 ml in tube—PM	EDTA	Plastic tube	Refrigeration
Blood stain	1 drop on FTA paper—AM 5 cm radius on cloth—PM	Air-dried	Envelope	Dry freeze
Swabs (oral/vaginal/rectal)	3–4 swabs	Air-dried	Plastic container	Dry freeze
Stain (blood, semen, saliva)	5 cm radius stain or scrapped off, if dried	–	Plastic container, envelope	Dry freeze
Seminal/vaginal fluid	1–20 ml or 1–2 drop	EDTA	Plastic tube	Refrigeration
Urine	60–100 ml	–	Plastic tube	Refrigeration
Saliva	A few drops	–	Plastic tube	Refrigeration
Hair	10–20 hair	–	Envelope	Dry freeze
Autopsy tissue	2 gm (spleen, muscle, etc.)	–	Plastic container	Dry freeze
Bone/tooth	Femur, humerus, sternum	–	Paper	–

Sometimes, the FSL person (along with kit) is accompanied for collection of blood for DNA profiling. So, if samples are collected and taken to the FSL on same day, then freezing is not required.

from tattoo marks, scar, congenital or acquired peculiarities, clothes and belongings with ornaments. But fingerprints and dental charting is the ideal method for identification.

Fingerprintings for Identification (details in separate heading of fingerprinting)
In Maharashtra, **fingerprinting** is under the control of CID of the state and **not done in**

FSL. In unknown persons, the fingerprints are taken by the police departments.

Materials Preserved But not Sent to FSL

1. **In dog bite cases**—for detection of Negri bodies in brain, the samples should be sent to Director, Haffkine Institute for Training, Research and Testing, Acharya Donde Marg, Parel, Mumbai–400012. Phone: 022–24160947, 24160961–61, Fax: 022–24161787.

2. **Histopathological examination** of tissue, detection of **diatoms, bone examination** for ascertaining age, sex, etc. **Biochemical** and hematological examination, and **microbiological examination are not done in FSL,** so such materials are not sent to FSL.

3. **For bone examination** in skeletonized or partially skeletonized body, the bones should be sent to the Professor and Head, **Department of Anatomy** (of authorized centers) Government Medical Colleges at Nagpur, Mumbai, Pune, Aurangabad, Solapur. However, in some states like MP, UP, Chhattisgarh, etc. the bones are examined in the Department of Forensic Medicine usually at medicolegal institute.

4. **For entomological examination:** Live as well as dead eggs, larvae, maggots are collected in two vials. Half to be preserved in ethyl alcohol or formaline and other half should be kept alive to be reared out without any preservative. Medicolegal Institute, Bhopal has carried out such examination to determine time since death.

MODE OF PRESERVATION, PACKING AND DISPATCH OF VISCERA

1. The collected viscera is preserved in a clean **wide mouth standard glass** or **preferably plastic** bottles **of ~1 liter capacity.** Blood is preserved in 30 ml bottle or plastic capped tubes of 5 ml. Sometimes bottles are supplied by the forensic science laboratory either in cleaned conditioned or it is to be cleaned with sulphuric acid—chromate solution, rinsed with distilled water and dried.

2. V1, V2, V3, etc. should be preserved separately. The additional material should be preserved in separate bottles.

3. However, **bone, hair, nails, clothes, etc. are packed in polythene packet or plain paper.** But polythene bags or plastic containers are not used in volatile poison (which diffuse through it) and in corrosives poison (which corrode it). Lungs should be **preserved in nylon bags** for **volatile substance.**

3. The tissues are open/cut into small pieces before preservation.

4. The **preservative is added to each bottle, so as to completely dip the viscera** (otherwise the exposed portions will decompose). A sample of preservative (100 ml rectified spirit or 25 gm common salt) is separately kept in a bottle and sent for analysis to exclude the possibility of contamination with poison.

5. However, container should not be filled completely and **one-third of the container should be kept empty,** so as to accommodate the gases liberated due to decomposition of viscera.

6. The bottle is made **air tight** by putting a lid on it. The lid is then **covered with** a piece of cloth, which is tied with string or is stuck with tape.

7. The bottle is then **properly labeled** and the ends of string/tape are **sealed.** The label contains the PM number; date and time of PM; name, age and sex of deceased; the viscera preserved; the preservative used and signature of medical officer.

8. All sealed bottles containing viscera/materials are **handed over to** the concerned **police** constable immediately, **after taking receipt.**

9. The forwarding **viscera form** requesting the chemical analyzer to examine the viscera/material, is **filled by the doctor and sent to FSL along with the viscera.** In the forwarding forms/letter to the chemical analyser, the **specimen of seal** and copy of label on the material should

be included along with the outward number, reference number and description of articles.

10. The **police then submitted** the sealed viscera bottles and sealed viscera form to the concerned chemical analyzer.

At some places where **viscera box** is being provided by chemical analyzer's office, these sealed bottles are first kept in the viscera box. The box is then closed and locked. Cloth is tied on the lock and it is sealed. A label is put on the box mentioning the content of the box. The key of the box, viscera form, and a sample seal on a piece of paper corresponding to the seal used on bottles, lock and viscera form are kept in an envelope which is sealed and sent with viscera box.

Resealing/relabeling: Sometimes the police bring back the viscera bottle stating that the seal of the bottle is detached or bursting of viscera bottle requesting to transfer the viscera to other bottle or resealing of viscera bottle. Sometimes the label is missing or soiled with the bottle contents, requesting to change the label. In such case viscera bottles once sealed should not be resealed or transfer to other bottle, nor the new label be prepared. It is always better to **advice the police to prepare a panchnama of the damaged viscera bottle** and submit the viscera bottle after proper sealing/labeling to the chemical analyser's office with a copy a panchnama at the earliest. **To avoid soiling**/tampering of the label, it is to be coated with transparent cello adhesive tape or using plastic coated labels written by permanent marker pen.

DISPOSAL OF VISCERA NOT TAKEN BY POLICE

Viscera collected and preserved for chemical analysis should be **handed over to police** or investigating officer **immediately** after completing the autopsy. However, if the viscera are not collected by the police/investigating officer for a period of **3 months** after autopsy without any information, then it can be disposed off.

It can also be disposed off
a. After taking written permission from magistrate or police.

b. When informed by the police/investigating officer in writing that the case is closed or viscera are not required.

c. When informed by the police/investigating officer in writing about disposal of viscera.

INTERPRETATION OF RESULT OF CHEMICAL ANALYSIS

a. Poison not found in bottles 1 and 2: Poison not detected or it was not a case of poisoning.

b. Poison found in bottle 1 and absent in bottle 2: Poison **not absorbed** or locally acting poison; death is not due to poisoning or poisoning may be postmortem.

c. Poison found in bottle 2 and absent in bottle 1: **Poison absorbed**, if poison is ingested, it is more than 2–6 hours before, may be **poisoning by other routes**, if the level is as that of fatal poisoning—death is due to poisoning.

d. Poison found in bottles 1 and 2: Poison partially absorbed.

REASON FOR NON-DETECTION OF POISON IN VISCERA

Sometimes poison may not be detected on chemical analysis due to following reasons

1. Delay in the examination of viscera and decomposition.
2. Improper preservation.
3. Tampering of preserved viscera.
4. Early disintegration or neutralization of the poison.
5. **Denaturation of protein**—example snake venom and bacterial toxins.
6. Use of wrong analytical technique.
7. Small amount of poison in viscera or small amount of sample for analysis.
8. Lack of suitable chemical test for certain poison.
9. Complete metabolism of the poison in the body.
10. Removal/detoxification of poison during treatment.
11. Poison vomited or excreted out completely.
12. Delayed death after poisoning.

13. Lastly, due to the **unavailability of the standard** of specific poisons it will not be detected even if consumed. Example: **Vegetables and drug poison**. Also, there are various sub-types of insecticidal poison, if the person consumed some particular poison whose **standard is not available** with FSL, then that particular **poison will not be detected**/analyzed **in spite of the presence of poison** in stomach at autopsy.

Court question—about CA report and opinion in poisoning: In most of the admitted poisoning cases and other poisoning cases of vegetable/animal source, the poison is not detected on CA (Negative CA Report). In such cases the court will ask the autopsy doctor about the cause of death and the reason for non-detection of poison in the viscera.

In an **admitted case of poisoning**, it is advised **not to keep opinion reserved** for pending chemical analysis, where the findings of poisoning were absent due to prolonged admission or gastric lavage or treatment. Rather, the **opinion** should be given at autopsy as "**PM findings are consistent with death due to poisoning**" in absence of any other findings suggestive of other cause of death. **Even in brought death or spot death of poisoning,** the opinion should be given at postmortem examination, if there are findings suggestive of poisoning in the stomach (like kerosene/insecticidal smell with hemorrhagic/eroded mucosa) or other specific findings to particular poisons (like fangs mark in snakebite).

In cases of poisoning, the opinion about cause of death **(death due to poisoning or PM findings are consistent with death due to poisoning)** is usually possible at autopsy either by way of positive findings of poisoning, or by way of exclusion of findings suggestive of other cause of death. The chemical analysis in such cases reveals only the type of poison, but in many cases it may not reveal any poisons on general and specific chemical testing. Similarly, in food poisoning cases, the toxin will not be detected on CA due to denaturation of toxin.

In snakebite cases, the **opinion (death due to snakebite)** should be given at postmortem examination. Chemical analysis is almost always negative in such cases due to denaturation of venom. The **death** is usually due to **poisonous snakebite**, but **can also be possible in non-poisonous snakebite due to fear.**

ALTERNATIVE TO ROUTINE VISCERA IN POISONING CASES

In **antemortem cases**, stomach wash, blood and urine are preserved in separate bottles for chemical analysis in case of poisoning. But in **postmortem cases,** routine viscera from the dead body are preserved in two separate bottles and blood is preserved in third bottle for the detection of poison or intoxicants. However, the purpose of detection of poison or intoxicant will be accomplished even if only the gastric content or washing (with normal saline) is sent in place of stomach and intestinal loop with content; blood in place of liver and spleen; and urine in place of kidneys. Moreover, there is no added advantage of sending routine viscera for CA. Thus, the alternative to routine viscera may be:

1st bottle	Gastric content or gastric washing with normal saline/plain water (100 ml or whole if less is available)
2nd bottle	Blood from heart—10 ml
3rd bottle	Urine—100 ml

FINGERPRINTING

As already mentioned **fingerprinting** is under the control of CID of the state and **not done in FSL.** In medicolegal deaths of unknown persons, the fingerprints are taken by the police departments; and analyzed by fingerprint expert. The study of fingerprinting as a method of identification is also known as dactylography, which is a process of taking the impression of papillary ridges of the fingertip.

Types of fingerprint and their percentage in population

Loops: 65%	Whorls: 25%
Arch: 7%	Composite: 2–3%

Method of fingerprinting: Fingerprints are taken with the help of printer's ink on non-glazed papers, after cleaning and drying the finger tips. It may be taken in two ways and are useful when the person is available.

1. **Plain method:** In this method, the inked finger is brought in contact with the paper and pressed gently. It is more clear and helps to check ridge pattern at a particular place, if the rolled impression is blurred at that place.

2. **Rolled method:** In this method, one side of the inked finger tip is gently pressed on the paper and rolled onto the other side without lifting finger. Maximum area of the impression is obtained and offer better study of the pattern of ridges, but sometimes may be blurred.

Fingerprints from the Dead Body

1. A few hours after death, tip of the fingers may get shrivelled in a dead body and may mask the picture. So to avoid this, **soak the fingers in alkaline solution first and then take the print as mentioned above.**

2. Fingerprints can be taken from even the **highly decomposed bodies**, either from the **peeled off epidermis** of the fingers or **from the dermis** when epidermis is lost.

3. Sometimes in dead bodies, the **skin and subcutaneous tissues of all the fingertips are dissected out** at the request of investigating officer and kept out in *weak alkaline solution* or normal saline **in ten different small clear bottles with markings** of initials of finger like RT, RI, RM (Right Thumb, Right Index, Right Middle), etc. respectively.

4. Sometimes in highly decomposed bodies, the skin of hand may be peeled off completely and come out as a 'gloves' that may also be **preserved completely.** In this, fingerprints can be made by inserting the technician finger into the 'skin glove', inking the area to be printed and rolling.

Plastic fingerprinting are the fingertips impressions left on soft materials like dust, soap or wax. The fingerprints which are not visible as such but made visible are called **invisible fingerprinting or latent fingerprinting.**

Method of development and lifting of fingerprinting: The fingerprints which are not visible, are made visible by using various developing agents and the use of these agents depends on the type of surface needed to be searched for fingerprint.

a. **Physical/powder method:** For hard and non-absorbent surface (like glass, porcelain, painted or sun-mica covered surface, metallic articles) but light or dark surface, following powders are used:
   i. Light/white surface—black powder is used
   ii. Dark/black surface—grey powder/aluminum powder is used
   iii. Multicolored surface—fluorescent type of powder is used
   iv. Dragon's blood (a natural powder) may be used for both surfaces.

Magnetic brush and powders are used to increase the efficiency in development of latent prints. The magnetic brush marks with magnetic powders are available in many colors like grey, black, red, yellow, etc.

Lifting of fingerprinting: Latent fingerprint on the paper or small articles can be preserved after development as such. But when they are on large immovable hard surface, the print can be lifted for preservation after being developed. Two types of lifting medium employed are:
- Transparent cello/adhesive tape in 1.5 or 2 inch width roll.
- Opaque rubber lifter.

b. **Chemical methods:** For soft absorbent surface (like paper, cardboard, clothes, etc.), iodine vapor, silver nitrate and ninhydrin are used.

Mechanism: Fingertips are usually layered with sebaceous secretion like other parts of the body. While committing crimes or due to nervous tension there is sweating from the pores of the skin and it occurs even from the fingertips. This perspiration consists of 98% water with traces of salts like NaCl, sulphates, phosphates, carbamates, lactic acid, fatty acid, glucose and urea. The chemical used for development reacts with these salts to produce visible prints against the background.

The following methods are used

i. **Iodine method:** The iodine fumes reacts with the fatty acids of the print and appear yellowish brown or brownish.

ii. **Silver nitrate method:** It reacts with NaCl to form silver chloride, which is an unstable white substance that darkens, when exposed to light breaking into silver and chlorine that appear reddish brown.

iii. **Ninhydrin method:** It reacts with amino-acid and gives purple reddish brown stains. All the above methods are used for old prints.

iv. **Osmium tetraoxide method:** It is reduced to free osmium that is dark in color in presence of fatty substance.

Finder (fingerprint reader): It is a computerized automatic fingerprint reading system which can record each fingerprint data in half seconds. The light reflected from a fingerprint can be measured and converted to digital data which is classified, codified and stored in the computer.

Primary classification system of scoring: Scores are allotted for the presence of whorls in different finger of each hand.

Presence of whorls in finger	Scoring
Right thumb (RT)/right index (RI)	16
Right middle (RM)/right ring (RR)	08
Right little (RL)/left thumb (LT)	04
Left index (LI)/left middle (LM)	02
Left ring (LR)/left little (LL)	01

The scores are then arranged as follows and one is added for the purpose of calculation.

$$\text{Scores} = \frac{RT + RM + RL + LI + LR + 1}{RI + RR + LT + LM + LL + 1}$$

$$= \frac{16 + 8 + 4 + 2 + 1 + 1}{16 + 8 + 4 + 2 + 1 + 1}$$

The score of numerator is multiplied with denominator. So, $32 \times 32 = 1024$ scores are possible, if whorls are present in all fingertips.

Federal Bureau of Investigation (FBI): USA maintains record of more than two crores fingerprints by systemic maintenance of separate files on the basis of presence of whorls in the finger. In 60% of the world population, there is no whorl in any finger, so according to primary classification, the score is one. On the basis of this scoring, 1024 divisions are made which are called **'pigeon holes'**. Depending on the scoring, final identification of any fingerprint is made by comparison.

Comparison Between Two Fingerprints

Different countries have developed their minimum number of points of comparisons for establishing complete identity of person. These are: France:16, Australia: 12, Japan: 12–14, Canada: 10–16, Interpol: 12, US: 7–12, Spain: 10–12, New Zealand: 8–12, Isreal: 10–12 and India: 9 point.

Point of comparison between two fingerprints is as follows

1. Ridge pattern
2. Ridge endings
3. Missing ridge
4. Gap in two ridges
5. Ridge breaking
6. Ridge bifurcation
7. Ridge reunion
8. Dot in the ridge gap
9. A stud in the ridge
10. An island formation
11. A lake formation
12. Dot in a lake
13. Union of two ridges
14. Presence of scar
15. Starting of new ridge in between two ridges
16. Distance between delta and core
17. Number of ridges between delta and core
18. Direction of any particular ridge.

DNA FINGERPRINTING

The technique of DNA fingerprint was first developed by Sir Alec Jeffreys of Leicester University, UK in 1984 and developed in India in 1987. It was successfully used in sensational cases like Rajiv Gandhi assassination, famous Tandoori case and recently Madhumita murder case.

DNA fingerprinting can be done by two techniques

i. Restriction fragment length polymorphism
ii. Polymerase chain reaction (PCR).

In above techniques, there is determination of sequence of bands on part of DNA strands within chromosomes.

Centers for DNA Fingerprinting

Initially it was done only in 'center for cellular and molecular biology' (CCMB), Hyderabad. Previously, all the samples had to be sent to Hyderabad from all regions of India. Now in Maharashtra, new center for DNA fingerprint is established in **Regional Forensic Science Laboratories at Mumbai and Nagpur.** These centers also provide the kit for collection, preservation and dispatch of samples with prescribed forms.

Materials used in DNA Profiling (Table 2.4)

DNA fingerprinting can be done from a wide range of biological specimens in both living and dead person. Biological specimens like blood, bone marrow, semen, hair root sheath, skin and any body tissue, fluid or secretion that contain nucleated cells are used. And cigarette butts, envelops, chewing gum and other articles which can contain saliva are amenable to PCR. Since DNA is very stable, the test can be done on very old stains (aged/dried stains) or specimens (mutilated/decomposed bodies).

Collection, Preservation and Dispatch of Samples for DNA Fingerprinting

Routinely, 1.5 ml of blood is collected in two plastic tubes (with EDTA) and a drop of blood in FTA paper provided by FSL (from mother, baby and alleged father separately) (Fig. 2.2).

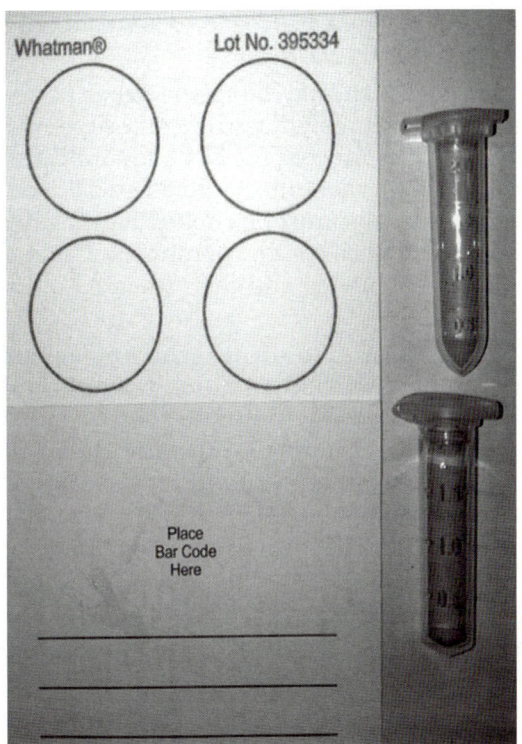

Fig. 2.2: Tubes and FTA paper for DNA profile

Autopsy samples can be used except in highly decomposed bodies, where nuclear chromatin is destroyed by putrefaction.

1. Blood

As red blood cells have no nuclear DNA, sufficient blood must be obtained to extract DNA from leukocytes. The blood sample of 2–5 ml is taken in EDTA containing plastic (not glass) tube. It should be frozen solid in deep freeze or the ice-making compartment of an ordinary refrigerator.

Blood stains should be rubbed with cotton or wool swab moistened with water. This swab is then air-dried without heat and frozen. Dried bloodstains on hard surface can be scraped off with a scalpel and sent as cold as possible.

2. Seminal and Vaginal Fluid/Swabs

Liquid fluid found in the vagina or elsewhere should be recovered with a fine pipette placed in a small plain tube and frozen solid. Seminal stains on small items of fabric or any other small objects may be frozen or kept as cool as possible during transit.

Mouth swab may be taken either to seek semen in suspected oral intercourse or to obtain buccal mucosa for DNA identification. In the latter case, the yield is small, so at least 3–4 swabs must be rubbed hard against inside of the cheek or the mouth lining scraped with an instrument and then smeared onto a swab.

Swabs from mouth, vagina and rectum should be air-dried as quickly as possible but not heated. They should then be stored in deep freeze unless sent straight to the laboratory. As with blood, suspect **dried seminal stains** on hard surface may be **scraped off** and dispatched dry to the laboratory.

Bulk clothing cannot be frozen and should merely be kept cool. They should be sent to the laboratory as soon as possible using strong paper bags and not impervious polythene, which encourages mould formation. Alternatively damp swabs may be taken off from suspect stains, which are then dried and frozen.

3. Hairs

Whatever, the source of hair, they are of no use for DNA profiling unless nucleated root or follicle cells are present in sufficient numbers. The keratinized shaft contain no DNA extractable material. Thus, hair shed naturally may have little or no root material and it is essential to have to **plucked hair** from the living or the dead. At least 10–20 hair are required, these should be placed in a small plastic bag and frozen. **However, where facilities for mitochondrial STR** are available, DNA profiling can be done with **any part of the hair.**

4. Autopsy Tissue Samples

At least 2 gm of tissue should be cut from the parenchyma of an organ and placed in small plastic tube with no fixative or preservative. These should be frozen solid. Spleen is said to be one of the best organs for DNA recovery, though liver, muscle and kidney may also be used. In decomposed or skeletonized body, molar tooth or bone (usually femur) should be preserved for DNA profiling.

5. For Paternity Disputes

DNA matching can be done by collecting amniotic fluid/chorionic membrane or by collecting blood from the umbilical cord and matching with suspected biological father. Recently, it can also be done by just collecting maternal blood for fetal cells.

Medicolegal Application

Here, the band of DNA is matched with the suspected source or individual.

1. Murder
2. Sexual offence
3. Paternity/maternity disputes
4. Mixed babies in hospitals
5. Identification of mutilated, dismembered or burnt bodies: The DNA fingerprinting obtained from such remains can be compared with those of close blood relatives of the deceased.
6. Missing person can be identified if his parents or children are available.

DIATOMS ANALYSIS IN DROWNING (IN REMOTE ORGANS AND TISSUE)

Revenstorf in 1904 was the first to attempt the use of diatoms as a test for drowning, though he stated that Hoffman in 1896 was the first to discover them in lung fluid. An excellent review of the diatom controversy was published by Peabody in 1980.

The basic concept is that when a living person is drowned in water containing diatoms, many **diatoms will penetrate the alveolar walls and will be carried to distant target organs** such as brain, kidneys, liver and bone marrow.

Diatoms belong to the class of plant known as Diatomaceae and consist of a box or 'frustule' composed of two valves, which fit together to enclose the cytoplasmic contents. These are the **unicellular algae,** which have inert silicon coating around them. These are present in all natural water sources. There are at least 10,000 species of diatoms. If diatoms are observed in the tissue of distant organs, then it goes strongly in support of death due to drowning, but there are certain fallacies.

Sample Used for Detection of Diatoms

1. Distant organ tissue like bone marrow, brain, kidneys: By acid digestion.
2. Test water where victim was drowned: Sedimentation, centrifuge and microscope examination.
3. Control water sample from place of testing: Sedimentation, centrifuge and microscopic examination.

Test: For tissue and bone **(sternum/femur)**

1. Bone marrow is exposed by cutting a small portion of bone or by crushing it.
2. Small portion (~10 ml) of marrow scooped out into a test tube/crushed tissue—TT.
3. Acid digestion: Add concentration HNO_3 solution in TT for 24–48 hrs.
   Heat the solution till clear fluid is obtained.
4. Cool and centrifuge at 4000 rpm for 10 min.
5. Examine the sediment under microscope for diatoms.

Method to Detect Diatoms from Water (Not <30 Liters) Sent by Police

1. Immobilize the container/bucket containing water for 4–7 days.
2. Take out 30 ml of sediment with the help of pipette.
3. Centrifuge the fluid at 4000 rpm for 10 min.
4. Examine the sediment under microscope.

Result: Presence of diatoms

Tissue	Test water	Control water	Result
+	+	–	True positive
+	+	+	False positive
–	+	–	False negative

Fallacies of Presence of Diatoms

1. **False negative:** Diatoms may not be observed in the tissue even in antemortem drowning and the water in which drowned contained diatom.

2. **False positive:** Even if drowning was not antemortem, similar diatom may be present in both the test sample and the control sample, if the victim was habituated to drink water from the same source.

Critics of diatom test

1. Diatoms are ubiquitous, being **present in soil, water and in air.**
2. Though entry into the body is thought to be mainly through lungs, **there seems no reason why they cannot penetrate the intestinal lining and gain access** to the bloodstream and to anybody tissue.
3. Certain fish contains large amount of diatoms that may enter the circulation and reach the tissue.
4. It is present in the tissue even when the cause of death is other than drowning.

In spite of the fallacies and critics, the greatest advantage of the diatom test would be that a positive diagnosis of drowning could be made even in the frequently putrefied bodies where no hope of anatomical recognition of drowning is possible. If diatoms are present in both tissue and control samples of water, then it can be presumed that death was due to drowning and occurred in that water. But still it is not conclusive in all cases. At present, the diatom test is used only as an indicative help and not as legal proof of drowning.

PRESERVATION OF MATERIAL FOR BIOCHEMICAL/HEMATOLOGICAL AND SEROLOGICAL ESTIMATION

1. **Blood:** 5–10 ml of blood is collected directly from heart during autopsy.

2. **Urine:** Obtained by catheter or suprapubic puncture with syringe and long needle before autopsy or by making incision on the anterior surface of bladder during autopsy. Preservative used is thymol 0.1 gm/100 ml urine.

3. **CSF:** Collected by lumbar or cisternal puncture.

4. **Vitreous humour:** It is obtained by using 20-gauge hypodermic needle. 1.5 to 2 ml crystal clear fluid is aspirated without exerting much pressure from outer canthus of each eye; the tip of needle is near the center of eyeball. Water is injected for cosmetic restoration of the eyeball after aspiration of vitreous fluid.

5. **Synovial fluid:** In supine position, the synovial fluid is aspirated by 18-gauge needle with 10 ml syringe by puncturing the supra-patellar pouch from lateral sides just below the patella and pushed directly backward.

6. **Pericardial fluid:** After removing sternum, the pericardial sac is cut by scissor. The pericardial fluid is then aspirated by taking care of contamination. There is increase in enzyme activity of gamma-glutamyl transferase, creatinine phospho-kinase, amylase and lactic dehydrogenase with increasing time interval.

Above Materials

It can be preserved in/for

1. Determination of time since death from the level of potassium in vitreous and synovial fluid; and from the level of enzymes in postmortem blood.

2. Different sudden/prolonged admitted cases like diabetes, uremia, hepatic failure, etc.

3. Poisoning deaths

a. Biochemical and Electrolyte Estimation

1. **In diabetes and hyperglycemia:** Serum glucose >600 mg/100 ml glucose in urine is diagnostic of **diabetic**. Level of >200 mg/100 ml in vitreous humour is significant for **hyperglycemia**; whereas presence of ketone bodies in vitreous is indicative of **diabetic acidosis.**

2. **In renal failure:** Well demonstrated level of urea and creatinine in vitreous is indicative of death due to **uremia. High serum or plasma potassium, uric acid, and phosphate** concentration usually indicate acute renal failure.

3. **Liver failure:** Raised serum bilirubin in postmortem sample is indicative of antemortem **jaundice.**

4. **Time since death:** It can be estimated from potassium level in vitreous and synovial fluid respectively as follows:

Death interval = 2.71 × potassium level − 20.19
Death interval = 2.83 × potassium level − 15.41

There is linear rise of potassium level with increasing time interval after death (Tumram, et al. Postmortem analysis of synovial fluid and vitreous humor for determination of death interval. Forensic Sci Int. 2011; 204:186–90).

b. Plasma Enzymes

1. **Time since death:** Peak levels of amylase and phosphatase are seen between 36 and 48 hrs after death. It is 48–60 hrs for transaminase and 4th day for lactic acid dehydrogenase.

2. **Fall in serum cholinesterase** level is useful indicator in **organophosphate or carbamate** insecticide poisoning.

3. **High plasma hepatic enzymes** are seen in poisoning due to **carbon tetrachloride, copper** salts, and paracetamol.

4. **Increase gamma glutamyl transferase** activity is seen in **chronic alcoholism.**

5. **Shock** coma and convulsions are often associated with non-specific **increase in plasma** or serum activities of enzymes such as **LDH, aspartate aminotransferase, and alanine aminotransferase.**

c. Hemolytic

1. **Blood clotting:** Prothrombin time and other clotting parameters are likely to be **abnormal** in acute poisoning with **hepatotoxic agents, rodenticides** containing anticoagulants, as well as certain types of snake, especially **vipers.**

2. **Hematocrit: Anemia** is seen in chronic **lead, arsenic, copper, mercury and iron poisoning.**

3. **Leucocyte count:** It is a feature of acute metabolic acidosis resulting from ingestion of **methanol and ethylene glycol.**

d. Serological Test

It is used in the following circumstances

1. **Infection:** For detection of antibodies like IgG for old infection and IgM for recent infection.

2. **Pregnancy test (hCG in urine):** For determination of suspected 1–2 months pregnancy in unmarried suicidal death.

3. **Abortion** cases up to 7–10 days of abortion for detection of hCG.

4. **Food poisoning/gastroenteritis:** For detection of toxin.
5. **Typhoid:** Widal test.
6. Antigen test for malaria.
7. **Dengue:** NS1 antigen.

PRESERVATION OF MATERIAL FOR MICROBIOLOGICAL TEST

Microbiological Investigation

It is useful in

1. **Food poisoning/gastroenteritis:** Swab from small and large intestine for staining and culture/sensitivity of the bacteria.
2. **Cholera:** Stool sample for hanging drop preparation (for demonstration of motility).
3. **Malarial parasites:** Peripheral smear, spleen impression for malarial parasite.
4. **Sexual offences:** Vaginal swab/fluid for detection of sperms and sexually transmitted disease; blood for STD/HIV.
5. **Sudden death after trivial injury:** Skin tissue from the site of injury/injection should be cultured in Robertson cooked meat media for detection of clostridium bacilli. Blood is preserved for detection of toxins.

The samples are sent to the microbiology or pathology department of Government Medical College or Virological Institute, if needed.

1. **Bacteriological examination:** All specimens must be collected under sterile condition. **Blood for culture** must be obtained before organs are disturbed.

   After opening **pericardial sac**, the anterior surface of right ventricle is seared with heated knife and 10 ml of blood is aspirated using sterile needle and syringe. The same technique may be used to remove material from other organs. The sample should be placed in sterile container.

   After opening **subarachnoid space** with sterile scalpel, a specimen is taken from a SA space by sterile swabs from which smears and cultures may be made.

   For **culture of splenic tissue,** the surface of the organ is seared with a hot spatula,

and the area is punctured with a sterile instrument and pulp is scraped from which smears and cultures may be made.

2. **Virological examination:** A piece of **appropriate tissue** or swab is collected under sterile condition and the sample is **freezed or preserved in 80% glycerol** in buffered saline. The specimen should be placed in a sterile container and sealed tightly.

3. **Protozoa and helminthes detection:** Fecal matter is examined for protozoa and helminthes. 5–10 gm feces is preserved without any preservative for **detection of protozoa and helminthes.** In cholera cases, **hanging drop** preparation is made from the faecal matter to examine the darting motility of vibrio cholera.

4. Smears for malarial parasite, blood dyscrasias, and sexually transmitted disease:
   Smears of brain cortex and spleen: Stained **for malarial parasite.**
   Smears of bone marrow (ribs/sternum): stained **for blood dyscrasias.**
   Smears from chancres and mucus patches: Stained or examined fresh by Darkfield **for STDs.**

PRESERVATION OF TISSUE FOR ENZYME HISTOCHEMISTRY

It is useful for

1. Determination of age of injury
2. To differentiate between antemortem and postmortem injury.

The injured tissue is stained for the presence of enzymes like:

- Alkaline phosphatase (peak at 4–8 hours),
- Acid phosphatase (4 hours),
- Aminopeptidase (1 hour), and
- ATPases (1 hour).

Small pieces of tissues of size $\frac{1}{2} \times \frac{1}{2}$ inches from the site of injury with non-injured tissue are excised. The tissue is then cut into two pieces, one part is kept in formalin solution for histology examination and other part is kept for enzyme histochemistry.

For enzyme histochemistry purpose, the tissue is kept in two ice packs and preserved in a thermos flask containing liquid nitrogen.

The sections of 15–16 microns thick are taken in frozen section cryostat. The section is then placed over the slide and fixed with 10% neutral formalin at 4°C for 5 minutes.

Then the slide is washed with distilled water and is placed in the jar containing different chemical for specific enzyme in the incubator at 37°C for 1 hour.

After treating with various chemicals, the tissue is then examined under microscope for staining of the tissue

PRESERVATION OF TISSUE FOR HISTOPATHOLOGICAL (HP) EXAMINATION

In some of the medicolegal cases, the tissue from the suspected pathology of the organ is preserved for histopathological examination. The microscopic examination of tissue not only helps to confirm the pathology on gross examination but also in a few other medicolegal cases while framing the cause of death.

The Tissue for HP Examination

It is preserved in

1. Pathological conditions
2. Injection deaths—part of the tissue at the site of injection is preserved to see local findings of anphylaxis
3. Electrocution/lightening cases
4. Dog bite cases
5. Poisoning and drug abuse case for degenerative changes in the target organs. (Patel F. Ancillary Autopsy—Forensic Histopathology and Toxicology. Med. Sci and law, 1995; 35: 25–30.)

The tissues are **preserved in 10% formalin or 70% ethanol.** For preservation of water soluble elements (such as mucus, glycogen, sodium urate crystals) **absolute alcohol is the** best preservatives.

Tissue size should not be more than 2 × 4 cm and 0.5–1.0 cm thick. Fixing fluid should be at least 25 times, the volume of tissue. A typical portion of affected area seen on gross examination should be removed along with adjacent normal tissue. It should be cut into pieces of about 1–2 cm thickness and fixed in 10% formalin or 95% alcohol.

The tissue should be preserved in a jar, labeled and sealed as soon as possible. It should be **dispatched** to the department of pathology directly or **usually through police** along with histopathology form (Fig. 2.3).

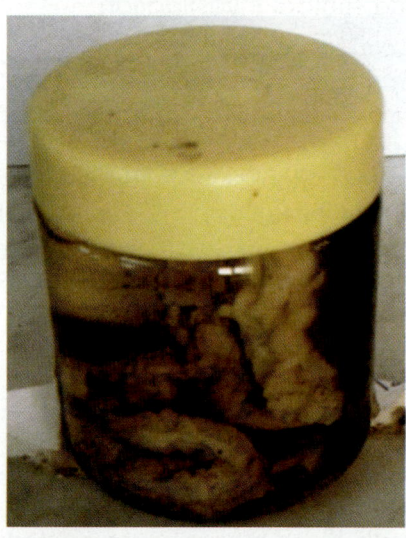

Fig. 2.3: Tissues preserved for histopathology

ORGAN/TISSUE PRESERVED FOR MUSEUM PURPOSE

There are two methods of preservation for museum purpose.

Method I

1. Firstly the tissue/organ is rinsed in cold water.

Then placed in Kaiserling-1 solution	
Sodium nitrate	01 gm
Potassium acetate	30 gm
Formalin	200 ml
Distilled water	1000 ml

- For 2–14 days depending upon the size of tissue (1 × 6 × 6 cm tissue kept for 2 days).

2. Washed in running water for 20 minutes.
3. Then placed in Kaiserling-2 solution (comprising 80% ethyl alcohol).

- For 10 mins–1 hr or until original color restored.

4. Then placed in vacuum desiccators filled with Kaiserling-3 solution:

Potassium acetate	100 gm
Glycerine	200 cc
Distilled water	1000 cc

And subject to a negative pressure of at least 50 mm Hg for 1 hr or more.

5. Mount the specimen in airtight museum jar filled with boiled Kaiserling-3 solution.

Method II: Restoration of natural color: Tissue fixed for 3–4 days in Kaiserling solution or formalin can be recolorized.

1. Fixed or fresh tissue are again fixed in following solution for 3–4 days.

Formalin	1000 cc
Common salt	300 gm
Distilled water	5000 cc

2. They are thoroughly washed in tap-water for 1–3 hrs.

3. Next treated with following solution for 2–3 days at least thrice.

Formalin	1000 cc
Distilled water	5000 cc
Sodium dithionite ($Na_2S_2O_4$)	100 gm
Potassium carbonate	30 gm
Pyridine	20 ml

4. Change the fluid or treat the tissue with above solution at least thrice.

5. They are finally mounted in glass or museum jar and filled with fresh solution.

Forensic Science Laboratory and Analytical Methods Including Psychoanalysis

3

Forensic science laboratories (FSLs) are the laboratories working under Union Government or State Government for the examination of physical evidences sent either by doctors after clinical examination/postmortem examination or recovered from the scene of crime in different criminal and civil cases. Thus, it helps to link the victim/accused to the crime or incident. As the person (Chemical analyser) working in FSL are using different analytical methods for the analysis of different physical evidences to link the suspect to the scene, they should be rightly called "Forensic Scientist" instead of "Forensic Expert".

Almost all the states have their FSL to carry out analysis of physical evidences. In Maharashtra, there are four FSLs at Mumbai (1958), Pune (1979), Aurangabad (1981) and Nagpur (1968). Two more laboratories have been started at Nashik (2004) and Amravati (2009).

FSL is having following sections for different purpose

1. **Toxicology section:** For chemical analysis of viscera and body fluids or suspicious articles.
2. **Serology:** For blood group estimation.
3. **Biological:** For identification of body fluids, hair and plant material.
4. **Molecular biology:** For DNA fingerprinting.
5. **Physical investigation:** For examination of trace materials.
6. **Ballistic and explosive section:** For examination of firearms and explosive material.
7. **Polygraphy section:** For Lie detection.
8. **Document analysis:** For examination of handwriting, type writing, forged documents and currencies.
9. **Photography section:** Evidences from various exhibits and materials.
10. **Narcoanalysis and brain mapping:** For extracting truth
11. **Mobile evidence collection unit:** For collecting different evidences from the crime spot directly under the supervision of police.

PHYSICAL EVIDENCE

It includes weapons, knives, blunt instruments, firearms, bullets, cartridge cases, wads, blood, seminal stains, saliva, epithelium, hair, poisons, fingerprints and foot/shoe prints, broken pieces of glass, vehicles paint, oil, grease, soil, clothes, documents, and cigarette butts, etc. It is useful to prove the crime and also connect it with the suspect.

Examples

1. In Poisoning

In poisoning, stomach wash, blood, urine, feces and vomitus apart from routine viscera at autopsy are sent for chemical analysis. In food poison, only the stomach contents are preserved without any preservative and should be sent to chemical analyzer for detection of toxin.

a. Chemical analysis of viscera/body fluids to know nature of poison.
b. Chemical analysis of food/utensils, bottle/clothes, etc.—provides corroborative evidence.

2. In Assault and Murder

In homicide, examination of certain object/material from the body or scene helps to detect crime and for identification of accused/victim.

a. Blood grouping from blood stains on victim, hair in victim's hand, saliva on cigarette butts for identity of assailant.
b. Clothes examination for identification.
c. Examination of weapon/object to detect crime.

3. In Burn Deaths

In this, the clothes and hair are sent to chemical analysis for detection of petroleum product (like petrol, kerosene).

However, examination of metallic objects, teeth and bones also helps in identification of the charred body.

4. In Sexual Offences

In this, the examination of different samples is collected for chemical analysis. It helps to know whether the offence has been committed and to identify the accused.

a. Examination of vaginal fluid, blood/seminal stains—to check whether crime has been committed.
b. Examination of hair, epithelium, blood grouping for identity of accused.
c. Examination of clothes—site of offence, identity of accused.

5. In Vehicular Accident

a. Blood for CA for alcohol detection (especially driver)
b. Blood grouping for identification/matching
c. Tyre marks to campare with the type of offending vehicle.
d. Grease, mud, blood, tissues, glass pieces, hair, paint, etc. on vehicle to indicate offending vehicle.
e. Examination of clothes/site to identify accused.

6. In Firearm Injuries

a. Examination of projectile (bullet/pellet) to know the nature and type of firearm.

b. Examination of markings on bullet—to know which gun was used in firing by comparison method.

7. In Explosion and Blast

a. Examination of the material/soil from the core of blast for detection of explosives material.

8. In Hanging/Strangulation

For matching of ligature material used in hanging and strangulation.

a. The fibers of ligature on the neck are taken by applying transparent cellotape over the mark and then stuck onto a clean glass slide. It is then compared with the fibers of ligature material used.
b. Also the epithelial tissue adherent over the ligature should be compared with the tissue of the victim.

9. Identification

Identification is the main concern in unknown, decomposed and skeletonized bodies. It can be known from fingerprints, footprints, clothes, tattoo marks, scar, or any acquired or congenital malformation. However, fingerprinting can be done by police person under CID crime.

10. Disputed Paternity/Identity

The cases can be settled by blood grouping and DNA fingerprinting.

11. Drug Addiction/Drug Trafficking/Drug Reaction

This can be known from detection of drugs in tissues and vials/specimen along with blood for CA.

ANALYTICAL METHODS USED IN TOXICOLOGY

In any particular case of poison, it is important either to know the nature/type of poison **(qualitative analysis)** or to know both type and concentration of poison in the body **(quantitative analysis).**

Qualitative Analysis

I. Bedside Tests

a. Color test
b. Other test

Bedside tests: A. color tests

Names of test	Procedure	Result	Indicates
1. Trinder's test:	2 ml urine + 100 ml Trinder's reagent and mix for 5 sec	• Violet/purple color • If turns darker	• **Salicylates** • **Negative test**
	Trinder's reagent: 40 g mercuric chloride in 850 ml water + 120 ml of aqueous HCl mixed with 40 g hydrated ferric nitrate diluted to 1 L with warm water. If the test sample is other than urine like stomach contents, etc. then it should first be hydrolyzed by heating with 0.5 mol/L HCl in boiling water bath for 2 mins, and neutralized with 0.5 mol/L sodium hydroxide		
2. Ferric chloride test:	2 ml urine + 1 ml of 5% ferric chloride solution	Persistent purple color	**Phenol, phenothiazines, phenylbutazone, or salicylates**
3. FPN test:	1 ml of test sample (urine/stomach content) + 1 ml FPN reagent	• Color from pink, red, violet to blue • Green/blue color	• Phenothiazines • Tricyclics
	FPN reagent: 5 ml ferric chloride + 45 ml perchloric acid + 50 ml HNO_3		
4. O-cresol test:	0.5 ml test sample + 0.5 ml concentration HCl → heat in boiling water bath for 10 mins and cool. Then add 1 ml aqueous O-cresol solution (1 gm/L) + 0.2 ml test mixture + 2 ml ammonium hydroxide (4 mol/L)—mix for 5 seconds	Blue or blackish color	**Paracetamol or phenacetin**
5. Dichromate test:	Urine + equal volumes of 10% sodium dichromate in 50% sulphuric acid	Orange to green color	**Alcohol**
6. Marquis test:	Gastric fluid + 3 ml concentration H_2SO_4 + 3 drops formalin	Purple color that gradually turns blue	**Opium/morphine**
7. Lee Jones test:	5 ml gastric fluid + a few crystals of $FeSO_4$ + 5 drops of 2% NaOH → boil and cool. Then add 8–10 drops of 10% HCl	• Greenish blue color • Purple color	• **Cyanide** • **Salicylates**
8. Reinsch test:	20 ml test sample in conical flask + 10 ml HCl + strip of copper → heat for 1 hr in a boiling water bath inside a fume cupboard. Copper is then removed and examined	• Silvery deposit • Black deposit • Purplish black	• **Mercury** • **Arsenic (dull black), or bismuth (shiny black)** • **Antimony**
9. Meixner test:	Dilute the test sample (stool/gastric content) with methanol and then centrifuge and filter. Put a drop or two on a piece of news paper/filter paper and dry it. Add a few drops of concentration HCl	Blue color within a few minutes	**Amatoxin present in mushrooms**
10. Forrest test:	0.5 ml test sample + 1 ml forrest reagent for 5 seconds	Yellow green color deepening to blue	**Imipramine and related compounds**
	Forrest reagent: 25 ml potassium dichromate + 25 ml H_2SO_4 + 25 ml perchloric acid + 25 ml HNO_3		

(Contd...)

Bedside tests: A. color tests *(Contd...)*

Names of test	Procedure	Result	Indicates
11. Ferrocyanide test:	50 ml of filtered stomach content + 100 ml HCl + 50 ml potassium ferrocyanide solution	Deep blue precipitate	Ferrous or ferric iron.
12. Ammonia test:	Test material in TT+ a few drops of NH_4OH	Deep blue precipitate	**Copper**
13. Dithionate test:	1ml of test sample + 0.5 ml of aqueous ammonium hydroxide (2 mol/L). Mix for 5 sec + 20 mg of solid sodium dithionate	• Blue to **blue black color** • Yellow-green color	• **Paraquat** • **Diquat**
14. Gutzeit test:	Test material in large TT + pure Zn + 3 drops of diluted HCU + potassium iodide. A plug of absorbent cotton wool is inserted in the upper part of TT and mouth of TT is covered with a filter paper moistened with concentrated solution of silver nitrate	• Filter turns yellow • Filter turn brown or black	• **Arsenic** • **Antimony**
15. Fujiwara test (1 ml each in all three test tubes):	**TT-A:** Sample + NaOH + pyridine **TT-B:** Putrified water + NaOH + pyridine **TT-C:** Trichloroacetic acid + NaOH + pyridine Heat in boiling water bath for 2 mins	A. Red/purple color B. No color C. Red/purple color	**Chloral hydrate, Chloroform, TC Ethylene**
B. Other tests:			
1. Isonitrile test:	A few ml gastric content +10 ml water +1 ml aniline + 2 ml of 20% NaOH— heat × a few minutes	Foul odor	**CCl_4, TCE, chloroform, chloral hydrate, chlorinated HC like OC**
2. Tensilon test:	In sudden paralysis, 10 mg edrophonium is given IV	• If dramatic recovery • If no recovery	• **Myasthenia gravis** • **Botulism**
3. Melzer's test:	Spores of mushroom are stained with 1 drop of Melzer's reagent and viewed under microscope	Spores turns to bluish black color	*Amanita phalloides* of toxic mushrooms
4. Nitric acid test:	5 ml adulterated mustard oil + 5 ml nitric acid → shake the test tube	Orange yellow color	**Argemone**
5. Rabbit eye test:	If a drop of stomach content (having datura) is put in rabbit's eye	Dilatation of pupil	**Datura**
6. Chemical test—alkali:	• Hydroxides + $AgNO_3$ • Carbonates + HCl	• Yellow precipitate • White precipitates	**Alkalies**
7. Chemical test—acid:	• $BaCl_2$ + test material • H_2SO_4 + $FeSO_4$ + test material • $AgNO_3$ + TM • TM + drop of phenolphthalein	• White precipitates • Junction-Brown ring • White curdy ppt • Pink + NaOH— disappear	• **H_2SO_4** • **HNO_3** • **HCl** • **Acetic acid**

TM: Test material; TT: Test tube

II. Thin Layer Chromatography (TLC)

TLC is a simple, and widely used, inexpensive qualitative technique, which involves movement by capillary action of a liquid phase through a thin, uniform layer of stationary phase (usually silica gel) held on a rigid support.

QUANTITATIVE ANALYSIS

If the positive result of any suspected poison is obtained from the qualitative analysis (chemical/bed side test), then its estimation is carried out by quantitative analysis. This can be done with the help of following methods:

1. Ultraviolet spectrophotometry (UVS)
2. Gas chromatography (GC)
3. High performance liquid chromatography (HPLC) and high performance thin layer chromatography (HPTLC)
4. Mass spectrometry (MS)
5. Radioimmunoassay (RIA)
6. Enzyme-mediated immunoassay technique (EMIT)
7. Atomic absorption spectrophotometry
8. Neutron activation analysis (NAA)

ANALYTICAL TECHNIQUES

1. Chromatography

It is a technique to separate mixture of substances, based on differences in the relative affinities of the substances for **two different media—one, a moving fluid (the mobile phase) and other, a porous solid/gel/liquid, coated on a solid support (the stationary phase or sorbent).** The speed at which each substance is carried along by the mobile phase depends upon its solubility and on its affinity for the sorbent. It is used to detect poisons and chemicals.

a. Thin Layer Chromatography (TLC)

In TLC, the stationary phase is a thin layer of absorbent, e.g. silica gel coated on a rectangular plate and the mobile phase is a solvent mixture. The sample is applied to a spot on the plate which is made to stand in solvent. As the solvent rises through the absorbent, the components of the sample are carried along at different rates and can be visualized as a row of spots, after the plate is dried and stained or viewed under UV light.

b. Paper Chromatography

It is similar to TLC. But the stationary phase is a sheet of special grade filter paper.

c. Column Chromatography

It is a type of chromatography using a sorbent packed in a column. The sample dissolved in a solvent, is poured on the top. Some

Comparison points	GC	HPLC	HPTLC
1. Stationary phase	Solid	Liquid	Solid
2. Mobile phase	Gaseous	Liquid	Liquid
3. Conditioning phase	–	–	Gas
4. Samples	Volatile	Non-volatile	Non-volatile
5. Sample	Invisible	Invisible	Visible
6. System	Closed	Closed	Open
7. Separating medium	Tubular column	Tubular	Planar (plate)
8. Analyzed at a time	1 sample	1 sample	up to 20 × 5
9. Automation	Full	Full	stepwise
10. Operation required	High temperature	High pressure	Room T and P
11. Sample clean up	Essential	Essential	Not essential
12. Maintenance	Medium	High	Low
13. Running cost	Medium	Very high	Low
14. Samples/shift	5–25	5–25	up to 100

components are retained in the column bound to the sorbent. They are then washed out in suitable solvents.

d. Gas Chromatography (GC)

It is a more sophisticated system of quantitative analysis. It offers a way of simultaneously separating, identifying, and measuring drugs and other organic poisons.

It is a type of chromatography in which the sample dissolved in a solvent is vaporized and carried by an inert gas through a column packed with a sorbent to any of the several types of detectors. Each component of sample, separated from others by passage through the column produces a separate peak in the detector output, which is graphed by a chart recorder. The sorbent may be an inert porous solid (gas-solid chromatography) or a non-volatile liquid coated on a solid support (gas liquid chromatography).

e. High Performance Liquid Chromatography (HPLC)

This is similar to GC, except that it is not restricted only to volatile compounds. It can be used to separate and analyze complex mixtures as well.

f. High Performance Thin Layer Chromatography (HPTLC)

This is the fastest of all chromatography methods. It can analyze about 100 samples of 5–10 different types per shift. It is a visual technique where the chromatogram (separated sample after chromatography) is visible. In this, the stationary phase is solid whereas in HPLC, the stationary phase is liquid. TLC is the method of choice for impurity analysis of pharmacopeias.

2. Electrophoresis (Electrochromatography)

It is a technique used to separate mixture of ionic solutes in an applied electric field. The speed at which the solutes are separated depends on the difference in their rate of migration. The original method in which the movement of the solvent is unrestricted is termed as **moving boundary electrophoresis**, because all the particles of a single species move at the same rate, maintaining a sharp boundary. This method involve a support medium such as paper, cellulose acetate, agarose gel, starch gel or polyacrylamide gel, which prevents convective motion of the solvent; this is called **zone electrophoresis**. The electrically charged protein components move on the phase plate. The plate is then treated with coloring agent which causes appearance of visible characteristic bands specific for a particular protein.

3. Spectroscopy

Every substance absorbs light of specific wavelength thus producing dark bands in specific zones. With the help of spectroscope, the light of specific wavelength is propagated through the medium/solution and then analyzed. Thus, it helps in the identification of various forms of hemoglobin.

4. Spectrophotometer

It estimates the quantity of coloring matter in the solution by the quantity of light absorbed after passing through the solution by means of spectrophotometer.

a. Colorimeter

Using filters, the light of specific wavelength is allowed to pass through the test substance, and the rays absorbed are detected.

b. UV/IR Spectrophotometry

This technique is based on the principle that many drugs when in solution will absorb Ultraviolet (UV)/infra red (IR) radiation. The degree of absorption depends on the chemical structure of the drug, its concentration in the solution, and the wavelength of the rays. The amount of UV/IR radiation that passes through the solution is measured by the photocell.

This technique is ideal to quantitative blood levels of paracetamol and salicylates, as well as urine levels of phenothiazines. A major disadvantage of UV spectrophotometry is the possibility of interference in multiple drug overdoses.

c. Mass Spectrometry (MS)

The testing material in minute amount is placed in high vacuum chamber, and is bombarded with electrons. The molecules of the material, lose electrons, get positively charged, and break into fragments, which get separated according to their mass in an electromagnetic field. The same is recorded as lines in a graph.

This is usually **combined with gas chromatography (GS-MS)**, and is considered to be the best technique for quantitative analysis of wide variety of chemicals, but its expense greatly restricts its use.

d. Emission Spectrophotometry

Every element on being excited emits light spectrum which can be separated and recorded by photography.

e. Atomic Absorption Spectrophotometry (AAS)

The element is vaporized and through this radiations from a light source are passed. This displaces the electrons of the atoms resulting in emission of energy which is recorded graphically.

This is the **best method for detecting inorganic elements (arsenic, lead, mercury, thallium, etc.).** However, it requires a large sample of blood for accurate analysis. The organic matrix is combusted and the metal forms a cloud of atoms, which absorbs a fraction of the radiation in proportion to the concentration of metal in the sample.

5. Neutron Activation Analysis (NAA)

It is based on the principle that many substances become radioactive when exposed to bombardment by neutrons. It can be used for the estimation of any of the 90 naturally occurring elements from antimony to zinc.

This is highly sophisticated and **expansive method of detection of a variety of inorganic elements** to analyze very small quantity of matter. **It is carried out in firearm cases to detect firearm residue.**

ACRO-Reaction Test

It is done in **electric current** death for **detection of metallic residue (pearls)** at the site of entry.

6. Radioimmunoassay (RIA)

It is slow and expansive method of detecting drugs in the blood, but is highly accurate. It involves mixing known quantities of drug specific antibody with known amount of radioactively labeled drug that allows analysis of the precipitate with a gamma counter. It is excellent for the **detection of drugs in extremely low blood concentration** (cannabis, LSD, paraquat, digoxin, etc.).

7. Enzyme-mediated Immunoassay Technique (EMIT)

It is a fast, expansive method with good accuracy. It works on the principle that the amount of drug present is proportional to the inhibition of an enzyme-substrate reaction.

A known quantity of a drug is labeled by chemical attachment to an enzyme. Drug specific antibodies added to the specimen bind the drug-enzyme complex thereby reducing enzyme activity. Free drug in the specimen competes with enzyme labeled drug and limits the antibody-induced enzyme inactivation. Enzyme activity correlates with the drug concentration in the specimen as measured by absorbance change resulting from the enzyme catalytic action on a substrate.

EMIT is preferred over other RIA methods because of its simplicity and speed in providing information on toxic drug concentrations.

There are two main disadvantages

1. Negative result does not exclude the ingestion of a drug that may be present in undetectable quantities.
2. Antibodies cross-reactions can produce false positive results.

8 Microscope

a. Comparison Microscope (Color Contrast Microscope)

It is an instrument which permits simultaneously viewing of parts of images of two separate specimens involving **two microscopes bridged together with a comparison eye piece** or one microscope, with two body tubes and lens systems.

b. Darkfield Microscope (Ultra Microscope)

It is a microscope with a central stop in the condenser, permitting diversion of light rays and illumination of the object, from the sides, so that details appear light against a dark background.

c. Electron Microscope

It is the microscope in which an electron beam, instead of light, forms an image for viewing, allowing much greater magnification and resolution. The image may be viewed on fluorescent screen or may be photographed.

d. Fluorescence Microscope

It is the microscope, used for the examination of specimens stained with fluorochromes, e.g. fluorescein labeled antibody which fluoresces in UV light.

e. Polarizing Microscope

It is a microscope, equipped with polarizer, analyzer and means for measurement of the alteration of the polarized light by the specimen.

f. Scanning Microscope/ Electron Microscope

It is a microscope, in which a beam of electrons scans over a specimen, point by point and builds up an image on the fluorescent screen of a cathode ray tube.

g. X-ray Microscope

It is a microscope in which a beam of X-ray is used instead of light, the image usually being produced on film.

9. Psychoanalytical Test

With the increase in crime incidence, the police interrogation techniques play a vital role in extracting the truth from the suspect. The scientific methods have been developed for extracting confession. Following are the scientific test used as police interrogation tools:

a. Lie detector or the polygraph test

b. P300 or the brain mapping test

c. Narcoanalysis or the truth serum test

d. The brain electrical oscillation signature (BEOS)

These psychoanalytical tests are also used to interpret the behavior of the criminal (or the suspect) and corroborate the investigating officers' observations.

a. Polygraph or Lie Detector Test

It is an instrument for simultaneously recording various physiological responses as represented by mechanical or electrical impulses, such as **respiratory movements, pulse wave, blood pressure and the psychogalvanic reflex.** Such phenomenon reflects emotional reactions which are of use in detecting deception. It is popularly known as Lie detector. The trace curve/graph is called as polygram.

It is based on the theory that when a person tells a lie in answer to a question and there is a fear that lie would be detected. The **emotion of fear results in stimulation of sympathetic nervous system** which results in certain physiological changes, some of which can be easily recorded.

It is an examination, which is based on an assumption that there is an **interaction between the mind and body and is conducted by various components or the sensors of a polygraph machine,** which are attached to the body of the person, who is interrogated by the expert. The machine **records** the blood pressure, pulse rate and respiration and muscle movements.

Polygraph test is **conducted in three phases—a pretest interview, chart recording and diagnosis.** The examiner (a clinical or criminal psychologist) prepares a **set of test questions** depending upon the relevant information about the case provided by the investigating officer, such as the criminal charges against the person and statements made by the suspect. The subject is questioned and the reactions are measured. **A baseline is established by asking questions whose answers the investigator know.** Lying by a suspect is accompanied by specific, perceptible physiological and behavioral changes and the sensors and a wave pattern in the graph expose this. **Deviation from the baseline is taken as a sign of lie.** All these reactions are corroborated with other evidence gathered. The polygraph test was among the first scientific tests to be used by the interrogators.

It was Keeler, who further refined the polygraph machine by adding a **psycho-galvanometer to record the electrical resistance of the skin.**

b. P300 or the Brain Mapping Test or Brain Fingerprinting

This test was developed and patented in 1995 by neurologist Dr. Lawrence A. Farwell, Director and Chief Scientist "Brain-wave Science", IOWA. Dr. Farwell has published that a Memory and Encoding Related Multifaceted Electroencephalographic Response (MERMER) is initiated in the accused when his brain recognizes noteworthy information pertaining to the crime. These stimuli are called the **target stimuli**.

In this method, called the "Brain-wave fingerprinting" the **accused is first interviewed** and interrogated to find out whether he is concealing any information.

Then **sensors are attached** to the subject's head and the person is seated before a computer monitor. He is **then shown certain images or made to hear certain sounds.**

The **sensors monitor electrical activity** in the brain and register P300 waves, which are generated **only, if the subject has connection with the stimulus,** i.e. picture or sound.

The subject is **not asked any questions.** In a nutshell, brain fingerprinting test matches information stored in the brain with information from the crime scene. Studies have shown that an innocent suspect's brain would not have stored or recorded certain information, which an actual perpetrator's brain would have stored.

The forensic science laboratory in Bangalore, is the first center in India, which conducts the brain-mapping or brain-fingerprinting test.

In the USA, the FBI has been making use of "Brain mapping technique" to convict criminals.

c. Narcoanalysis or Truth Serum Test

It is one of the scientific tools of interrogation for extracting confessions/truth after giving certain anesthetic and sedative drugs by putting a subject into a hypnotic state. This lowers a subject's inhibition in the hope that the subject will more freely share information and feelings.

Historical background

The term narcoanalysis was introduced in 1936 for the use of narcotics to induce a trance-like state wherein the person is subjected to various queries. The term *narcoanalysis* was coined by Horseley. Narcoanalysis first reached the mainstream in 1922, when Robert House, a Texas obstetrician used the drug scopolamine on two prisoners.

Narcoanalysis was rather unheard in India till recent past. It was first used in 2002 in the Godhra carnage probe. It was again in news in the Telgi stamp paper case, when Abdul Karim Telgi was subjected to the said test in December 2003 at a government hospital in Bangalore.

Principle and theory

This is based on the principle that **at a point close to unconsciousness, the person cannot resist questions and also will not be able to give false answers,** which he had been giving to conceal his crime. It is believed that if a person is administered a drug which suppresses his reasoning power without affecting memory and speech, he can be made to tell the truth.

The **underlying theory** is that a person is able to lie by using his imagination. In the narcoanalysis test, the subject's imagination is neutralized by making him semiconscious. The subject is not in a position to speak up on his own but can answer specific and simple questions. In this state, it becomes difficult for him to lie and his answers would be restricted to facts, he is already aware of. His answers are spontaneous as a semiconscious person is unable to manipulate his answers.

Drugs and dose

1. 0.5 mg of **scopolamine hydrobromide** SC followed by 0.25 mg every 20 minutes—

average 3–6 injections, till the stage is reached.

2. Sodium amytal or **sodium pentothal** 2.5–5% IV at the rate of 1 cc/minute, till the stage is reached.

3. 0.1 gm **sodium seconal** 1½ hours before induction, 45 minutes later 15 mg morphine sulphate and 0.5 mg scopolamine hydro-bromide subcutaneously.

The test

In India, the narcoanalysis test is done by a **team** comprising of an **anesthesiologist, a psychiatrist, a clinical/ forensic psychologist, an audio-videographer, and supporting nursing staff.** The forensic psychologist will prepare the report about the revelations, which will be accompanied by a compact disc of audio-video recordings. The strength of the revelations, if necessary, is further verified by subjecting the person to polygraph and brain mapping tests.

Procedure

i. The narcoanalysis test is conducted by mixing 3 gm of sodium pentothal or sodium amytal dissolved in 3000 ml of distilled water. Depending on the person's sex, age, health and physical condition, this mixture is administered intravenously along with 10% of dextrose over a period of 3 hours with the help of an anesthetist.

ii. The rate of administration is controlled to drive the accused slowly into a hypnotic trance, resulting in a lack of inhibition.

iii. The subject is then interrogated by the investigating agencies in the presence of the doctors.

iv. The revelations made during this stage are recorded both in video and audio cassettes. The report prepared by the experts is what is used in the process of collecting evidence.

This procedure is conducted in government hospitals after a court order is issued instructing the doctors or hospital authorities to conduct the test. Personal consent of the subject is also required.

Reliability

Although inhibitions are generally reduced, people under the influence of truth serums are **still able to lie** and even tend to fantasize.

Legal position

This type of test is **not admissible** in the law courts. However, the court **may grant limited admissibility after considering the circumstances** under which the test was obtained. It states that subjects under a semiconscious state do not have the mind set to properly answer any questions, while some other courts openly accept them as evidence.

Studies have shown that it is possible to lie under narcoanalysis and its reliability as an investigative tool is questioned in most countries. Narcoanalysis is not openly permitted for investigative purposes in most developed and/or democratic countries.

In the end, these tests can only assist police investigations.

Uses of narcoanalysis drugs

1. Used as "truth drugs" in police work for extracting confessions/truth. The usefulness of the suspect's revelations depends ultimately on their acceptance in evidence by a court of law.

2. The psychiatrist, on the other hand, using the same "truth drugs" in diagnosis and treatment of the mentally ill, is primarily concerned with psychological truth rather than empirical facts.

Different aspects of narcoanalysis test

The police believe that narcoanalysis as a scientific tool of interrogation:

1. It helps a lot in crime prevention and detection.

2. It also helps in getting clinching evidence and is an effective and non-hazardous method of inducing hypnosis.

3. If a criminal was put under narcoanalysis then he would reveal about the crime committed, where he had hidden the weapons used in committing the crime and why did he do it?

4. This would help in getting the motive for the crime and collect other evidence needed for prosecution.

5. Narcoanalysis is also considered by many to be a very scientific approach in dealing with an accused's psychological expressions, definitely better than third degree treatment to extract truth from an accused. The police in order to find out the truth and solve the mysteries of the crime must use the advances in science.

But on the other hand, doubts have been cast on its reliability and legal validity, and it suffers from certain **drawbacks**:

1. The person to administer them has to be a **highly qualified physician.**

2. It is always **difficult to determine the correct dose** of the drug, which varies according to the physical constitution of the subject, but also his mental attitude and will—power.

3. A wrong dose can send a subject into **coma or even cause death** thus resulting in legal complications.

4. If the subject is an abuser of other intoxicants/narcotics, narcoanalysis **could fail to disinhibit them on account of the property of "cross tolerance"** between pentothal sodium and other intoxicants. Thus, the subject could fake the state of semiconsciousness and tell lies, which are useful to him.

d. Brain Electrical Oscillation Signature (BEOS)

An Indian Scientist, Champadi Raman Mukundan as developed a technology called Brain Electrical Oscillation Signature test. The concept behind this electroencephalography (EEG) technology is that, it is able to show like as functional MRI, activated areas of the cortex which are then localized and the implications are determined. It deals with the experiential knowledge of the person. The Visual and Auditory Stimulus Programming (VASP) system allows recording and compilation of the probe like in different scenarios, marking events, etc. as well as creating video presentation for priming the subject. The probes are presented in a predefined manner by the VASP computer. They are sequentially interlinked and are designed after extensive interviews with the investigation officers and the suspects. Non-controversial information is used as 'control probes'. The 'neutral probes' are used for baseline correction. When the experiential knowledge is consistently present for relevant sequence of event, the test findings are said to be forensically significant.

Legal position: In Maharashtra, a lady (Mrs. Aditi Sharma) was convicted for murder of her husband in the court of law.

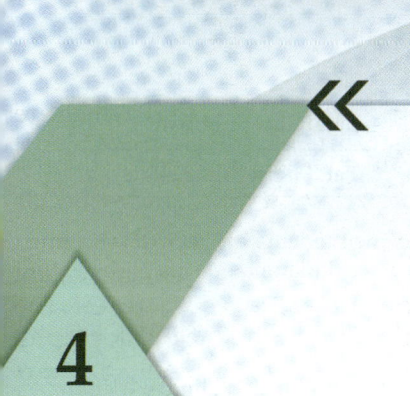

Corrosives

Corrosives are the substance which corrode and destroy the tissue with which they come in contact and when diluted they act as an irritants.

Action

1. Destruction and corrosion of all the tissues come in contact.
2. Coagulation of tissue protein
3. Fixation of tissues
4. Extraction of water from the tissues—hygroscopic
5. Convert hemoglobin into acid hematin
6. Carbonization of organic matter

Sulfuric acid	*Nitric acid*	*Hydrochloric acid*
Synonyms	**Synonyms**	**Synonyms**
Oil of vitriol, battery acid. **Chemically:** H_2SO_4	Red spirit of nitre, aqua fortis **Chemically:** HNO_3	Muriatic acid **Chemically:** HCl
Source Industries, commercial, laboratories	**Source** Industries, commercial, laboratories	**Source** Industries, commercial, laboratories, household
Uses Wet batteries, diatom test, fertilizer manufacturing, ore processing, oil refining	**Uses** Used by goldsmith, in explosives: Picric acid, nitrocellulose in fertilizer	**Uses** Cleaning of ceramic surface, preparation of chlorine, treatment of achlorhydria, in hemoglobin estimation, in leather processing
Properties 1. Colorless 2. Suffocating/choking odor 3. Non-fuming 4. Burning sour taste 5. Carbonises organic matter: It chars tissue and blackened organic matter 6. Oily, heavy and hygroscopic	**Properties** 1. Colorless/yellowish tinge 2. Pungent odor 3. Fuming 4. Burning sour taste 5. Xanthoproteic reaction: Nitric acid reacts with organic proteins to cause nitration of phenyl group and thus forms picric acid 6. Powerful oxidizing agent dissolves all metals except gold and platinum	**Properties** 1. Colorless 2. Odorless/irritating smell 3. Non-fuming 4. Burning sour taste
Clothes: Burns instantly, black	**Clothes:** Yellow staining	**Clothes:** Whitish or grey stain
Action: Locally corrosives	**Action:** Locally corrosives	**Action:** Locally corrosives

Fatal dose: 5–10 ml	**Fatal dose:** 12–24 hrs	**Fatal dose:** 10–15 ml
Fatal period: 12–24 hrs	**Fatal period:** 15–20 ml	**Fatal period:** 12–24 hrs

Clinical features

1. Intense burning pain, difficulty in speech and deglutition, dyspnea (edema of larynx), vomiting, thirst, excessive salivation with blood and mucous, hoarseness of voice (inflammation of epiglottis and larynx), Constipation, suppression of urine and dehydration followed by shock
   - The vomitus is strongly acidic mixed with altered blood (brown or black due to hematin), mucous and mucous membranes
2. There is erosion of mucosa from lips to stomach. There is also erosion of skin along line of trickling of acid from the mouth

Erosion: Blackish color	Yellowish color	Brownish color
3. **Teeth:** Chalky white	Yellowish	Not significant
4. **Perforation:** Common	Less common	Uncommon
	On inhalation—irritation of the eyes, lacrimation, photophobia, burning sensation in the throat, cough and dyspnea	In few, there may be convulsions, delirium and paralysis

Cause of death: Shock, perforation, peritonitis and laryngeal spasm, with infection and malnutrition.

Treatment

1. Emetics and gastric lavage are contraindicated (danger of perforation of stomach)
2. Drinking of plenty of plain water or wall scrapping or toothpaste
3. Use of weak solution of non-carbonated alkalies like CaO, MgO (4TSF in a pint of water or milk) and lime water, aluminum hydroxide
4. Demulcent drinks like milk, egg albumin, vegetable oil, ghee, butter, soap solution, etc.
5. Supportive
   For pain—morphine.   For thirst—ice sucking.   For fluid loss—IV fluids.
   For shock—corticosteriod. For edema glottis—tracheostomy and artificial respiration.
   Surface excoriations—washing and ointment applied. Perforations—laparotomy and surgical repair

Postmortem findings: It depends upon the concentration of corrosive and the period of survival.

A. In early deaths

Gross corrosion of skin and mucous membrane of mouth, tongue and lips with discoloration

Stomach: Wall—soft, swollen,
   Mucous membrane (MM)—desquamated, ulcerated, hemorrhagic with discoloration
   Contents—acidic, altered blood, mucous, epithelium shreds

Corrosion color: Blackish	Yellowish	Brownish
Gastric perforation Verycommon	Common	Uncommon
Peritonitis: Very Common	Common	Uncommon

B. In late deaths: Signs of repair; Scarring; Healed trickle marks

Medicolegal aspect of strong inorganic acids

1. **Suicide:** Mostly used for suicide
2. **Homicide:** Rarely used for homicide, especially on children. It is also used for Acid bath murder
3. **Accidental poisoning:** May occur in laboratory or goldsmith shop, mistaken with liquid paraffin or water
4. **Abortifacient:** Sometimes used to procure criminal abortion
5. **Vitriolage:** They are commonly used for throwing on body
6. Punishment for adultery/infidelity by putting acids in the vagina of a woman
7. **Forgery:** Hydrochloric acid is used to erase writings in an attempt at forgery

Material preserved	Material preserved	Material preserved
Routine viscera in rectified sprit	Routine viscera in rectified sprit	Routine viscera in rectified spirit
Stained scrapping— no preservative	Stained scrapping—no preservative	Stained scrapping—no preservatives
Clothes: No preservatives	**Clothes:** No preservatives	**Clothes:** No preservatives

Chemical test		
$BaCl_2 + H_2SO_4 \rightarrow BaSO_4$ (white ppt.)	$H_2SO_4 + FeSO_4 \underline{HNO_3}$ brown ring at the junction	$AgNO_3 + HCl \rightarrow AgCl$ (white curdy ppt.)

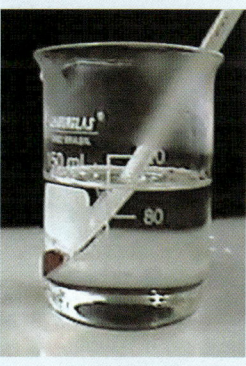 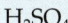

H_2SO_4

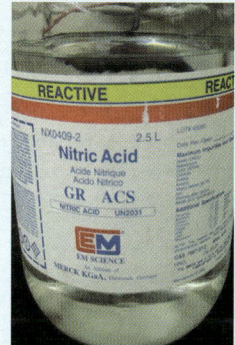

HNO_3

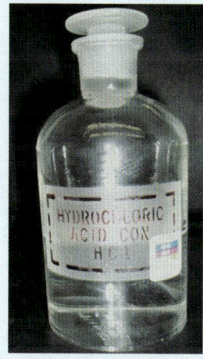

HCl

Vitriolage

Definition: It is defined as throwing of any corrosive substance (usually acids) on the body of the other person with the intension to cause injury, disfigurement or death. Since sulfuric acid (oil of vitriol) is commonly used, hence the name vitriolage. Old electric bulbs filled with acid are often thrown

Substances used: Sulfuric acid, nitric acid, hydrochloric acid, carbolic acid, sodium hydroxide, potassium hydroxide, and marking nut juice

Purpose: The purpose of vitriolage is to take revenge or it is done in a fit of anger or for jealousy

Features of vitriolage

1. Chemical burns: Characterized by
   a. Discoloration and staining of clothes and body
   b. Absence of vesicles/blisters
   c. Marks of trickling of an acid
   d. No red line of demarcation
   e. The chemical can be detected in the stains

2. Eye: Blindness, corneal destruction or conjunctival edema

3. Grievous injury: Due to
   a. Permanent privation of vision of either eye
   b. Permanent privation of hearing of either ear
   c. Permanent disfiguration of face or head
   d. Pain for more than 20 days so that the person cannot do his/her daily routine work

Cause of death: Neurogenic shock or infection

Treatment
1. Wash the area with soap and water
2. Apply magnesium oxide
3. Treat like a case of burns, using antibiotic and steroid ointments and eye drops

Medicolegal aspect
1. Grievous injury

Oxalic acid	*Carbolic acid*	*Acetic acid*
Synonyms: Acid of sugars	Phenol, phenic acid, phenyl alcohol	Glacial acetic acid (100% conc.), vinegar (4–8%)
Chemically: $C_2H_2O_4$	**Chemically:** C_6H_5OH	**Chemically:** CH_3COOH
Source Industries, commercial, laboratories, household (metal cleaning, stain remover), vegetables—onion, spinach, cabbage, radish, carrot, beet	**Source** Industries, commercial, laboratories, household (disinfectants), it is a coal tar derivative	**Source** Industries, commercial, laboratories, household (vinegar)
Uses 1. To erase writing in an attempt at forgery 2. For stain/rust removal 3. For calicoprinting 4. For metal/glass cleaning 5. In bleaches (esp., pulp wood)	**Uses** 1. Used as disinfectant/antiseptic 2. Accepted as snake repellant 3. In cosmetics/sunscreen, hair dyes, skin lightening preparations	**Uses** 1. Used in food 2. Medicinal use in superficial ear infection, jelly fish sting and bladder irrigation
Properties 1. Colorless, transparent, shining crystals (resemble $MgSO_4$ and $ZnSO_4$) 2. Odorless/irritating smell 3. Burning sour taste 4. Vaporizes on heating and sublimates on cooling	**Properties** 1. White small needle like crystals, on exposure to air, it becomes a light pink liquid 2. Sweetish pungent smell 3. Burning sweet taste 4. Hygroscopic 5. Though an acid it does not turn blue litmus red but forms salts with bases 6. Crude carbolic is **phenyl**, which is dark brown in color	**Properties** 1. Colorless liquid, when freezes becomes crystalline solid 2. Vinegar, pungent smell 3. Burning sour taste 4. Volatile liquid
Action 1. Locally corrosives 2. Systemic: It causes utilization of serum calcium to form oxalate. Hence, leads to hypocalcemia. 3. Nephrotoxicity—oxaluria	**Action** 1. **Locally:** Corrosion, necrosis and Gangrene of the local area. 2. **Systemic:** CNS—first stimulate and then depresses 3. Nephrotoxicity—carboluria	**Action** 1. Locally corrosives 2. Respiratory distress

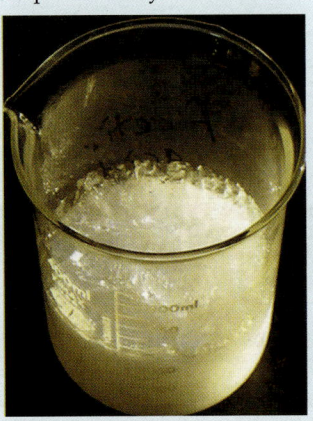

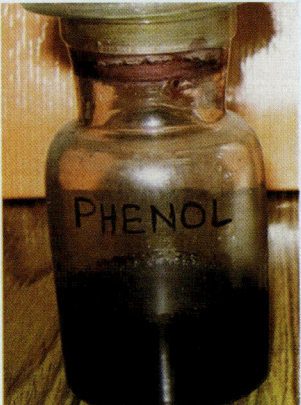

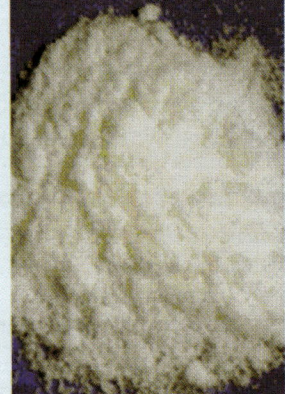

Fatal dose: 10–15 gm **Fatal period:** 2–12 hrs	**Fatal dose:** 10–20 gm **Fatal period:** 2–12 hrs	**Fatal dose:** Uncertain **Fatal period:** Uncertain
Clinical features **Locally:** There is corrosion of mucosa of mouth, tongue and lips. Skin—no corrosion, but redness due to irritation of skin.	**Clinical features** **Locally:** There is corrosion of mucosa of mouth, tongue and lips. Skin—reddened, necrosis and gangrene.	**Clinical features** **Locally:** There is corrosion of mucosa of mouth, tongue and lips. Skin—no corrosion

1. **GIT:** Intense burning pain, difficulty in speech and deglutition, dyspnea (edema of larynx), vomiting, thirst, excessive salivation with blood and mucous, hoarseness of voice (inflammation of epiglottis and larynx), **diarrhea** and pain at anus, suppression of urine and dehydration followed by shock. The vomitus is strongly acidic mixed with altered blood (brown, black or coffee color due to acid hematin), mucous and mucous membranes

2. **CNS:** Tingling and numbness, twitching of face and extremities, convulsions, finally collapse (due to hypocalcemia) 3. **Kidney: Oxaluria** characterized by oliguria, albuminuria, hematuria and presence of calcium oxalate crystals in urine (envelope/octahedral shaped crystals). Acute renal failure may occur due to toxic nephritis	2. **CNS:** Dyspnea, dizziness, delirium, convulsion, collapse, coma 3. **Kidney: Carboluria** characterized by oliguria, albuminuria, hematuria and presence of casts in urine, which on exposed to air for 20–30 sec turns greenish due to the oxidation of metabolic product of phenol like hydroquinone and pyrocatechol 4. These metabolites may also be deposited in cartilages and ligaments producing dark pigmentation—called **ochronosis** 5. Pupils constricted	2. **CNS:** Not specific 3. **Kidney:** Oliguria and hematuria 4. **RS:** Respiratory distress due to trickling of vomitus or leakage of acid
Treatment 1. Emetics 2. Gastric lavage with calcium lactate (2 TSF), chalk, CaO. Warm water should not be used since it will dissolve oxalic acid 3. Purgatives and demulcents 4. **Antidotes:** Orally, chalk, egg shells, lime or wall scrapping (all contain calcium carbonate) can be given (30 gm chalk powder for 20 gm oxalic acid), **or** 10 ml of 10% calcium gluconate is given IV 5. **Supportive:** IV fluids—25% glucose; acidosis—NaHCO$_3$	**Treatment** 1. Emetics 2. Gastric lavage with 20% glycerol or alcohol or vegetables oil 3. Demulcents 4. **Antidotes:** Magnesium oxide, Magnesium sulfate 5. **Supportive:** IV fluids—25% glucose acidosis—NaHCO$_3$ Digitalis for circulatory shock Artificial respiration + oxygen inhalation	**Treatment** 1. Emetics 2. Gastric lavage 3. Demulcents 4. **Antidotes:** Not specific 5. **Supportive:** IV fluids—25% glucose acidosis—NaHCO$_3$ Safeguarding respiration Artificial respiration + oxygen inhalation
PM findings 1. **Local:** Skin irritation due to mild corrosive action 2. MM of mouth/tongue-corroded, swollen/sodden, bleached	**PM findings** 1. **Local:** Skin necrosis, gangrene 2. MM of mouth/tongue-corroded, first appear greyish white 3. **Stomach:** **Wall:** Tough, thick, leathery	**PM findings** 1. **Local:** Nil 2. MM of mouth/tongue, lips-corroded 3. Stomach: Wall: Soft, swollen **MM:** Congested, desquamated, hemorrhagic

3. **Stomach:**
   Wall: Soft, swollen
   MM: Congested, desquamated, hemorrhagic, brownish streaks
   Contains: Brownish, blood mixed with mucus
4. All visceral organs congested
5. Kidneys are congested and loaded with calcium oxalate crystals
6. Visceral organs show cloudy areas due to deposition of calcium oxalate

brown,— **"Leather bottle appearance"**
MM: Congested, desquamated, hemorrhagic
Contains: Brownish, blood mixed with mucus + phenolic smell
4. All visceral organs congested
5. Kidneys are congested, enlarged and cortical hemorrhagic
6. Surrounding structure/organs appeared necrosed and hardening with greyish white staining of the viscera

Contains: Brownish, altered blood + mucus shreds + vinegar smell
4. All visceral organs congested
5. Kidneys are congested
6. Respiratory tract-congested, inflamed due to leakage of acid in RT. Lungs edematous

---

Preservation of viscera: V1 + V2
Preserved in: Rectified spirit

V1 + V2 preserved in saturated salt solution and **not in rectified spirit**

V1 +V2 preserved in saturated salt solution and **not in rectified spirit**

Medicolegal (ML) aspects
1. **Suicide:** Sometimes used for suicide
2. **Homicide:** Rarely used
3. **Accidental poisoning:** Mistaken with magnesium or zinc sulfate, in children.
4. Used to erase writings in an attempt at forgery

ML aspects
1. **Suicide:** Commonly used for suicide (household poison)
2. **Homicide:** Rarely used where it is mixed with rum
3. **Accidental poisoning:** Mistaken with drakshasava (Ayurvedic drug), usually in children, chronic exposure due to its use or industrial exposure
4. **Abortifacient:** Used to procure criminal abortion

ML aspects
1. **Suicide:** May be used for suicide (household poison)
2. **Homicide:** Rarely used— detectable smell
3. **Accidental poisoning:** Mostly in children when taken by mistake, chronic industrial exposure

---

Chemical test
$BaCl_2$ + oxalic = barium oxalate crystals

Chemical test
Ferric chloride + phenol = blue color substance

Chemical test
A. acid + drop of phenophthalein → pink color + drop of 0.1 N $NaOH$ → pink color disappear

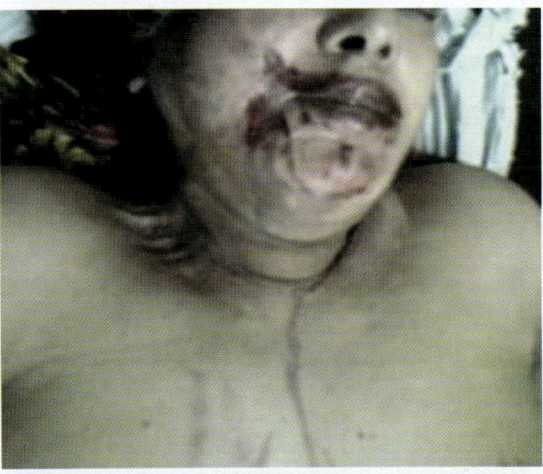

Fig. 4.1: Corrosion around mouth in carbolic acid

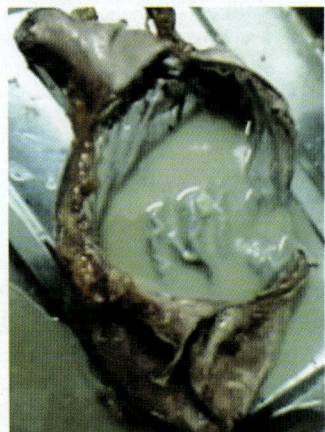

Fig. 4.2: Stomach in carbolic acid: Tough, thick and leathery bottle appearance

Differences	Oxalix acid	Magnesium sulfate (epson salt)	Zinc sulfate
1. Taste	Sour	Bitter	Bitter
2. Reaction	Acidic	Neutral	Acidic
3. On heating	Vaporizes	–	–
4. With $NaCO_3$	Effervescences, no ppt.	White ppt.	White ppt.
5. Stain	Removed	–	–
6. Figure			

ALKALIES

Hydroxide: Ammonium (NH_4OH), potassium (KOH, caustic potash), sodium (NaOH, caustic soda), calcium [$Ca(OH)_2$].

Carbonate: Ammonium [$(NH_4)_2CO_3$], potassium [K_2CO_3], sodium [Na_2CO_3, washing soda].

Lye: It is a mixture of caustic soda and washing soda, used for washing purpose.

Source: Industries, laboratories.

Uses: As chemicals, bleaching agents, used in medicines.

Properties

- Most of these occur as white powder.
- Odorless
- Burning irritating taste
- Ammonium hydroxide is a liquid, having ammoniacal smell.

Mechanism of Action

Locally: Act as corrosives. They dissolve the protein and saponify facts, hence cause deeper burns.

- Precipitates protein
- Hygroscopic—absorbs water from tissue.
- Combine with fats to form alkaline soaps (saponification of fats)
- Combine with protein to form alkaline proteinates (causes **liquefaction** necrosis).

Fatal dose: Variable (NaOH and KOH—5 gm, NH_4OH—30 gm, K_2CO_3—15 gm, Na_2CO_3 and $(NH_4)_2 CO_3$—30 gm).

Fatal period: About 24 hrs. NH_3 inhalation—immediate.

Clinical Features

a. Intense burning pain in mouth and throat and abdomen with **acrid, caustic and soapy taste,** difficulty in speech and deglutition, dyspnea, vomiting, thirst, excessive salivation with blood and mucous, hoarseness of voice, diarrhea, suppression of urine and dehydration followed by shock.

b. The vomitus is **strongly alkaline** mixed with altered blood (brown or black due to hematin), mucous and mucous shreds. Stool is mixed with blood and mucus.

c. There is erosion of mucosa from lips to stomach, reddish brown color.

There is also erosion of skin **(greyish, soapy)** along line of trickling of alkalies from angle of the mouth.

d. Perforation may occur
e. With ammonia vapors—congestion and watering of eyes, sneezing, coughing and choking. There may be edema glottis, pneumonia and death.

Treatment

1. Emetics and gastric lavage are contraindicated (danger of perforation of stomach).
2. Drinking of plenty of plain water.
3. Use of weak vegetable acids like 3–5% acetic acid (vinegar), citric acid (lime/orange juice), 0.5% HCl
4. Demulcent drinks like milk, egg albumin, vegetable oil, ghee, butter, soap solution, etc.
5. Supportive:
   • For pain—morphine.
   • For thirst—ice sucking.
   • For fluid loss—IV fluids.
   • For shock—corticosteriod.
   • For edema glottis—tracheostomy and artificial respiration.
   • Surface excoriations—washing and ointment applied.
   • Keep airway patent, in ammonia inhalation-oxygenation
   • Antibiotic to prevent infection.
   • Perforations—laparotomy and surgical repair

Cause of death: Shock, perforation, peritonitis and laryngeal spasm, infection, stomach, esophageal stricture.

PM Findings

Gross corrosion of skin with soapy, greyish discoloration. Corrosion of mucous membrane of mouth, tongue and lips with brownish discoloration present.

Stomach

Wall: Soft, swollen,

MM: Desquamated, ulcerated, hemorrhagic, brownish (alkali hematin)

Contents: Alkaline, altered blood, mucous, epithelium shreds

Gastric perforation leading to peritonitis

In late deaths: Signs of repair with scarring present.

Medicolegal Aspects

Poisoning by alkali is rare.

1. **Suicide:** Is rare.
2. **Homicide:** Is rare.
3. **Accidental poisoning:** Sometimes may occur due to mistaken for medicine, by children, or due to ingestion while pipetting the fluid usually in laboratory.
4. **Vitriolage:** They are commonly used for throwing on body, usually caustic soda.

Chemical Test

Hydroxides + $AgNO_3$ → yellow precipitates
Carbonates + HCl → white precipitates

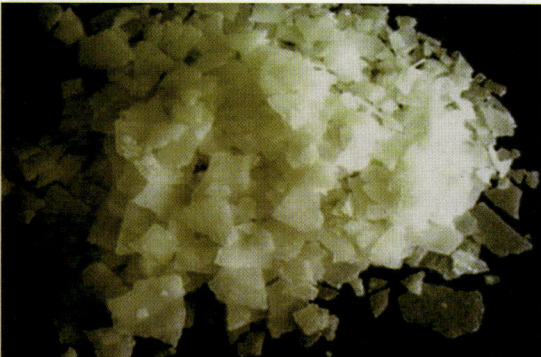

Fig. 4.3: Sodium hydroxide (caustic soda)

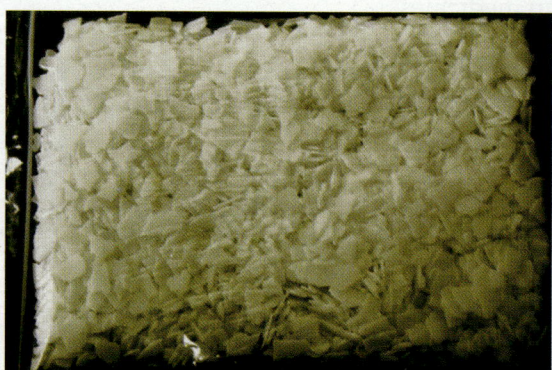

Fig. 4.4: Potassium hydroxide (caustic potash)

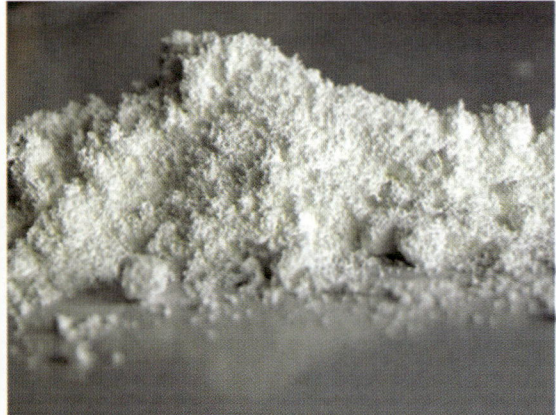

Fig. 4.5: Sodium carbonate (washing soda)

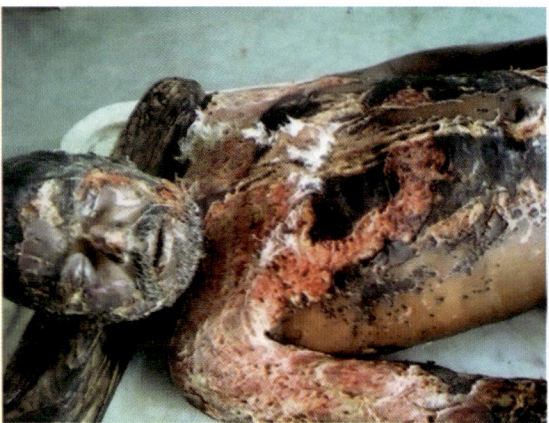

Fig. 4.6: Burns due to fall of sulfuric acid

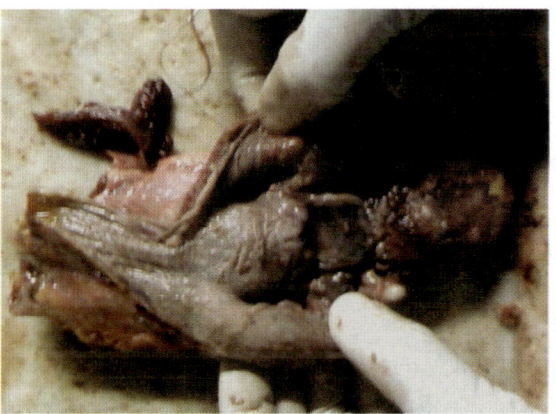

Fig. 4.7: Corrosion of tongue, epiglottis and esophagus due to consumption of acid

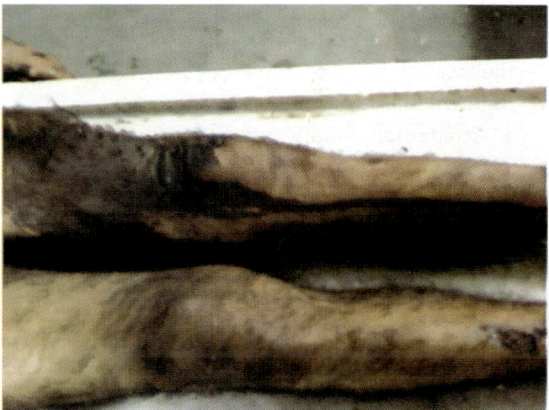

Fig. 4.8: Trickling mark of acid over legs

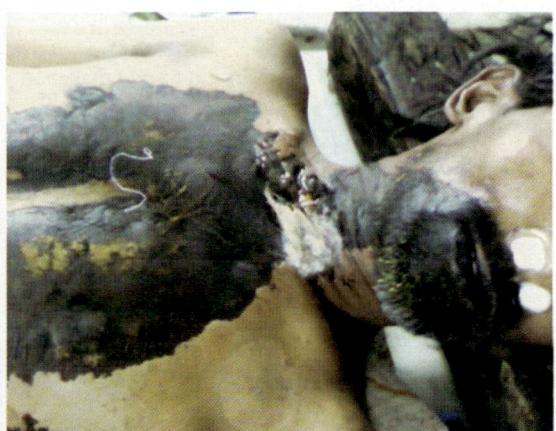

Fig. 4.9: Blackish corrosion of skin due to consumption of sulfuric acid

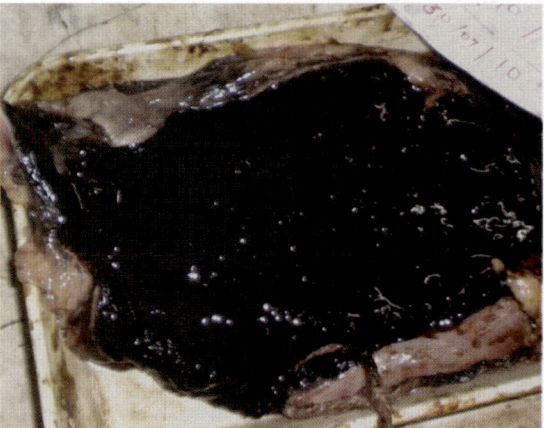

Fig. 4.10: Blackish corrosion of stomach in sulfuric acid poisoning

Irritants: Mechanical and Non-metallic Inorganic Poison

5

MECHANICAL IRRITANT

1. *Glass powder/broken glass pieces*

Bigger pieces can cause injury and hemorrhage in GIT. But smaller pieces fortunately do not get adhered to the wall of GIT and rather pass out the whole length of the tract by peristaltic movement

Medicolegal aspects

a. **Accidental:** Usually with jam, jelly, etc. contaminated with broken piece of their container. It also occurs to showmen while performing their show and may face problem

b. **Homicidal:** May be used, where it is mixed with food/drink

2. *Hair and fibers*

They may stuck on the wall of stomach and intestine and may cause irritation (inflammation and pain)

Medicolegal aspects

a. It is usually seen in the psychotic patient, where there is a collection of mass of hair in the stomach. This condition is called as 'Trichobazoar'

b. Homicidal: Very rare, where it is mixed with food

3. *Diamond dust or powder*

It is really harmful due to the presence of minute spike on the surface of the diamond powder. These spikes get stuck and impregnated the wall of intestine and cause perforation, hemorrhage, inflammation and peritonitis

Medicolegal aspects

a. **Accidental:** Poisoning may occur due to chronic exposure to diamond cutters

b. **Homicidal:** Used in ancient period by slow poisoning the king

c. **Suicidal:** Rarely used

4. *Metallic chips/nails and pins*

Minute piece do not pose any problem but bigger piece may cause injury, hemorrhage and perforation of GIT. But the sharpness of the corner of metal piece is reduced due to the action of digestive enzymes

Medicolegal aspect

Accidental: Mostly to children and also to magician (showmen) while performing their show

Treatment of mechanical irritant poisoning

1. Bulky foods like banana, mashed potato, boiled rice, etc.

2. Demulcents: Starch, milk, barley water, oil, ghee, butter, egg albumin, etc.

3. Surgical intervention if required

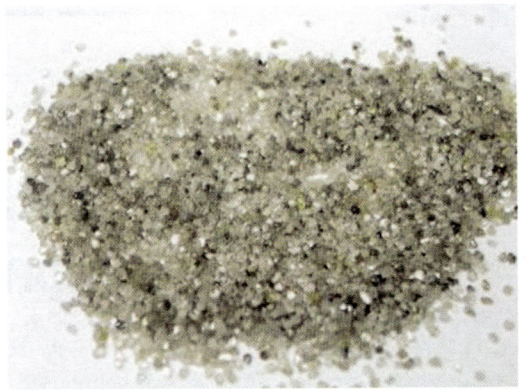
Fig. 5.1: Diamond powder

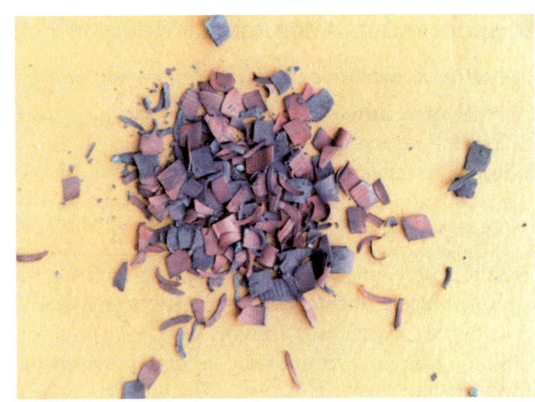
Fig. 5.2: Metallic chips

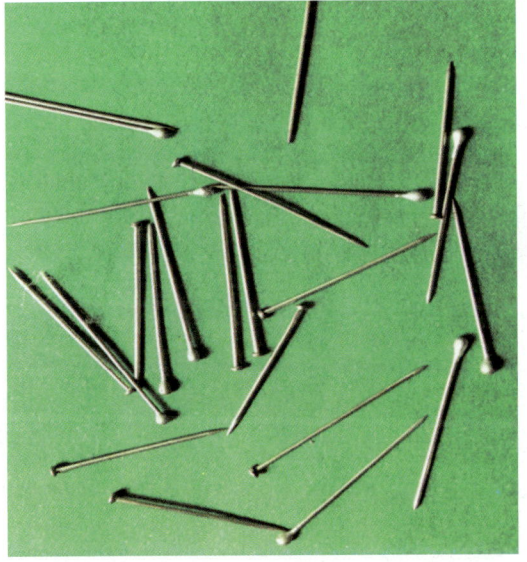
Fig. 5.3: Nails/pins

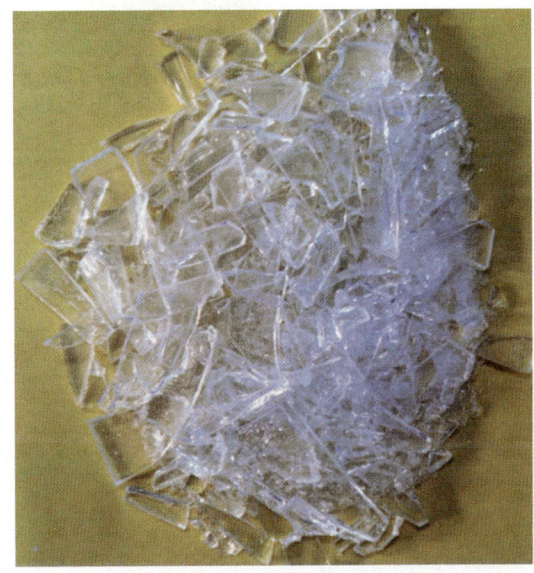
Fig. 5.4: Glass pieces

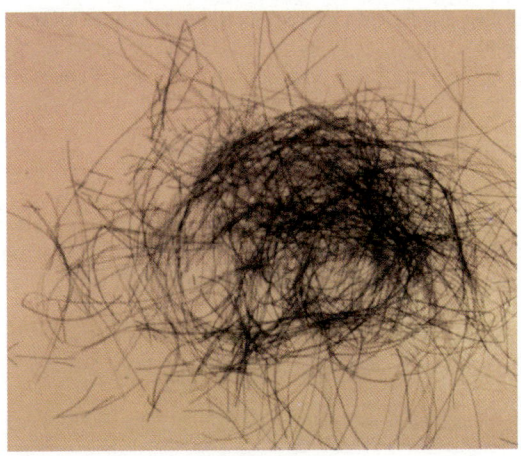
Fig. 5.5: Hair

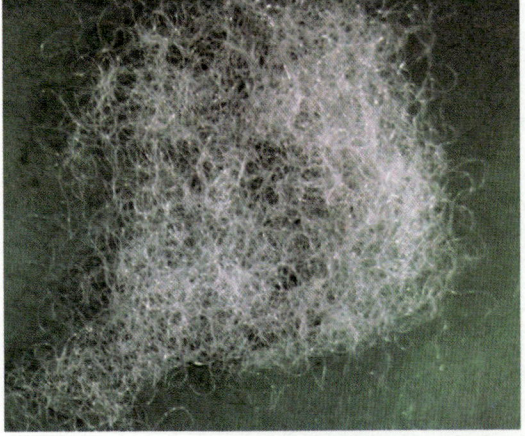
Fig. 5.6: Fibers

Phosphorus: It is a non-metallic inorganic chemical irritant.

Properties and uses: It exists in 2 forms—white or yellow and brown or red.

1. White or yellow phosphorus
Crystalline, translucent, waxy, cylindrical, highly toxic, garlicky smell and taste, luminous in dark, ignites at 30°C on exposure to air, so it is stored under water/kerosene

Uses: It is used in chemicals, fertilizers, manufacture of phosphates and organophosphorus compounds, rodenticide, insecticide, fireworks and gunpowder (smoke bombs and incendiary bullets), i.e. firearm ammunition

2. Red or brown phosphorus: It is prepared when white phosphorus is heated at a temperature of 280°C, in the atmosphere of nitrogen
Non-toxic, odorless, tasteless, non-luminous, inert, non-fuming

Uses: It is used on the sides of matchbox, where it is mixed with glass. It is also used in matchstick head, where it is mixed with potassium chlorate ($KClO_3$) and antimony sulfide (AnS)
Before 1931, white phosphorus was being used for the manufacture of Lucifer Matches, but due to its toxicity, it was banned in 1931 and present day safety match came into being

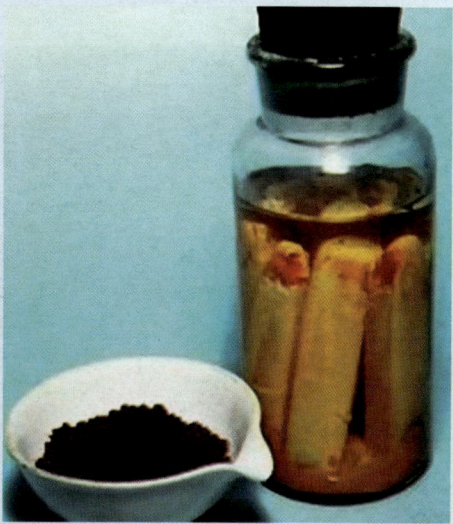

Fig. 5.7: Brown and yellow phosphorus

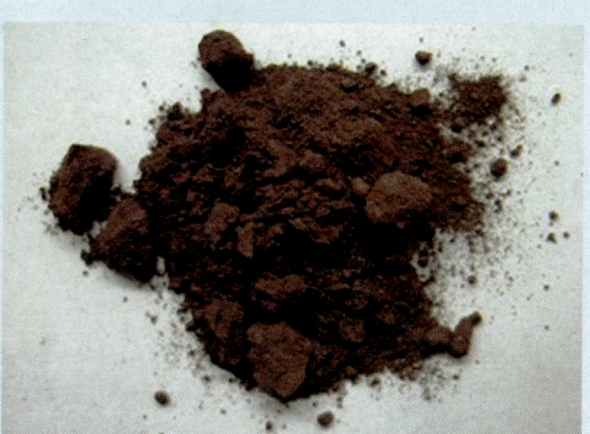

Fig. 5.8: Brown phosphorus

Mechanism of action
Locally, it destroys the tissue with which it comes in contact. It is a **protoplasmic poison**, hampers tissue oxidation and causes fatty infiltration and **necrosis**
1. **In acute poisoning:** It causes hepatic dysfunction resembling ischemia known as **necrobiosis**, which results in disturbance in carbohydrate and fat metabolism
2. **In chronic poisoning:** There is excessive bone formation at the epiphyseal end (sequestration) with necrosis
3. Phosphine (PH_3) causes respiratory distress

Fatal dose: 50–100 mg

Fatal period: Variable, 12 hrs to 1 week

Absorption, metabolism, excretion
Absorbed through mucous membrane, quickly when stomach is empty or contains fatty foods. After absorption, it is distributed in all the organs and metabolized to hypophosphate and excreted through urine. Small part is excreted as such through feces and respiration

Clinical manifestation depends upon
1. Dose,
2. Period of exposure,
3. Nature/type of poison, and
4. Routes: Contact/ingested/inhaled

I. *Acute phosphorus poisoning*	II. *Chronic phosphorus poisoning*
Local: Necrosis of epidermis of skin after 1–2 days of its contact. Burned when ignited and becomes ulcerated (very painful and heals slowly) **GIT:** Burning pain, vomiting, diarrhea, garlicky smell, intense thirst, salivation, and abdominal pain, followed by dehydration 　　Vomitus is dark, garlic smell, luminescence 　　Stool is dark, garlic smell, luminescence **CNS:** Headache, insomnia, vision impaired, deafness, restlessness, delirium, tremor, convulsion, coma **Liver:** Jaundice, pruritis, bleeding points, with hepatosplenomegaly **Kidney:** Oliguria, albuminuria, hematuria, with sugar and bile salt present Bleeding from gums, nose, in skin, and under surface of visceral organs **Priapism** (painful persistent erection of penis)	**It occurs due to** i. Exposure/inhalation of fumes in industries where phosphorous is used ii. Consumption of sea fish containing high quantity of phosphorus—Minimata disease There is a **triad** of manifestation 1. **GIT/general disturbances:** Nausea, vomiting, loss of weight/appetite, pain in abdomen, alternate constipation and diarrhea, irritability, fatigability, lack of interest/concentration, weakness 2. **Cirrhosis of liver** 3. **Phossy jaw:** It is the necrosis of mandible and sequestration (due to increased bone formation) and discharge of foul smelling pus by sinus formation. It is seen in 3% of industrial worker exposed to phosphorus. It is characterized by: 　　Pain/swelling/loosening of teeth with osteomyelitis and necrosis of lower jaw with multiple sinuses discharging foul smelling pus. 　　Failure of dental socket to heal when teeth fall. Inflammation of mucous membrane showing small reddish areas. Osteomyelitis and necrosis of the jaw with multiple sinuses discharging foul smelling pus
Cause of death: Shock, circulatory failure, hepatic and renal failure	**Cause of death:** Infection, pyemia and weakness due to dysphagia
Treatment 1. Emesis 2. Stomach wash with **antidote:** 　　0.1% $CuSO_4$ (forms copper phosphide) 　　0.1% $KMnO_4$ (oxidizes phosphorus to phosphates) 3. **Demulcents are contraindicated** because they dissolve phosphorus 4. Non-fatty purgatives—$MgSO_4$ 5. Restriction of fats, demulcents, morphine due to liver damage 6. **Symptomatic** 　**Dehydration or shock:** IV fluids and glucose, vitamin K, B-complex and vitemin C. 7. For external lesion: Washing, covered with wet cloth and application of bland and antibiotic ointment	**Treatment** 1. Prevent further exposure 2. **Regular dental care:** Mouth wash with $NaHCO_3$ 3. Plenty of oral calcium 4. Protect liver 5. Prevent intercurrent infection 6. Use of exhaust fans 7. Working area sprayed with turpentine oil vapor
PM findings: Acute phosphorus 1. Locally, skin-necrosis, ulcerated 2. Mucous membrane of mouth eroded 3. Gum swollen with bleeding points 4. GIT stomach wall—soft, swollen; 　MM—eroded, desquamated, hemorrhagic; 　Contents—dark, garlic smell, luminous	**PM findings:** Chronic phosphorus 1. Phossy jaw 2. Liver cirrhosis 3. Poor oral hygiene

5. **Liver:** In early stage, it is **enlarged**, soft, friable, greasy due to **fatty degeneration (necrobiosis)**.
    In late stage it is **shrunken**, leathery, gritty, dirty yellow due to **necrosis (acute yellow atrophy)**

6. Yellowish discoloration of skin and petechial hemorrhage

7. **Kidneys:** Tubular degeneration

8. Fatty degenerative changes in heart and kidney

Medicolegal aspects

1. **Suicide:** Not preferred (due to painful death)

2. **Homicidal:** Not used (due to its smell and taste)

3. **Accidental poisoning:** Children are attracted by luminosity, or when they chew the match stick heads or side
   • Also occurs due to industrial exposure
   • And through consumption of rat poison tablet containing phosphorus

4. **Abortifacient:** Used both locally or general administration

5. **Arson:** It is used for causing outbreak of fire without being suspected. For this, phosphorus is wrapped in moist cow dung or moist rag and is kept/thrown on the roof of a house. When dung/rag become dry, the phosphorus gets ignited, producing fire on the thatched roof

6. To destroy undesired letters that has been posted

7. It is also used to create smoke screen in war field so as to infiltrate in the enemy side

8. **Greek fire:** Phosphorus dissolved in carbon disulfide may be thrown on one's face/body with malicious intention is known as Greek fire

HALOGENS: Chlorine, bromine, fluorine, iodine.
ACTION: Very irritable to GIT/RT.

Iodine

Physical characteristics: Solid, bluish-black crystals emitting violet vapors.

Uses

1. In radiopaque dyes.

2. For dressing, e.g. tincture of iodine, Lugol's iodine, or povidone iodine.

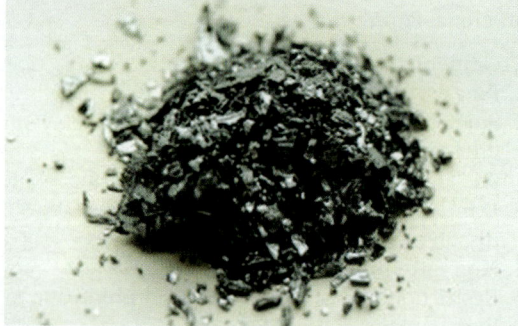

Fig. 5.9: Iodine crystals

Clinical manifestation: Iodine poisoning

I. Acute poisoning	II. Chronic poisoning (iodism)
There may be sudden death due to anaphylaxis in sensitive people	It results due to excessive consumption of drugs contain iodine
Burning pain in upper GIT	Headache, nausea, vomiting and diarrhea.
Vomiting—is blue or violet with smell of iodine.	Increased nasal and bronchial secretions, salivations, conjunctivitis, parotitis, erythematous patches and ulcers on the skin.
Sometimes diarrhea	
Uremia	Death may be immediate in case of anaphylaxis
Shock	

Fatal dose: Approx. 2 gm.

Fatal period: Normally 24 hrs

Mechanism of action
- Irritation of GIT and RT
- It also precipitates proteins

Sudden death: A few people are hypersensitive to iodine

Treatment
- Emetics
- Gastric lavage

Antidote: Starch solution and sodium thio-sulfate

Postmortem findings
- **Mucosa of upper GIT:** Inflamed
- Stomach contents are blue and emit smell of iodine
- Degeneration of heart, liver and kidney

Medicolegal aspects
- **Suicide:** Rare
- **Homicide:** Rare
- **Accidental poisoning:** When taken by mistake
- **Vitriolage:** It is used for vitriolage.

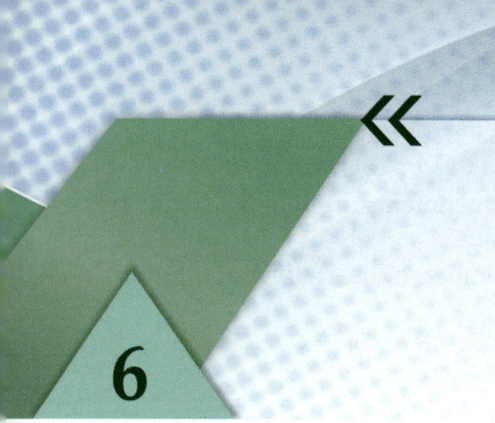
Irritants: Inorganic Metallic Poison

These are the inorganic metallic compounds causing local irritation to the GIT. It includes toxic compounds of the metals. From the forensic point of view, important inorganic metallic poisons include compounds of arsenic, lead, copper and mercury.

Arsenic	Lead
Pure metallic arsenic is not poisonous and not absorbed through GIT	Pure metallic lead is absorbed through GIT
Source Industrial, commercial, domestic, agricultural. Soil, water, sea fish, crustaceans, tobacco, beer, cigar/cigarette smoke	**Source** Industrial, commercial, domestic
Uses Calicoprinting, fruit spray, depilatory and cosmetic agents, coloring agents—toys, paints, insecticidal, weed killer, rodenticide, in fly paper and fly powder, in medicine—as Fowler's solution in intermittent fever, general tonic, syphilis	**Uses** Water pipes, batteries, paints, hair dye, vermillion, petrol, glass blowing on the surface of ceramic articles
Toxic compounds The common poisonous preparations of Arsenic with (common names) are: 1. **Arsenic trioxide** (sankhya, somalkhar): White amorphous powder, colorless, odorless, tasteless, sparingly soluble in water 2. **Arsenic hydride** (Arsine) (AsH_3): Highly toxic gas, burns with blue flame, garlic smell 3. **Copper arsenite** (Scheele's green) and **copper acetoarsenite** (Paris green): Greenish color powder 4. **Arsenic trisulfide** (orpiment, multani mitti, harital)—bright yellow solid 5. **Arsenic bisulfide** (Realgur)—brick red powder 6. **Arsenic trichloride:** Highly toxic liquid having pungent smell and irritant to eyes	**Toxic compounds** The common poisonous preparations of lead with (common names) are: 1. **Lead acetate, lead sub-acetate**—white crystalline salt, sweet astringent taste 2. **Lead carbonate**—white fine dusty powder used in paints 3. **Lead tetraoxide** (vermillion, sindoor)—scarlet crystalline powder (used on Hanuman idol) 4. **Lead sulfide** (surma, kajal)—black powder 5. **Lead monoxide**—brick red 6. **Tetraethyl lead** (added to petrol) 7. **Other:** Lead chloride, lead nitrate, lead chromate, lead bromide, lead iodide

Lead poisoning may occur by:
1. Ingestion,
2. Inhalation, and
3. Absorption through skin. Lead is 10 times more poisonous when inhaled.

Mechanism of action	**Mechanism of action**
1. Inhibits sulfhydryl group of enzymes thereby interfering with cell metabolism and oxidation 2. Uncouple the mitochondrial oxidative phosphorylation 3. Locally, it may cause necrosis, sloughing and gangrene	1. Inhibits sulfhydryl group of enzymes thereby interfering with cell metabolism and oxidation 2. Spasm of capillaries 3. Fixation of lead in brain and peripheral nervous system
Absorption, distribution, and excretion Absorbed through mucous membrane of GIT, intact skin, or through other natural orifices. Deposited in liver, kidneys, bones, hair, nails. Excreted through urine, hair and nail. Small amount is also eliminated through feces, saliva, bronchial secretions, and milk	**Absorption, distribution, and excretion** Usually absorbed through GIT. Lead dust/fumes through respiratory track. Lead tetraoxide/tetraethyl lead through skin. Lead is a cumulative poison and deposited in bones, liver and kidneys. It is excreted through urine, bile and nails
Fatal dose: White arsenic = 200 mg. **Fatal period:** 24 hrs to 1 week	**Fatal dose:** Lead acetate = 20 gm. Lead carbonate = 30 gm. **Fatal period:** 24 hrs to 1 week

Acute arsenic poisoning
Burning sensation, metallic taste, difficulty in speech and swallowing, excessive salivation, thirst with abdominal pain, vomiting, diarrhea with painful defecation and micturition
This is followed by dehydration, muscle cramps, convulsion, collapse, and coma
    Vomiting initially contains stomach contents mixed with blood and finally mucoid, watery with streaks of blood
    Diarrhea initially contains foul smelling fecal matter mixed with blood and finally colorless, odorless mucoid and watery **like rice-water stool of cholera** (due to rupture of vesicles formed under the mucosa)
    Scanty urine containing blood and albumin
    There is jaundice, anemia, hepatomegaly
Inhalation of fumes: Cough, frothy sputum, breathlessness, cyanosis, pulmonary edema, congestion of eyes and ulceration of cornea
	Acute lead poisoning
	Burning sensation, metallic taste, difficulty in speech and swallowing, excessive salivation, thirst with abdominal pain, vomiting, diarrhea with painful defecation and micturition. This is followed by dehydration, muscle cramps, convulsion, collapse, and coma
	    Vomiting—curdy white (lead chloride)
	    Diarrhea—black (lead sulfide)
	    Scanty urine containing lead, albumin, copro-porphyrin 3 (**red colored urine**).
	CNS manifestations: Headache, insomnia, drowsiness, dizziness, muscular cramps, tremor, convulsions, collapse, coma, rarely paralysis

Treatment
1. Emesis
2. **Stomach wash:** With freshly prepared ferric oxide (45 ml $FeCl_2$ + 15 gm MgO)—filtering the ppt.
3. Demulcent
4. **Purgatives:** Magnesium sulfate
5. **Antidotes:** BAL/ferric oxide
6. **Supportive**
    Shock/dehydration—IV fluids
    Liver protection—vitamin/amino acids
    Renal failure—dialysis
    Pain—morphine
    Blood transfusion, if required
	Treatment
	1. Emesis
	2. **Stomach wash:** With magnesium/sodium sulfate (forms insoluble lead sulfate)
	3. Demulcent
	4. Purgative
	5. **Antidotes:** Mg/Na sulfate or calcium edetate or penicillamine
	6. **Supportive**
	    Shock/dehydration—IV fluids
	    Liver protection—vitamins D, and C/amino acid
	    Renal failure—dialysis
	    Pain in abdomen—morphine
	    Abdominal colic—calcium gluconate and atropine

Antidote

1. **Physical:** Demulcents.
2. **Chemical:** Freshly prepared **ferric oxide** precipitate (prepared by adding 45 ml ferric chloride and 15 gm magnesium oxide then filtering the precipitate). Dose is 15 gm ppt in glass of water. It forms ferric arsenite—which is a harmless salt
3. **Pharmacological: BAL**, given 3 mg/kg as 10% solution in arachis oil with benzyl benzoate, deep IM, 4 hourly for 2 days, and 12 hourly till 10th day. (It forms BAL—arsenic complex that is excreted out by the kidney)

Antidote

1. **Physical:** Demulcents
2. **Chemical:** Sodium sulfate and magnesium sulfate
3. **Pharmacological: Calcium edetate** $CaNa_2EDTA$ (calcium disodium ethylenediaminetetra-acetic acid), 1 gm per day as slow IV drip as 3% solution in saline. It excretes lead from circulation and bones

PM findings

MM of mouth/esophagus—inflamed.

Stomach: 'Red-velvety appearance'
Wall—soft, swollen
MM—inflamed, hemorrhagic, and reddened
Contents—blood with mucous shreds present arsenic powder or watery fluid mucoid and blood streaks
Surrounding viscera—soft, inflamed, congested.
Visceral organs congested

Large intestine: Contains mucoid, watery material
Heart—subendocardial hemorrhage
Hemorrhages on larynx, trachea, lungs and abdominal organs
Usually, it retards decomposition. In decomposed body, yellowish discoloration occurs in stomach and surrounding tissue due to the formation of arsenic sulfide (arsenic + H_2S = arsenic sulfide)

PM findings

MM of mouth—inflamed

Stomach
Wall—soft, swollen
MM—congested, greyish, sometimes eroded
Contents—curdy white material
Visceral organs congested
Large intestine: Stools are black

Chronic arsenic poisoning: It occurs due to:
1. Industrial or agricultural exposures.
2. Contaminated food or drinks.
3. Arsenical medicines
4. Consumption of repeated small doses.
5. In West Bengal, there is adulteration of water with arsenic

Clinical features: It may be specific and non-specific findings.
The stage 1 includes non-specific findings whereas rest includes specific findings

Chronic lead poisoning (**plumbism**, also known as saturnism): It occurs due to:
1. Inhalation of dust/vapors in people working in factories/industries (e.g. paint industry, plumbing, glass—blowers, electric wire industries, batteries, toys, hair-dye and gasolene industries)
2. Contaminated food and drinks with lead (stored/cooked in tins or lead vessels)
3. Prolonged use of vermillion, dye and cosmetic containing lead
4. One who handled petrol
   Clinical features: It is Chronic **LEAD** Poisoning.

Chronic arsenic poisoning
Stage I: General loss of health and gastrointestinal disturbances
   Irritability, fatigability, lack of interest and concentration, loss of weight and appetite, abdominal pain, alternate constipation and diarrhea, gums inflamed and tooth loosened

Chronic lead poisoning
C → Constipation, colicky pain
The colic is intermittent, spasmodic and relieved by pressure and is associated with constipation
L → Lead line (**Burtonian line**—bluish discoloration over gingival surface of gums)

Stage II: Nasolacrimal and bronchial catarrhal changes

Inflammation of conjunctiva, with watering from eyes and nose, photophobia, hoarseness of voice, cough with expectoration. (Features as of common cold)

Ulceration of nasal mucosa

Stage III: Cutaneous/keratin involvement

i. **Pigmentation of skin:** Rain-drop appearance—pin-point brownish pigmentation of the skin. MiIk rose complexion—generalized brownish pigmentation due to vasodilatation Dark pigmentation with thickening of palm and soles

ii. **Nails**—brittle, 'Mee's lines' present (transverse, white streak at growing part of nail)

iii. **Hair**—dry, alopecia, pigmented (yellow or brown)

Stage IV: Neurological involvement

Headache, irritability, fatigability, lack of interest and concentration

Tingling and numbness, tremor, cramps, muscle weakness and paralysis

Other manifestations

Liver damage—jaundice, pruritis

Kidney damage—albuminuria, hematuria, renal failure

Bone marrow aplasia and **basophilic stippling of RBC**

E → Encephalopathy—due to inactivation of MAO. It leads to irritability, fatigability, lack of interest/concentration, delirium, convulsion, collapse, coma.

A → Alopecia, anemia with punctate basophilia. Anemia is due to:

i. Impaired hemesynthesis.

ii. Increase fragility of RBC due to loss of potassium due to increase cell permeability

iii. Antithrombin effect of lead leads to defective clotting

There is also **basophilic stippling of RBC** due to condensation of iron containing RNA near mitochondria. The RBC shows dark blue spots due to metabolic products of porphyrin.

Other features seen on peripheral smear examination are:

a. Reticulocytosis

b. Decreased platelets

c. Increased monocytes

d. Anisocytosis

e. Poikilocytosis

D → Degenerative effect, lead deposited. Degenerative effect on:

Reproductive system—leads to sterility.

CVS in arteries—hypertension.

Kidneys—chronic interstitial nephritis.

Peripheral nerves—peripheral neuritis.

Eye changes—retinal stippling and optic atrophy leading to blindness.

Lead is deposited beyond the epiphysis of growing end of long bones leading to abnormal development in children **(lead osteopathy)**.

P → Pallor (facial pallor due to vasospasm).

P → Palsy—due to degeneration of nerves and atrophy of muscles leads to tingling numbness, weakness, tremors, cramps, etc. and ultimately leads to wrist drop and foot drop due to paralysis of extensor muscles of wrist and foot

(**Blue line of gums** is also seen in mercury, copper, silver, iron, bismuth and thallium poisoning).

Treatment: Chronic arsenic poisoning
1. Prevention of exposure
2. BAL/penicillamine
3. Vitamin B complex
4. Supportive

Treatment: Chronic lead poisoning
1. Prevent further exposure
2. Antidote: Calcium versenate—1 gm/day slow IV drip or BAL/penicillamine
3. Potassium iodide—(1–2 gm) removes lead from bones
4. Potassium citrate—removes lead from circulation
5. **Supportive:** Magnesium sulfate—for constipation Atropine sulfate for severe colic NaHCO$_3$, vitamin D, calcium diet

PM Findings

Dehydration, jaundice, anemia

PM Findings

Emaciated

Degenerative changes in thoracic and abdominal organs and nerves Bone marrow aplasia **Keratin/cutaneous changes:** Skin pigmentation, Mee's line in nails, alopecia	Blue lining over gums Alopecia Evidence of anemia Degenerative changes in liver, kidney, heart Bone marrow aplasia
Laboratory investigation **Urine:** Arsenic level of >100 microgram/day is suggestive of poisoning. It becomes positive within 6 hrs of poisoning and continuous for about 2 wks. **Hair and nails:** Arsenic level of >100 microogram/day is suggestive of poisoning **Blood:** Basophilic stippling of RBC present	**Laboratory investigation** **Blood:** Lead level of >50 microgram per day **Stool:** Lead level of >75 microgram per day X-ray shows higher density beyond epiphysis

Interpretation of arsenic in exhumed body
In dead bodies recovered from graves, there is the possibility that either the arsenic from the body percolates to the soil or arsenic from the soil may imbibe the body. Hence, the presence of arsenic should be interpreted very carefully in exhumed body:
1. Arsenic absorbed during life usually consists of soluble salt forms
2. If arsenic has gone from the body to the soil, then not only the concentration of arsenic will be more in the body, the concentration in soil below the body will be more than the soil on both sides of the body and over the top of the body

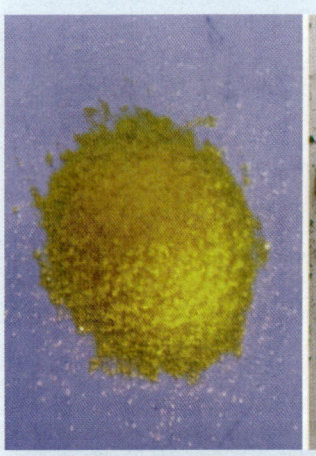 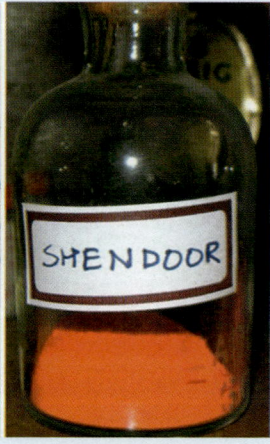 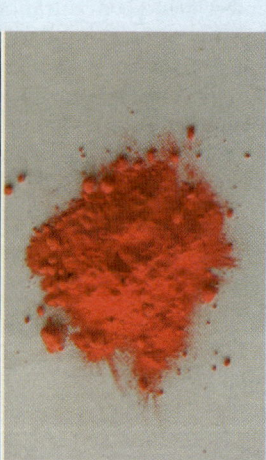

Arsenic trisulfide	Copper arsenite	Lead tetraoxide	Lead monoxide

Medicolegal aspects: Arsenic
1. Suicidal: Not preferred due to painful death.
2. Homicidal: Earlier it was the most popular and considered as ideal homicidal poison and signs and symptom resembles that of cholera. But it has got great disadvantages that it is detected not only in decomposed body but also in the body ash and there is also chemical test to detect the poison
3. **Accidental due to**
   i. Consumption of contaminated food and drinks,
   ii. Exposure while in agricultural field, or in industries
   iii. **Its abuses**
4. Abortifacient for procuring criminal abortion
5. Cattle poison and as stupefying poison

Medicolegal aspects: Lead
1. Suicide: Rare—long, painful
2. Homicide: Rare, detection in CA
3. Accidental: Due to chronic exposure, to children
4. Abortifacient: Sometimes used to procure abortion
5. Cattle poison

Preservation of viscera
1. Routine viscera
2. Additional viscera like hair, nails and ends of long bones are also preserved. A serial analysis of hair and nails gives an idea of successive dosages of arsenic consumed (rate of growth of hair—1 cm per month, and nails—0.3 cm per week). Hair examination proved the death of Napoleon to be due to chronic arsenic poisoning

Preservation of viscera
1. Routine viscera
2. Additional viscera like nails and ends of long bones are also preserved.

Abuses of arsenic
a. It is used as **love philter**—it increases the affection towards the giver. In ancient days, the wives used to administer arsenic to their husband to gain attraction of the husband in the wake of unhealthy competition amongst the wives
b. **Aphrodisiac purpose**—it gives a sense of well-being and is used to increase sexual desire
c. It is also used to **improve the dark** complexion
d. **Arsenophagists**, are the person who takes arsenic daily. They can tolerate unbelievable amount of arsenic without much harm. It leads to tolerance and addiction

Differential diagnosis of arsenic poisoning
1. Bacterial food poisoning—the manifestations of vomiting and diarrhea are delayed by 6–36 hrs in bacterial food poisoning while they occur within 15–30 min in arsenic poisoning
2. Cholera—the manifestation starts with diarrhea and not with vomiting as in arsenic poisoning. The differences between arsenic poisoning and cholera are:

Points	Arsenic	Cholera
1. Start with	Vomiting	Diarrhea
2. Vomitus contains	Blood and mucus	Mucus only
3. Metallic taste	Present	Absent
4. Motive	Present	Absent
5. Restricted to	Individual	Not restricted, affects many
6. Lab test	On chemical analysis, arsenic present	On hanging drop—darting motility of bacteria present

Mercury	*Copper*
Pure metallic mercury is not poisonous as it is not absorbed through GIT. Mercury is a liquid metal, heavy, silvery and non-adhesive. Poisoning occurs if the finely divided particles or vaporized mercury is swallowed, inhaled or rubbed on the skin	Pure metallic copper is not absorbed through GIT and not poisonous

Source	**Source**
Industrial, commercial, domestic	Industrial, commercial, domestic, agricultural

Uses	**Uses**

1. As preservatives
2. Vermillion
3. BP apparatus
4. Thermometer
5. Medicine
6. **Snake tablet (mercury thiocyanate)** in Diwali
	Copper sulfate is used as:
	a. Emetic agent
	b. Antidote for phosphorus
	c. Other uses
	  1. Paints
	  2. Laboratory test for fragility of RBC
	  3. Coloring agents—used to impart color to peas, vegetable
	  4. It is used as fungicide, and pesticide
	  5. Household appliances—copper utensils

Toxic compounds

Common poisonous compounds of mercury are:

1. **Mercuric chloride** (corrosive action)—colorless crystalline powder, odorless, burning metallic taste, highly toxic. Used in medicines, laboratories, industries, and as preservatives. *Mercurous chloride (ras kapoor) is non-toxic, used as purgatives.*
2. Mercuric **cyanide**—used in medicine
3. Mercuric **sulfide**—[vermillion, sindoor, kumkum, kunku]—scarlet red crystalline powder
4. **Phenyl mercuric acetate**—used as fungicidal agent and preservation of seeds
5. **Other:** Mercuric nitrate, mercurous nitrate, mercuric methide, mercury fulminate, mercury thiocyanate and mercurochrome

Toxic compounds

Common poisonous compounds of copper are:

1. **Copper sulfate** ($CuSO_4$—blue vitriol, blue stone)— greenish blue crystals/powder, odorless, metallic taste, soluble in gastric juice, absorbed in water
2. Copper **subacetate** (verdegris)
3. Copper **chloride**—white crystals
4. Copper **carbonate**—white dusty powder

Mechanism of action

1. Mercury combines with sulfhydryl (SH) group of enzymes and thus depresses the cellular enzymatic mechanisms

Mechanism of action

1. Inhibits sulfhydryl (SH) group of enzymes thereby interference with cell metabolism and oxidation
2. It precipitates proteins

Fatal dose

Mercuric chloride = 400–500 mg
Fatal period: A few hrs to 3–7 days

Fatal dose

Copper subacetate = 15 gm
Copper sulfate = 30 gm
Fatal period: A few hrs to 3–7 days.

Absorbtion, distribution, and excretion

Absorption through GIT. The vapors and salts are also absorbed through RT, vagina (in vaginal douche), and bladder. Distributed in liver, spleen, kidney, bone and brain (in phenyl mercuric acetate). Soluble forms get deposited in liver, spleen, kidney, intestines, heart, muscles and lungs. Excreted in urine, bile, feces and body secretions

Absorbtion, distribution, excretion

Absorbed through GIT
Distributed in liver, spleen, and kidney
Excreted in urine, bile, feces

Acute mercury poisoning

Local: Skin—corrosion.
MM of mouth and tongue: Corroded and is greyish-white in color
Burning sensation, metallic taste, difficulty in speech and swallowing, excessive salivation, thirst with abdominal pain, vomiting, diarrhea with painful defecation and micturition. This is followed by dehydration, muscle cramps, convulsion, collapse, and coma
Vomiting contains mucous with altered blood and shreds of mucosa
Diarrhea is blood stained with necrosed mucus shreds of colon
Scanty urine containing blood and albumin
General: Headache, tremor, deafness, scotoma, loss of memory, loss of appetite, fatigue
On inhalation of vapors: Salivation, stomatitis, cough, dyspnea, conjunctivitis, corneal ulceration and nephrotoxicity

Acute copper poisoning

Anemia: Due to increase fragility of RBC causes hemolysis
Burning sensation, metallic taste, difficulty in speech and swallowing, excessive salivation, thirst with abdominal pain, vomiting, diarrhea with painful defecation and micturition. This is followed by dehydration, muscle cramps, convulsion, collapse, and coma
Vomiting is greenish blue—**turns to deep blue with ammonia/NH_4OH**
Diarrhea is greenish blue
Scanty urine containing blood, albumin
Liver damage: Jaundice

Treatment

1. **Emesis:** By lukewarm $NaHCO_3$ solution, Ipecacuanha
2. **Stomach wash:** Sodium formaldehyde sulfoxylate
3. **Demulcent:** egg albumin, milk, gelatin, etc.
4. Purgatives, high colonic lavage
5. Antidote
6. Supportive:
   Shock/dehydration—IV fluids
   Renal failure—$NaHCO_3$/peritoneal, or hemodialysis
   Exchange tranfusion

Antidote

a. **Physical:** Egg albumin (forms mercuric albuminate), demulcents, charcoal
b. **Chemical:** 5% solution of sodium formaldehyde sulfoxylate with 5% $NaHCO_3$
c. **Pharmacological:** BAL or penicillamine

PM findings

1. Skin and MM of mouth, tongue, esophagus— corroded and **greyish white**.
2. **Stomach:** Wall—soft, swollen
   MM—desquamated, hemorrhagic, ulcerated, necrosis and greyish white/black
   Contents—altered blood and mucus shreds.
3. **Intestines:** Congested, ulcerated, and sometimes gangrenous.
4. **Kidney:** Swollen, nephritis.
5. **Liver:** Congested, central necrosis and cloudy swelling
6. **Heart:** Sub-endocardial hemorrhages

Chronic mercury poisoning

(Hydrargyrism): It occurs due to:
1. Chronic exposure to people working in industry and laboratory
2. Injudicious medical administration, multiple repeated small doses
3. Contaminated food, drinks, and sea fish. Mercury is methylated under sea water and consumption of such fish causes chronic poisoning.
   (Minimata disease)

Clinical features

Skin: Contact dermatitis, penetrating ulcers on fingers, nails and knuckles.
GIT and general manifestaion: *metallic taste,* irritability, fatigability, lack of interest and concentration, loss of weight and appetite, alternate constipation and diarrhea, abdominal colic, *anemia*

Treatment

1. **Emesis:** There is no use of emetics. (Copper salts are potent emetics).
2. **Stomach wash:** With 1% Pot. ferrocyanide
3. Demulcent
4. **Purgatives:** Castor oil
5. Antidotes
6. Supportive:
   Diuretics
   Shock/dehydration—IV fluids.
   Liver/renal damage—vitamin, AA, dialysis
   Exchange transfusion

Antidote

a. **Physical:** Demulcents (forms copper albuminate with proteins)
b. **Chemical:** Potassium ferrocyanide (forms insoluble cupric ferrocyanide)
c. **Pharmacological:** Penicillamine or BAL

PM findings

1. MM of mouth, tongue and esophagus—greenish blue lining
2. **Stomach:** Wall—soft, swollen
   MM—desquamated, hemorrhagic, congested, greenish blue lining
   Contents: Greenish blue
3. **Intestines:** Hemorrhages and ulcerations, greenish blue lining
4. Greenish—blue froth at mouth and nostrils.
5. **Liver:** Jaundice

Chronic copper poisoning

It occurs due to hemocromatosis:
1. Chronic industrial exposure
2. Consumption of vegetables colored with copper sulfate
3. Consumption of contaminated food and drink (stored/cooked in copper utensils—Wilson disease)

Clinical features

GIT and general manifestaion *metallic taste,* irritability, fatigability, lack of interest and concentration, loss of weight and appetite, alternate constipation and diarrhea, abdominal colic, *anemia*
Gums: Blue lining or greenish blue line (Clapton's line), unhealthy

Buccal cavity: Suggestive of gingivitis, glossitis, salivation, loosening of teeth

Gums: Blue line, inflammation, ulceration and necrosis

Acrodynia: Redness, swelling, vesiculation and desquamation of palm, soles, fingers and toes with pink cheeks, nose, hands and feet **(pink disease)**

Mercuriolentis: Deposition of mercury in lens (brownish discoloration of eye) leading to restricted field of vision

Mercurial erethism, i.e. disturbed personality characterized by irritability, fatigability, lack of interest/concentration, insomnia, anxiety, loss of memory, delusions, hallucinations and tremors (**Hatter's shakes**/glass blower's shakes) affecting fingers, tongue, face, arms and legs

Kidney: Uremia, nephritis

Muscular weakness and paralysis of limbs and atrophy. Body **secretions**—greenish blue

Blood picture altered and presence of premature cells in peripheral blood. Contact dermatitis

---

Treatment

Prevent further exposure

Antidotes: BAL

General/oral hygiene

Treatment

Prevent further exposure

Antidotes: Penicillamine

General and oral hygiene

PM findings

Skin: Contact dermatitis, penetrating ulcers.

Gums: Blue line, inflammation, ulceration and necrosis

Signs of acrodynia, mercuriolentis

Degenerative changes in kidney/liver—necrosis

PM findings

Gums—blue lining and unhealthy

Blood pictured altered and presence of prematured cells

Liver/kidney—degenerative changes

Preservation of viscera

1. Routine viscera
2. **Additional viscera:** Bones, teeth, hair and nails are preserved

Preservation of viscera

1. Routine viscera
2. **Additional viscera:** Bones, teeth, hair and nails are preserved

---

Medicolegal aspects: Mercury

1. **Suicidal:** Rare—painful suffering
2. **Homicidal poisoning:** Rare—chemical test
3. **Accidental poisoning** is common and mainly due to:
   i. Excessive use of medicines (diuretics; mercury ointments)
   ii. Consumption of bleaching creams, or **snake-tablet** (mercuric thiocyanate) used in Diwali.
   iii. Consumption of food contaminated with preservative and sea fish
   iv. Chronic industrial or agricultural exposure
4. **Abortifacient:** Sometimes used for criminal abortion

Medicolegal aspects: Copper

1. **Suicidal:** Mostly but deaths are less due to vomited out of poison
2. **Homicidal poisoning:** Uncommon
3. Accidental poisoning may occur because
   i. Copper salts are used as fungicide
   ii. Also used to retain green color of vegetables
   iii. Contaminated food/drink stored in copper vessels
4. **Abortifacient:** Sometimes used to procure abortion
5. Cattle poison

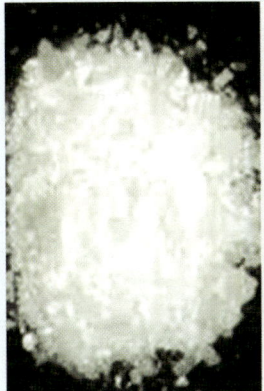
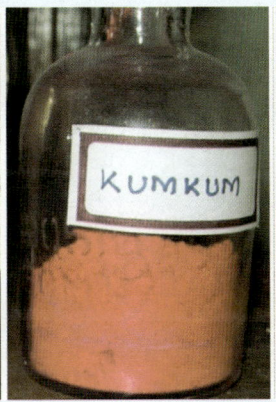
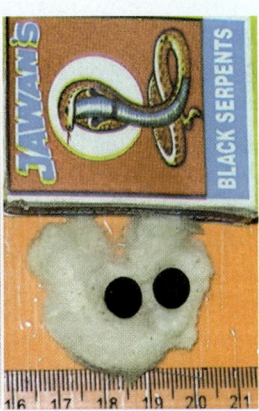
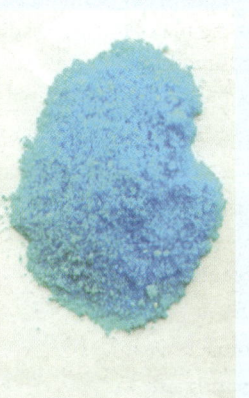

| Mercury chloride | Mercury sulfide | Mercury thiocyanate | Copper sulfate |

Chemical tests for metallic poisons

1. **Marsh's test**

   Test material is placed in a hydrogen generator. If the material contains arsenic, then arsine is formed which comes out through the narrow mouth of a generator and burns with a blue or greenish flame and gives garlicky smell. If the porcelain plate is at the top of the flame then greyish metallic arsenic is deposited, which is soluble in hypochlorite solution

2. **Reinsch's test: Test material (20 ml of stomach content) in test tube + 5 ml of conc HCl + clean copper foil.** Heat test tube (TT) for 5 minutes:

   - If the test material contains arsenic, mercuric or antimony, then there is greyish deposite on the surface of copper foil
   - Remove the foil and washed with water, alcohol and acetone to make it free from any other substance. The foil is then placed in a clean dry TT and heated in a slanting position
   - If the deposit over the copper coil is of arsenic, then on heating, there is formation of arsenic trioxide, which sublimated and deposited on the inner upper cooler surface of the TT as a white substance

3. **Gutzeit test: Test material in large test tube + pure zinc + 3 drops of dil HCl + potassium iodide** (to remove SO_2 and H_2S if formed). A plug of absorbent cotton wool is inserted in the upper part of TT and mouth of TT is covered with a filter paper moistened with concentrated solution of silver nitrate. If the test material contains:

   i. Arsenic, then filter paper turns yellow, which on addition with water turns black

   ii. Antimony, then filter paper turns brown or black

4. **Ammonia test for copper**

   Test material in TT + a few drop of $NH_4OH \rightarrow$ deep blue precipitate

Potassium toxicity (hyperkalemia)	Iron toxicity
Types: 1. Exogenous due to	**Poisoning is due to**
1. High dose of potassium therapy	1. Consumption of ferrous sulfate tablets
2. Poisoning with $KMnO_4$/potassium iodate	2. IV injection of iron preparation
Fatal dose: 12–15 gm Endogenous toxicity due to renal failure	**Fatal dose:** 10–15 tabs

Clinical features
  I. **When taken orally**
     Potassium iodate: Orally—GIT irritation. After absorption—causes liver, kidney, bladder and retinal damage
	Clinical features
	Same as arsenic poisoning with **diarrhea (offensive stool).** Scanty urine containing bilirubin, bile salts and urobilinogen
	Liver: Jaundice—centrilobular necrosis

Potassium permanganate: Orally—gastroenteritis, edema of glottis, respiratory distress
Intravaginally—gross ulceration and necrosis/perforation of vaginal wall

Blood: Increase iron bind with transferrin

II. Systemic: Tingling, numbness and weakness of limbs and fingers and toes with paralysis

III. ECG: Elevation of T-waves

Treatment	Treatment
Emesis	Emesis
Stomach wash	Stomach wash: $NaHCO_3$
Demulcent	**Demulcent**
Antidote: Calcium chloride/calcium gluconate (Dose = 1 gm IV)	Antidote: Desferrioxamine/EDTA/penicillamine
	Deferiprone—50–100 mg/kg orally daily in 2–4 divided dose
	Symptomatic: Dialysis, blood transfusion

PM findings

GIT—irritation

Visceral organs—congestion

PM findings

GIT—irritation

Pulmonary hemorrhage, petechial hemorrhage

Liver—centrilobular necrosis

Kidney—tubular necrosis

Medicolegal aspects

Suicidal: Rare

Homicidal: Not possible—high dose

Accidental: Mistaken with other

Abortifacient

Medicolegal aspects

Suicidal: Usually by females

Homicidal: Very rare

Accidental: Overdose, prolonged IV therapy

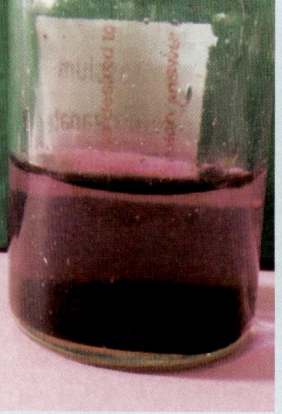

$KMnO_4$ powder and solution

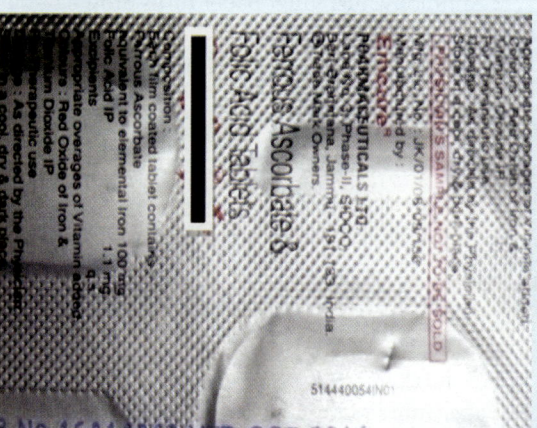

Ferrous tablet

Autopsy Photo of Metallic Poisons (Courtesy—Dr. Nitin Barmate)

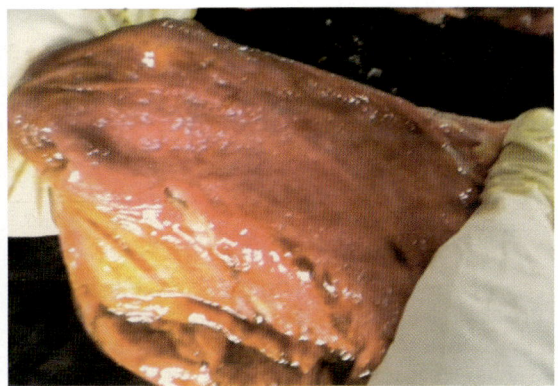

Fig. 6.1: Stomach in sindoor poisoning—mercury

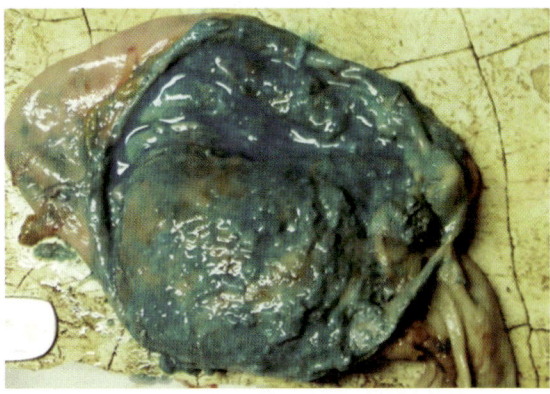

Fig. 6.2: Stomach in paint poisoning

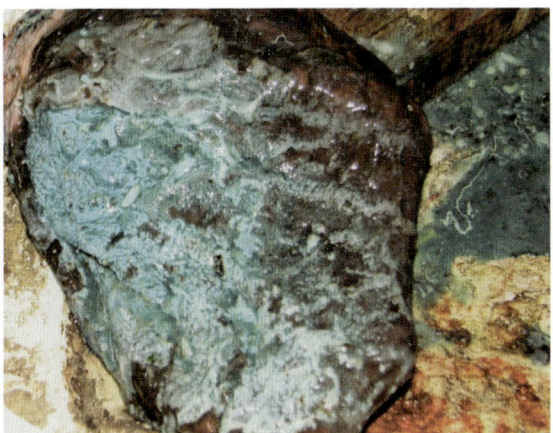

Fig. 6.3: Stomach in copper sulfate poisoning

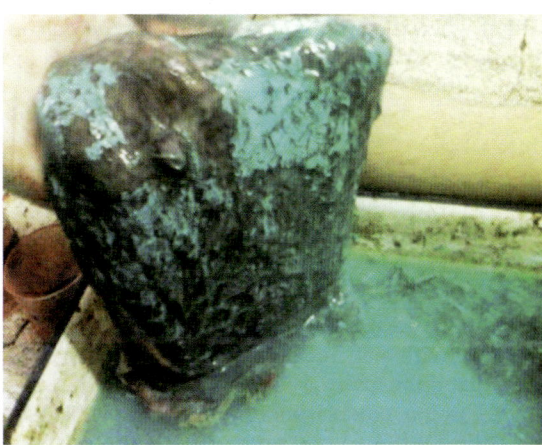

Fig. 6.4: Stomach in copper arsenite poisoning

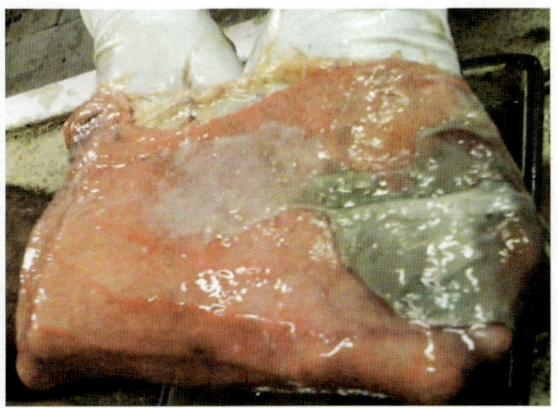

Fig. 6.5: Stomach in lead poisoning

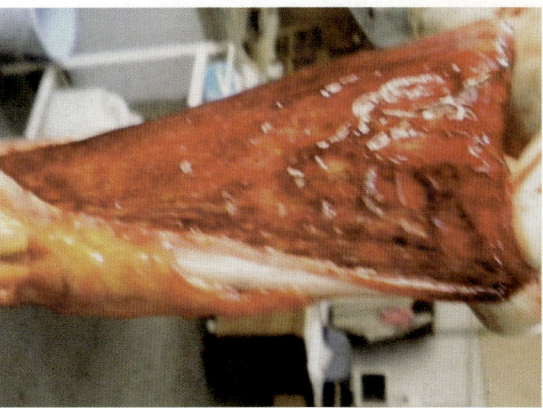

Fig. 6.6: Stomach in metallic poisoning

Agricultural Poison: Pesticides

7

Agricultural poisons are the organic irritant poisons that are used in the agricultural field. They are commonly called pesticides. Pesticides are compounds that are used to kill pests, which may be insects, rodents, fungi, nematodes, mites, ticks, molluscus, or unwanted weeds and herbs, which causes much harm to the production and storage of agricultural foods.

Pesticides are used as aerial spray mixed with suitable liquid or dust as their vehicle or mixed with soil. When sprayed in air, absorption in the plants occurs through leaves and stems. When mixed with soil, absorption occurs through the roots of the plant without causing any harm to the plants.

But when the insect sits on the plant, the poison acts as a contact poison and is absorbed through their exoskeleton or when the insect eats the leaves of the plant, it consumes the poison along with the leaves.

Classification of agricultural poisons				
Insecticidal	Herbicidal	Fungicidal	Rodenticidal	Others
Organophosphorus		Organochlorine	Carbamate	Pyrethroid

I. **Insecticides:** Compounds which kill insects and related species

Insecticidal poisons are classified into various groups and are mentioned in different tables along with their generic names and brand names

1. **Organophosphorus compounds**
   Malathion, monocrotophos (nuvacron), HETP, TEPP, OMPA, quinolphos, dimethoate, chlorothion, diazinon, phorate
2. **Organochlorine compounds**
   Endosulphan, chlordane, BHC, gammahexachloro-cyclohexane (lindane) DDT, methoxychlor. Toxaphen
3. **Carbamates:** Propoxur (baygon), carbaryl
4. **Pyrethrins and pyrethroids:** Allethrin, cypermethrin, dexamethrin

II. **Herbicides:** Compounds which kill weeds or herbs. Example: 12% sulfuric acid, potassium cyanide, sodium chlorate, sodium arsenite.
   • Acrolein, dalaphon, paraquat, diquat, atrazine, propazine, simazine, targa super (Quizolofeb), Glycel (Glyphosate)

III. **Fungicides:** Compounds which kill fungi and moulds. Example: Phenyl mercuric acetate, thiocarbamates, hexachlorobenzene, sodium azide—captan, captafol, bavistin, vitavax, Jatayu (Chlorothalonil), index (Mycobutanil), Dhanuka (Mancozeb), Benofit (Benomyl)

IV. **Rodenticides:** Compounds which kill rats, mice, moles and other rodents. Example:
   a. **Inorganic preparations:** Zinc phosphide, aluminium phosphide, arsenic, barium carbonate, phosphorus, thallium
   b. **Organic preparations:** Fluoroacetate
   c. **Convulsant:** Strychnine
   d. **Anticoagulants:** Warfarin
   e. **Others:** Vacor, alpha-naphthyl-thiourea, cholecalciferol, bromethalin, fluoroacetamide, sodium monofluoroacetamide, and red squill

V. **Others**
   a. **Nematicides:** Kill nematodes (i.e. worms)
      Example: Ethylene dibromide
   b. **Acaricides:** Kill mites, ticks, and spiders
      Example: Azobenzene, chlorobenzilate, tedion, and kelthane
   c. **Molluscicides:** Kill molluscous such as snails and slugs. **Example:** Metaldehyde
   d. **Flowering stimulants:**
      Example: Dinitrobenzene-Combi-flowers
   Miscellaneous pesticides: Compounds of lead, copper, and mercury, nicotine; hydrogen cyanide, methyl bromide, naphthalene, tetrachloroethylene, trichloroethane, dinitro-phenol, dinitrocresol, dinitrobutylphenol, pentachlorophenol, chlorfenson, and chloralose

Table 7.1: Agricultural poisons: Organophosphorus compound poisons

Group	Chemical name	Trade/market name of organophosphorus compounds	Clinical features	Treatment
Alkyl	1. Chlorfenvinphos 2. **Chlorpyriphos**	Birlane, Chlorfenvinphos Agrofas 20, Blase, Chlorofos 20, Chlorguard, Coroban 20, Durshban, Gilphos, Hyban 20, Pyriban, Ruban 20, Tafaban, Trishul 20 EC, Hilban-20, Sacban-20, Rickcare-50	**I. Parasympatho-mimetic** a. **Muscarinic:** **(SLUDGE**—Salivation, Lacrimation, Urination, Dyspnea, Gastro-intestinal distress—N, V, AP, D. Extramiosis sweating, bronchoconstriction) or **(DUMBELS**—diarrhea, urination, miosis, bronchospasm, emesis, lacrimation, salivation)	1. Remove patient from source of exposure 2. Remove all clothing 3. Thorough skin wash with soap and water 4. If ocular exposure has occurred, copious Eye irrigation with normal saline or Ringer's solution, or tap water 5. In case of ingestion, **stomach wash with** NS/KMnO$_4$ solution
	3. **Dimethoate**	Agrodimet 30, Cygon, Agromet 30 EC, Bangor 30 EC, Corothate, Cropgor 30, Cygon, Devigor, Dimethoate, Dimex, Entogor, Hexagor, Hygro 30, Rogor, Milgor, Paragor, Vikagor, Parrydimate, Ramgor, Rogar, Tagor, Vijaygor, Awant, Daksha, Dhawa		**6. IV atropine 2 mg/15 min (adult) and 0.05 mg/kg/15 min (children) till full atropinization**
	4. Indoxacarb 5. Malathion	Agromal, Cython, Finit, Kathion, Licel, Maladan, Malathion, Malazene, Sulmithion, Veg Fru, Malatox		7. IV PAM 1–2 gm in 100–150 ml 0.9% normal saline over 30 min (30 mg /kg), then every 6–12 hrs for 24–48 hrs
	6. **Monocrotophos**	Anacron, Azodrin, Biphos, Corophos, Entophos, Guardian, Hycrophos, Macrophos, Microphos, Monocil, Monolik, Monocron, Monokem, HICIL, Monophos, Nuvacron, Poryuphos, Shrimono, Totamonr, Yuromono	b. **Nicotinic** Fasciculation, weakness, hypertension, tachycardia and paralysis	8. Maintenance of airway and O$_2$ inhalation or artificial respiration
	7. **Quinolphos**	Agroquin, Agroquinol, Anuphos, Bayrusil, Ekalux, Flash, Hyquin, Kilex, Quinal, Quinguard, Shakti 25 EC, Solux, Vikalux, Dhanulux	**II. CNS: Depression** Headache, dizziness, restlessness, twitching of face and tongue, slurred speech, convulsions	9. IV fluids 10. Diazepam 5–10 mg IV slowly to control convulsions every 15 min (max dose—30 mg)
	8. Temephos/fox 9. Triazophos	Teme Guard, Abete, Farmicos, Abate 50 EC Hexban, Hexban 20 EC, Hostatnion, Kranti, Ninza, Sutathion, Tackle, Tricon, Trizer, Trizocel		**In children:** 0.2–0.5 mg/kg every 5 min to max 5–10 mg
	10. Others	HETP, TEPP, OMPA, Demeton, Trichlorfon, Isopestox		11. Antibiotics.
Aryl	1. **Diazinon** 2. Methyl parathion 3. **Parathion** 4. Others	Agroziron, Basudin, Bazanon, Ditaf, Suzinon, Zionosul 50 Dhanumar, Paradol, Paradol 2 DP, Folidol, Kilphos Paraoxon, Chlorothion,		
Others	1. Acephate	Acemil, Agrophate, Asataf, Hythane, Starthene,		

(Contd...)

Table 7.1: Agricultural poisons: Organophosphorus compound poisons (*Contd...*)

Group	Chemical name	Trade/market name of organophosphorus compounds	Clinical features	Treatment
2.	Ethion	Demite, Dhanunit, Ethion, Ethiosul 50, Force, Mit 50, Miticil, RP-thion, Tafethion, VegFru, Fosmite		12. Prevention of further exposure for a few weeks
3.	Fenitrothion	Accothion, Agrothion, Danathion, Fenicol, Fenitrosul 50, Folithion, Sumithion, Tik 20, Vikathion		13. Prophylaxis
4.	Fenthion	Agrocidin, Baytex, Fenthiosul, Lebaycid		
5.	Formothion	Anthio		
6.	Glyphosate	Weed off		
7.	Methyl Demeton	Hexasystox, Hymox, Knock out, Metasystox		
8.	Phenthoate	Agrofen, Delsan, Elsan, Guard, Phentox Dragnet, Fortan, Glorat, Luphate,		
9.	**Phorate**	Phoratox, Thimet, Volphor, Veg Fru Foratox, Umet, Starphor-10G		
10.	**Phosphamidon**	Agromidon 85, Bangdon 85, Cildon, Delphamidon, Dimecron, Directon, Entecron 85, Phamidon, Phosul, Sudon, Vimidon		
11.	Primiphos methyl	Acetellic		
12.	Thiometon	Agrothimeton, Ekatin		
13.	Trichlorphon	Dipterex		

Table 7.2: Agricultural poisons: Organochlorines compound poisons

Group	Chemical name	Trade/market name of organochlorines compounds	Clinical features	Treatment
1. Cyclodienes and related compounds	1. Aldrin	Agroaldrin, Alcrop, Alditon, Aldrex, Aldrin 30, Mildrin 30, Tarmahit 30, **Endrin**	1. **GIT:** Nausea, vomiting, hyperesthesia / paresthesia of mouth and face, diarrhea	1. Decontamination: (Same measures as described under organophosphate poisoning must be undertaken)
	2. Endosulphan	Agrosulfan, Endohit, Hildon, Hexosulfan, **Thiodan**	2. **CNS:** Headache, vertigo, myoclonus, rapid and dysrhythmic eye movements, mydriasis, weakness, agitation, confusion, and convulsions	2. Stomach wash
	3. Heptachlor	Agrochlor D5, Agrodono, Heptachlor, Heptaf 50, Heptar, Heptox		3. IV diazepam, phenytoin, or phenobarbital in usual doses to control convulsion
	4. Chlordane	VegFru Heptex, Agrodane 20 EC, Chlordane, Mitox 20 EC, Sudarshan 5 EC, Termex, VegFru Chlortox	3. **Other:** Fever, aspiration, pneumonitis, renal failure	4. **Cholestyramine** resin: 16 gm/day for several days mixed with fruit juice and given orally (4 gm, 6th hourly) before meals. It is a non-absorbable bile acid binding anion exchange resin and is effective in **enhancing the fecal excretion** of organo-chlorine compounds
2. Benzene Hexachloride compounds	1. BHC (Benzene hexachloride)	Agrobenz D10, Agro BHC, Gamazene, Gammexane, Haxaman, Hexidol, Hilblich 50WP, Kargo BHC, Premodol 10EC, Solchlor, Sudarshan, Sulbenz 50		5. Calcium gluconate
	2. Gamma-hexachloro-cyclohexane (lindane)	Agrodane, Bexarid, Emscab, Gab, Gamaric, Gamascab, Lindane 20, Lindex, Scarab, Linsuline, Lintaf, scabex, Scaboma, Rasayan lindane, Ultrascab, Standard lindane.		6. Cold sponging for hyperthermia
3. DDT and analogues	1. DDT (Dichloro-diphenyl-trichloroethane	DDT, Sudarshan 50, Didinex 25 EC, Ramdit		7. Airway maintenance
	2. Methoxychlor	Ranodit, Soltax, Suldit 50, Sunbrand, Tafarol, Tafidex		8. IV fluids
4. Toxaphene and related compounds	Toxaphene Dicofol	Kelthane		9. **Contraindication:** Do not give **adrenaline or atropine** unless absolutely necessary. Also do not give **oil based cathertics/ demulcent**
				10. **PAM does not play any role in organochlorides poisoning**

Table 7.3: Agricultural poisons: Carbamates and pyrethroids compound poisons

Chem constituents	Trade/market names	Clinical features	Treatment
Carbamates compounds			
1. Propoxur	Baygon, Protox bait.	Salivation, lacrimation, sweating, vomiting, diarrhea, slow pulse, low BP, weakness, twitching, convulsions. (S/s similar to OP compounds poisoning, but symptoms are less severe and of shorter duration)	1. Remove clothing and thorough skin wash with soap and water
2. Carbendazim	Bavistin, Carbistin 50, Glizim, Kilex, Carbendazim 50, Spot free, Zen		2. Stomach wash with NS/KMnO$_4$
3. Carbofuron	Agrofuron 3 G, Carbocil 3, Furadan 3 G, Hexafuran, VegFru, Diafuran		3. **IV atropine** 2 mg /15 min (adult) and 0.05 mg/kg/15 min till full atropinization
4. Methomyl	Lannate, Duonate		4. IV diazepam 5–10 mg slowly to control convulsions
5. Triallate	Avadex		5. Maintenance of airway and O$_2$ inhalation or artificial respiration
6. Carbaryl	Agrovin, Agroyl, Bangvin 30, Caravet, Hexavin, Kevin 50, Kilex Carbaryl, Sevin 50, Sujacarb, Sulfarl 50		6. IV fluids
7. Carbaryl + g BHC	Sevidol		7. Antibiotics
8. Aldicarb	Temik		8. **Inj. PAM is contraindicated in cases of poisoning with carbamate compounds**
9. Aminocarb	Metacil		
Pyrethrins and pyrethroids			
1. Allethrin	Baygon mats, Pynamin forte.	1. **Skin contact** Dermatitis, blistering	1. **Skin contact** Decontaminate with soap and water
2. D-allethrin	Baygon knock out aerosol, Baygon power mats, Good night mats, Hit insect repellant.	2. **Eye contact:** Irritation	2. **Eye contact** Irrigate with normal saline or water for 10–15 min.
3. **Cypermethrin**	Agrocyper, Basathrin, Bilsif, Challanger, Cilcord,Cybil, Cymbush, Cymet, Cymperm, Cyper, Cannon, Cyperguard, Cyperhit, Cyperin, Cypermethrin sandoz, Cypermil, Cypersul, Cyrux, Gilcyp Tech, Hilcyperin, Ustad, Hypowder, Hycper, Motal, Parathrin, Ralathin, Ramceper, Ripcord, Shakti, Sicerin,Vegfrucott, Starcyprin, Superkiller-25, Tackle	3. **Inhalation:** Increase nasal secretion, sneezing, coughing, dyspnea, sore throat, wheezing	3. **Systemic poisoning: stomach wash** with NS/KMnO$_4$ or activated charcoal
4. Decamethrin	Decamethrin	4. **Ingestion** Hypersecretion, nausea, vomiting, salivation, paresthesia, vertigo, fasciculation, hyperthermia, altered mental status, cramp, spasm, convulsions, pulmonary edema, coma	4. Oxygen and ventilator support
5. Deltamethrin	Decis, Hexit, K-Othrin		5. Bronchodilator for bronchospasm
6. Fenvalerate	Agrofen, Caovalerate, Fencidin, Fenhit, Fenkill, Fenval, Fighter, Gilfen, Parafen, Starfen, Sumicidin, Sumitox, Trumpcard.		6. Diazepam for convulsions
7. Fluvalinate	Marvik		7. **Do not give oil based cathertics/demulcent. Atropine is given only if needed for hyper-secretion and pulmonary edema**
8. Permethrin	Ambush, Lee, Permasect, Permethrin, Pounce		8. **Oximes (PAM): No role in T/t**
9. Pyrethrum	Tortoise mosquito coil		9. Adrenaline and antihistaminic for allergic reaction
10. Alpha methrin	Alpha guard, Farssa, Axis		10. **Mats and coils:** Wait and atch, symptomatic treatment

Organophosphates

Organophosphorus compounds are deadly toxic to human beings and also most effective as insecticidal agents. Hence, they are most popular and most widely used insecticides in India

They are broadly classified into two main groups:

a. Alkyl group—**chloropyriphos, dimethoate**, indoxacarb, malathion, **monocrotophos, quinolphos, temefox**, triazophos
b. Aryl group—parathion, methyl parathion, **diazinon, chlorothion**
c. Others—**phorate**, methyl demeton

Organochlorines

Organochlorine pesticides are one variety of chlorinated hydrocarbons. There are 4 distinct categories of these pesticides:

1. DDT and analogues—e.g. **DDT** (dichloro-diphenyltrichloroethane), and methoxychlor
2. Benzene hexachloride group—e.g. benzenehexachloride (**BHC**), and gamma-hexachloro-cyclohexane (**lindane**)
3. Cyclodienes and related compounds—e.g. aldrin, dieldrin, **endosulfan (thiodan), endrin**, isobenzan, chlordane, chlordecone (kepone), heptachlor, mirex (dechlorane)
4. Toxaphene compounds—e.g. toxaphene

Physical appearance

These compounds are available as dusts, granules, or liquids. Some products need to be diluted with water before use, and some are burnt to make smoke that kills insects. Kerosene and turpentine oil is used as a solvent

Physical appearance

These compounds are available as dusting powders, wet powders, emulsions, granules, and solutions. They are insoluble in water but soluble in kerosene and ethyl alcohol. DDT is a white crystalline, slightly volatile solid having a faint smell, highly soluble in benzene, chloroform; moderately soluble in kerosene and slightly in ethyl alcohol

Uses

Mainly used in agricultural field as insecticide.

Uses

1. Insecticide at home (also in gardens and in agricultural fields), used to kill bedbugs, mosquitoes, lice, flies, and fleas
2. Gamma benzene hexachloride is used in the treatment of scabies and head lice. It is available as topical ointment, cream, or lotion

Fatal dose

Highly toxic: Parathion/systox: 15 to 30 mg
Phosdrin/pestox: 200 mg
TEPP: 5 gm
Moderately toxic: Diazinon – 10 to 25 gm
Mildly toxic: Chlorthion, malathion, dipterex –25 to 60 gm

Fatal dose

DDT, lindane: 15 to 30 gm
Chlordane: 5–7 gm
Aldrin, dieldrin, endrin: 2 to 5 gm

Fatal period: 30 min to 3 hourss

Fatal period: Within 24 hours

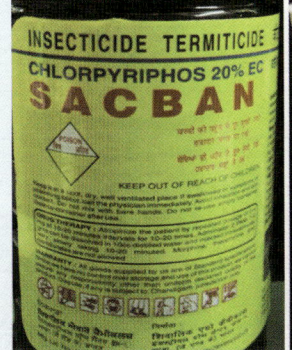
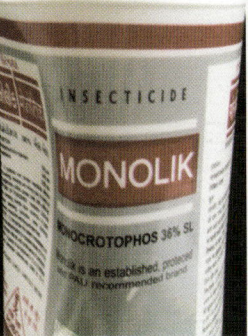
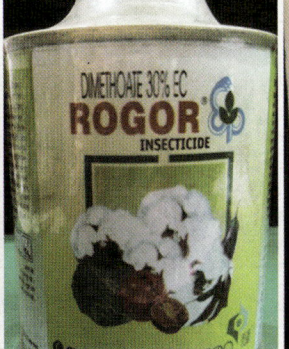
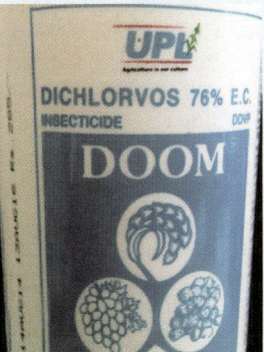

Absorption, fate, excretion: OP
Absorbed through mucosa of GIT, RT, and through skin and through direct injection

Parathion is first stored in the body fat and is slowly released in the circulation. It is metabolized first to paraoxon and then to paranitrophenol, which is excreted through urine

Malathion is metabolized in liver by esterase and is excreted through urine

Absorption, fate, excretion: OC
Absorbed transdermally, orally, and by inhalation. Dry powders (except dieldrin) are only poorly absorbed through GIT and are not absorbed through the skin. But when hydrocarbons are dissolved in kerosene and other solvents, they are all rapidly absorbed through skin and mucous membrane. Chlordane being liquid is absorbed through the skin too

Most of the hydrocarbons are metabolised slowly and deposited mainly in the body fat and also in liver, kidneys and brain for prolonged periods. They are excreted through urine, milk, and feces

Action
Organophosphates have action both on ANS as well as CNS
  1. On ANS, they **inhibit** the **acetylcholinesterase** enzyme by phosphorylation of serine moiety at myoneural junction and synapses of ganglion. As a result, there is **accumulation of acetylcholine** producing parasympatho-mimetic action. The action is both muscarinic (post-ganglionic) and nicotinic (pre-ganglionic)
  2. On CNS, the action is depression

Action
1. DDT and analogues affect the sodium channel and sodium conductance across the neuronal membrane especially of the axon
2. They also alter the metabolism of serotonin, norepinephrine, and acetylcholine
3. The cyclodienes and lindane appear to inhibit the GABA-mediated chloride channels in the CNS
4. CNS stimulant and death by overstimulation

Clinical features
Acute poisoning: Poisoning may occur through ingestion, inhalation, or absorption through skin.
  A. **ANS:** Parasympathomimetic action:
    1. Muscarinic effects—nausea, vomiting, diarrhea, abdominal colic, salivation, lacrimation **(increased tears which may be red due to porphyrin)**, profuse sweating, **Constriction of pupils,** bronchoconstriction (with increased bronchial secretion, wheezing and dyspnea, cough, pulmonary edema), garlicky smell in breath, muscle weakness, slow pulse, bradycardia, hypotension, and urinary incontinence (urination)*
    2. Nicotinic effects—fasciculation, weakness, hypertension, tachycardia, and paralysis.
  B. **CNS effects:** CNS depression
    Restlessness, headache, dizziness, drowsiness, delirium, tremor, twitching of face and tongue, slurred speech, ataxia, and convulsions

Clinical features
Acute poisoning
1. **GIT:** Nausea, vomiting, diarrhea, hyperesthesia or paresthesia of the mouth and face with peculiar smell
2. **CNS:** Confusion, headache, dizziness, vertigo, tremor, twitching, convulsion, myoclonus, rapid and dysrhythmic eye movements, **dilatation of pupils,** weakness, and agitation
3. **Other systems:** Fever, aspiration pneumonitis, renal failure

* Often summarized in the mnemonic (**DUMBELS**—**D**iarrhea, **U**rination, **M**iosis, **B**ronchospasm, **E**mesis, **L**acrimation, **S**alivation) or **SLUDGE**—**S**alivation, **L**acrimation, **U**rination, **D**yspnea, **G**IT distress (N, V, AP, D), **E**xtra-miosis, profuse sweating, muscle weakness, slow pulse, fall in HR and BP, and bronchoconstriction

Note: In the diagnosis of organophosphate poisoning, history and clinical manifestation plays an important role. Every effort should be made to extract information regarding name, type, or trade name of consumed poison from every possible source (patient, relatives, and friends).

Chronic poisoning: OP

It usually occurs as an occupational hazard in persons who are engaged in pesticide spraying of crops. Route of exposure is usually inhalation or contamination of skin

Following are the main features:

1. **Polyneuropathy:** Paresthesias, muscle cramps, weakness, gait disorders
2. **CNS effects:** Drowsiness, confusion, irritability, anxiety, psychiatric manifestations

Diagnosis

1. **Decrease in serum cholinesterase** level by 30% of the normal level
2. P-nitrophenol, a metabolite of OP compounds (e.g. parathion, ethion), is excreted in the urine
3. Thin layer chromatography (TLC)
4. Ancillary investigations

Treatment: *See* Table 7.1

PM findings

1. Characteristic odor (garlicky) near mouth
2. Frothing at mouth and nose—blood stained
3. Cyanosis of extremities
4. **Constricted pupils**
5. It resists decomposition and can be easily detected even in putrefied bodies
6. Stomach—garlicky or kerosene/turpentine like odor of solvent and content, mucosa-congested, hemorrhagic
7. Pulmonary and cerebral edema
8. Froth in the respiratory tract
9. Visceral organs are congested

Chronic poisoning: OC

It occurs due to long-term exposure to some of these compounds results in cumulative toxicity. There may be vague neurological symptoms and toxic rash in the skin

There may be irritability, fatigability, lack of interest and concentration, loss of weight/appetite, tremor, ataxia, abnormal mental changes, oligospermia

There is increased tendency to leukemias, thrombocytopenic purpura, aplastic, anemia, and liver cancer

Diagnosis

1. Abdominal X-ray may reveal the presence of certain radiopaque organochlorines
2. Organochlorines can be detected in serum, adipose tissue, and urine by gas chromatography

Treatment: *See* Table 7.2

PM findings

1. Characteristic odor near mouth
2. Discharge of blood stained froth from nose and mouth
3. Cyanosis and s/o asphyxia
4. **Dilatation of pupils**
5. Detected even in putrefied bodies
6. Stomach—chlorinated or kerosene/turpentine smell of solvent and content, mucosa-congested, hemorrhagic
7. Lungs—congested, edematous, subpleural hemorrhagic spots
8. Froth in the respiratory tract
9. Visceral organs are congested, brain—edema.
10. Liver, kidneys, adrenal—fatty degeneration

A useful postmortem finding in insecticidal poisoning case infested with flies at mortuary is that some of these flies after settling on decomposed body may subsequently die and found on the body

ML aspects

1. **Suicidal:** Common in India both rural and urban areas
2. **Homicidal:** Not occur due to detectable smell of solvent. However, a few cases have been reported
3. **Accidental:** Mainly to manufacturer, packers, sprayers in the fields, and also due to contaminated food grains

ML aspects

1. **Suicidal:** Common, more in rural areas
2. **Homicidal:** Very rare where the smell of kerosene is masked by alcohol
3. **Accidental:** Usually in children, and one who handle the poison

Mechanism of action in organophosphorus

$$\text{Acetylcholine} \xrightarrow[\text{enzyme}]{\text{Acetylcholinesterase}} \text{Acetic acid + choline}$$

OP → inactivates the Ach-esterase enzyme by the process of phosphorylation.

Thus, there is **decrease in the level of serum cholinesterase enzyme** and an **accumulation of acetylcholine at the nerve ending** resulting in the interference at the passage of nerve impulse across the myoneural junctions and synapses of the automatic ganglions

Diagnosis in OP compounds poisoning

1. Decrease in red cell and serum cholinesterase level: For the purpose of estimation of cholinesterase level, blood should be collected only in heparinized tubes. Alternatively, samples can be frozen

   a. If the RBC cholinesterase level is less than 50% of normal, it indicates organophosphate toxicity. However, a very low cholinesterase level does not always correlate with clinical illness. False decrease of RBC cholinesterase level is seen in pernicious anemia, hemoglobinopathies, anti-malarial treatment, and blood collected in oxalate tubes

   b. Decrease of plasma cholinesterase level less than 50% of normal is a less reliable indicator of organophosphate toxicity, but is easier to assay and more commonly done. Because it is a liver protein, plasma cholinesterase activity is depressed in cirrhosis, neoplasia, malnutrition, and infections

2. **Urinary P-nitrophenol test:** P-nitrophenol is a metabolite of some organophosphates (e.g. parathion, ethion), and is excreted in the urine

   Procedure: Steam distill 10 ml of urine and collect the distillate. Add sodium hydroxide (2 pellets) and heat on a water bath for 10 minutes. Production of yellow color indicates the presence of p-nitrophenol. The test can also be done on vomitus or stomach contents

3. Thin layer chromatography (TLC)

4. Ancillary investigations:

   a. Blood sugar level—increases

   b. Leukocytosis

   c. High hematocrit

   d. Anion gap acidosis

Treatment for organophosphates

a. **Atropine:** It blocks the muscarinic manifestations of organophosphates

   Dose: 1 to 2 mg IV or IM (adult); 0.05 mg/kg IV (child); every 15 minutes until the endpoint (atropinization) is reached, i.e. drying up of tracheobronchial secretions. Pupillary dilatation and tachycardia are not reliable indicators of the end point. After that the dose should be adjusted to maintain the effect for at least 24 hours

b. **Pralidoxime (pyridine-2-aldoxime methiodide; 2-PAM):** Pralidoxime competes for the phosphate moiety of the organophosphorus compound and releases it from the acetylcholinesterase enzyme, thereby liberating the cholinesterase

   Availability: 500 mg PAM tabs for oral use; inj PAM-A of 500 mg in 20 ml for IV use

   Dose: For adults—1 gm in 100 ml of normal saline, given IV for 30 minutes as a loading dose. This can be repeated after 1 hour, and followed by 500 mg TDS IV for next 1–2 days

   For children—20 to 40 mg/kg to a maximum of 1 gm/dose given IV, and repeated every 6 to 12 hours for 24 to 48 hours

c. **Prevention of further exposure:** Patient should not be re-exposed for at least a few weeks

d. **Prophylaxis:** Use protective clothes; spraying against direction of wind flow and move backward; No smoking, eating, drinking at workplace; spraying not >2 hr/day for >6 days/week; intermittent medical check up

Stomach in Insecticidal Poisoning (Courtesy—Dr. Barmate/Dr. Tumram)

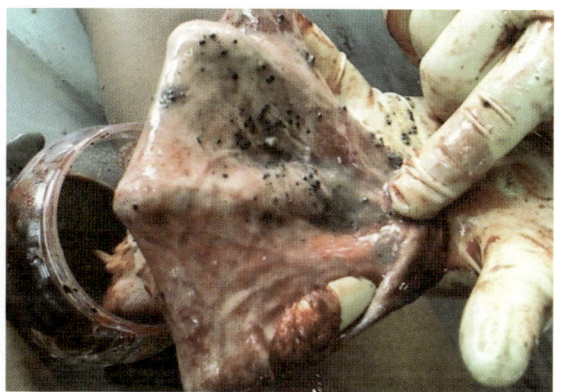

Fig. 7.1: Phorate poisoning (OP)

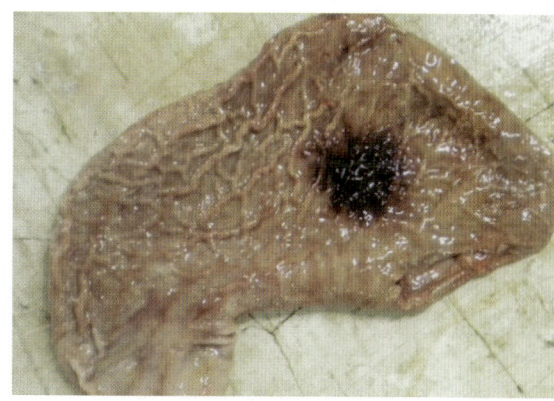

Fig. 7.4: Dimethoate-Rogar poisoning (OP)

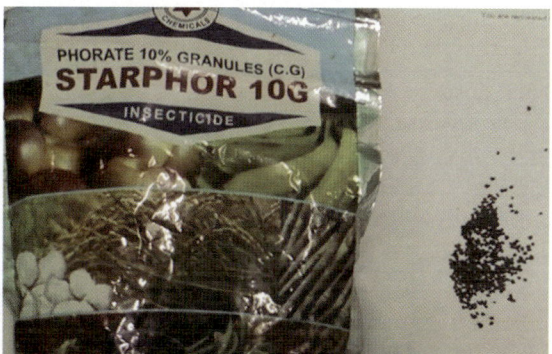

Fig. 7.2: Phorate granules

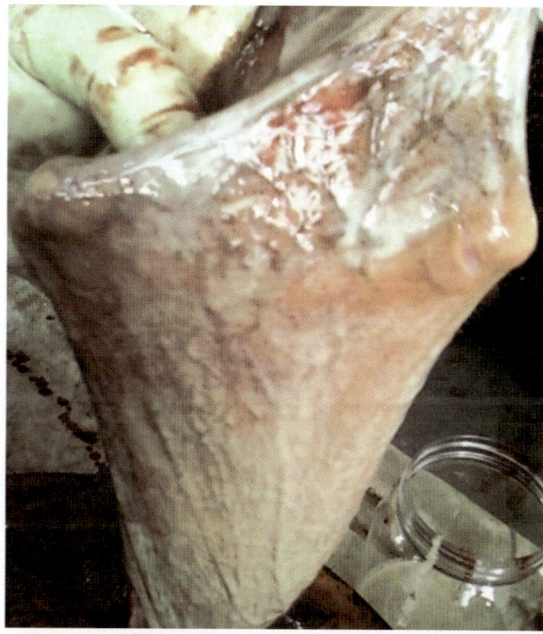

Fig. 7.5: Endrin poisoning (OC)

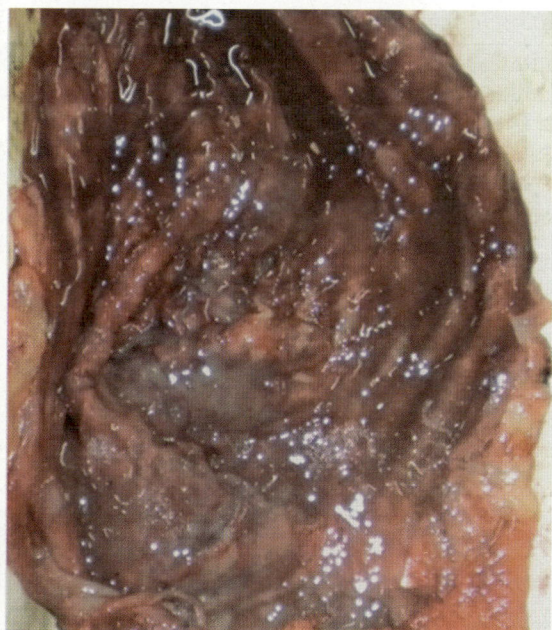

Fig. 7.3: Monocrotophos-Nuvacron poisoning (OP)

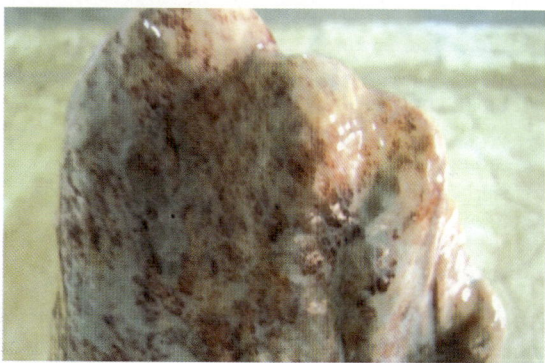

Fig. 7.6: Endosulphan-thoidane poisoning

Carbamates	*Pyrethrins and pyrethroids*
They are as popular as organophosphates in their role as insecticides and share a number of similarities include pyrethrum and piperonyl butoxide.	Pyrethrins are active extracts of the Chrysanthemum plant (*Chrysanthemum cinerariaefolium*), and Pyrethroids are synthetic analogues and number over 1000 varieties which are used as insecticides to incapacitate or "knock out" insects. Most mammals are resistant since they can rapidly metabolize and detoxify these agents.
Properties They are available as liquids, sprays, dusts and powders	**Properties** They are available as liquids, sprays, dusts, powders, mats, and coils
Uses Apart from insecticidal use, these are used to kill insect and ants in household spay	**Uses** These compounds are used as insect repellants and insecticides in household sprays, mosquito coils, and mats They are also used to prevent pest infestation in granaries, and in agriculture as pesticides
Fatal dose The following are extremely or highly toxic: Carbaryl, carbofuran, methomyl, propoxur. The following are moderately/slightly toxic: Aldicarb, carbendazim, triallate **Fatal period:** Uncertain	**Fatal dose** Pyrethrum has an LD50 of over 1 gm/kg. Most cases of toxicity are actually the result of allergic reactions **Fatal period:** Uncertain
Action Carbamates (like organophosphates) are inhibitors of acetylcholinesterase, but carbamylate the serine moiety at the active site instead of phosphorylation. This is a reversible type of binding and hence symptoms are less severe and of shorter duration	**Action** Like DDT, pyrethroids prolong the inactivation of the sodium channel by binding to it in the open state. Type II agents are more potent in this regard, and also act by inhibiting GABA-mediated inhibitory chloride channels
Clinical features The clinical manifestations of carbamate poisoning are very **similar to organophosphate poisoning.** Salivation, lacrimation, sweating, vomiting, diarrhea, slow pulse, low BP, weakness, twitching, convulsion	**Clinical features** 1. **Skin contact:** Dermatitis, blistering 2. **Eye contact:** Irritation 3. **Inhalation:** Rhinorrhoea, sore throat, wheezing, dyspnea 4. **Ingestion (large doses):** Paresthesias, nausea, vomiting, vertigo, fasciculation, hyperthermia, altered mental status, seizures, pulmonary edema, coma
Diagnosis 1. Blood cholinesterase **level is decreased** 2. X-ray may reveal the presence of certain radiopaque carbamates 3. Carbamates can be detected in serum, adipose tissue and urine by gas chromatography	**Diagnosis** 1. Blood cholinesterase **levels are normal** 2. ECG may demonstrate ST-T changes, sinus tachycardia, and ventricular premature beats 3. Thin layer chromatography

Structurally, pyrethroids are of 2 types

Type I pyrethroids do not contain a cyano group, e.g. permethrin

Type II pyrethroids contain a cyano group, e.g. deltamethrin, cypermethrin, fenpropathrin, fenvalerate

Table 7.4: Use of atropine and oximes in the treatment of different groups of insecticidal poisoning

Insecticidal groups	Atropine	Oximes
1. Organophosphorus	Antidote	Antidote
2. Organochlorines	Do not give	No role in treatment
3. Carbamates	Antidote	Contraindicated
4. Pyrethroids	Given only if needed	No role in treatment

Other Pesticides

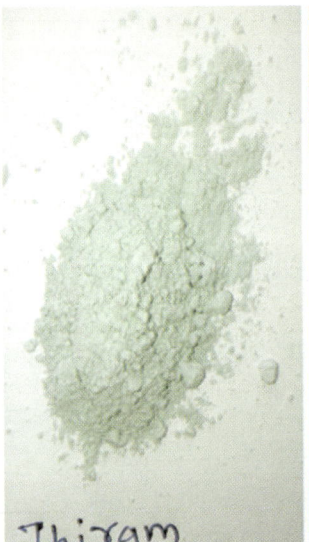

Fig. 7.16: Fungicidal (Devithiram)

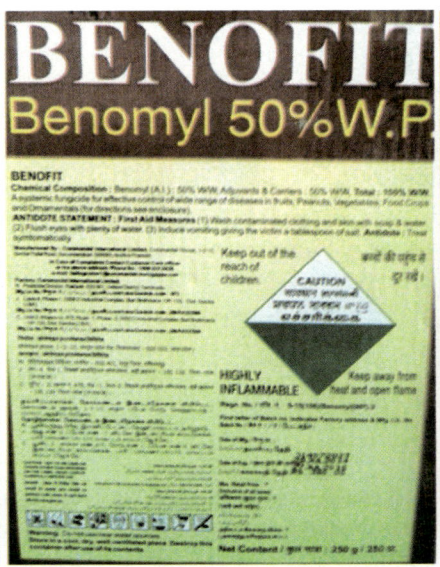

Fig. 7.17: Fungicidal (Benomyl)

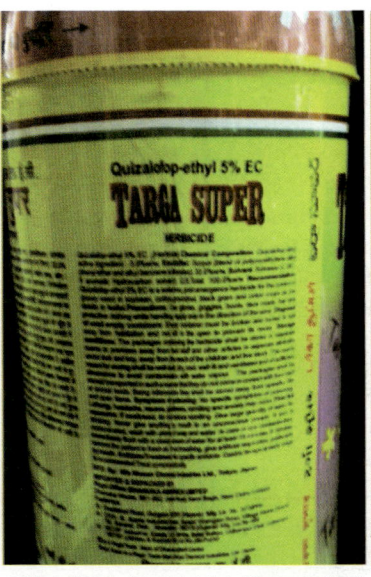

Fig. 7.18: Herbicidal (Quizolofeb)

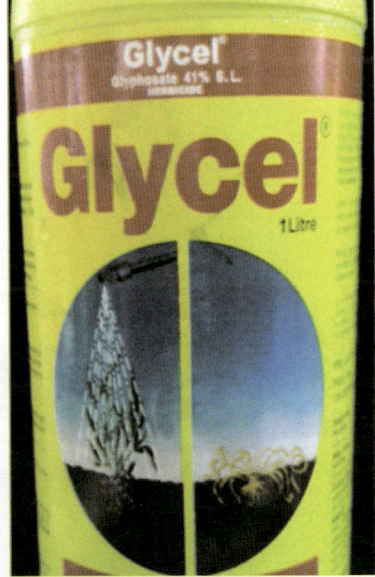

Fig. 7.19: Herbicidal (Glyphosphate)

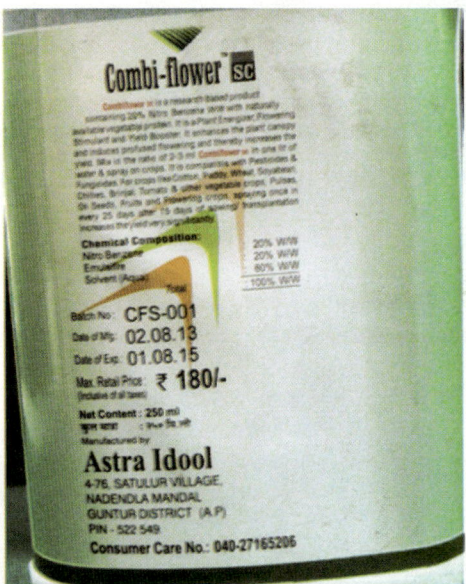

Fig. 7.20: Flowering stimulant (Nitrobenzene)

8

Vegetable Irritants

Vegetable irritants include *Abrus precatorius*, *Ricinus communis*, *Croton tiglium*, **Semicarpus anacardium**, **Calotropis**, *Plumbago rosea*, **Capsicum**, **Ergot, etc.** It does not include all poisons of vegetable origin like Datura, cannabis, strychnine, etc.

Toxalbumin is the toxic protein present in some of the vegetable irritants. The action resembles the action of bacterial toxin. Example: Ricin, Abrin, Crotin, Snake venom.

It is antigenic in nature and capable of producing specific antibodies when injected into the body. It causes agglutination, haemolysis and cell destruction.

Abrus precatorius	*Ricinus communis*	*Croton tiglium*
Synonyms: Rati, Gunj, Kunch, Crab eyes, Precatorius beans, Lucky beans	**Synonyms:** Castor, Arandi	**Synonyms:** Croton, Jamalgota
Toxic parts: Seeds. **Seeds:** Small beautiful, bright red, glossy, with black head, and weigh 102 mg	**Toxic parts:** Seeds. **Seeds:** Small/big (2 varieties) brownish oval glossy seeds with yellowish marking	**Toxic parts:** All part of plant (max. conc. in oil and seeds) **Seeds:** Small dark brown oval matt/dull dusty seeds
Uses 1. Decoration purpose 2. To weigh gold by goldsmith 3. Have hair promoting factor 4. Antifertility effects 5. Leaves used in paan masala	**Uses** 1. Purgatives 2. Ayurvedic medicine—for arthritis 3. Bland oil 4. Cream for sole crack	**Uses** 1. Strong purgatives 2. Ayurvedic medicine—for arthritis 3. For creating comedy scenes
Active principle: Abrin	**Active principle:** Ricin castor oil—nontoxic	**Active principle:** Crotin, crotonoside croton oil—highly toxic
Action **Local:** Irritation CVS depressant Viper bite like action	**Action** Local: Irritation CVS depressant Viper bite like action	**Action** **Local:** Irritation CVS depressant

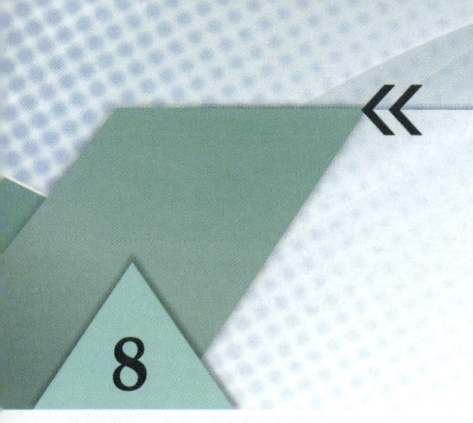

Abrus precatorius	*Ricinus communis*	*Croton tiglium*
Fatal dose: 1–2 seeds **Fatal period:** 12 hrs to 3 days	6–8 seeds 12 hrs to 3 days	6–8 seeds 12 hrs to 3 days

Clinical features
1. Local
  a. At the site of injection by *sui*—local severe reaction in the form of inflammation, edema, swelling, oozing, necrosis with evidence of hemolysis
  b. Conjunctivitis
	Clinical features
	1. Local
	  a. At the site of injection—local severe reaction in the form of inflammation, edema, swelling, oozing, necrosis with evidence of hemolysis
	  b. Conjunctivitis
		Clinical features
		1. Local: At the site of contact of oil to skin—erythema and blister formation
		
		–

2. Burning pain in mouth/throat, difficulty in speech and deglutition, increase salivation, abdominal pain, nausea, vomiting, diarrhea, dizziness, dyspnea, dilatation of pupil, flushing of face, cold calmy skin, rapid pulse, fall in BP, with muscular weakness, cramps, tremor, convulsion, collapse, coma		
Treatment 1. Local: Wash with soap water, application of bland ointment. 2. Stomach wash 3. Demulcent 4. Supportive 5. Antiabrin	**Treatment** 1. Local: Wash with soap water, application of bland ointment. 2. Stomach wash 3. Demulcent 4. Supportive	**Treatment** 1. Local: Wash with soap water, application of bland ointment. 2. Stomach wash 3. Demulcent 4. Supportive
PM findings Not specific 1. Local reaction with presence of spike/sui/sutari 2. GIT—inflamed, hemorrhagic, crushed seeds may be present 3. Organs—congested, petechial hemorrhage present	**PM findings** Not specific 1. Local reaction with presence of injection mark 2. GIT—inflamed, hemorrhagic, crushed seeds may be present 3. Organs—congested, petechial hemorrhage present	**PM findings** Not specific 1. Local reaction at the site of contact with oil 2. GIT—inflamed, hemorrhagic, crushed seeds may be present 3. Organs—congested, petechial hemorrhage present
ML aspects 1. Suicidal: Often used 2. Homicidal: Through parentral route using *sui*. 3. Accidental: Children are attracted towards the seeds 4. Abortifacient 5. Arrow poison 6. Cattle poison 7. Dust used to malingerers to produce conjunctivitis	**ML aspects** 1. Suicidal: In villages 2. Homicidal: Rare 3. Accidental: Usually in children 4. Abortifacient 5. Dust used to malingerers to produce conjunctivitis	**ML aspects** 1. Suicidal: Not common 2. Homicidal: Very rare 3. Accidental: Mistaken with castor oil 4. Abortifacient: Using oil, root 5. Arrow poison

Preparation of *sui* from *Abrus precatorius* seeds

It is prepared by crushing the seeds of Abrus along with datura seeds and chloral hydrate to make it in a powder form, from which paste is formed. *Sui* (needles) of size 1.5 cm × 1 cm is prepared from the paste. These *suis* are then dried and used to kill cattle by keeping it front of the bamboo stick used to push cattle and also used for homicide purpose by keeping it in between the finger and then slapped over cheek or other parts of body.

Semicarpus anacardium	Calotropis	*Plumbago rosea*
Synonyms Marking/dhobi nut, bhela, bhilwan, biba	**Synonyms:** Rui Gigantae—Akand: *Purple* flower Procera—Madar: *White* flower	**Synonyms** Lal chitra
Toxic parts All parts of plant (max. conc. in juice, seeds) Seeds: Black large heart shaped seeds.	**Toxic parts** All parts of plant (max. conc. in juice, stem, leaves) Seeds: Datura like seeds with cotton fibers at one point in the spindle/crescent shaped fruit having purple or white flowers	**Toxic parts** All parts of plant (max. conc. in root)
Uses 1. Abdominal pain 2. Ayurvedic medicines 3. Marking over clothes (brownish oily juice yields from the pericarp of seeds turns black on exposure to air, so used to inscribe identification number over clothes)	**Uses** 1. Depilatory agent 2. Ayurvedic medicines—by quack 3. Keeps snakes away from area. 4. Flower used for worshipping god (lord Hanuman/Shiva)	**Use** Ayurvedic medicines—quack
Active principle Semicarpol, Bhilawanol	**Active principle** Calotropin, calotoxin uscharin, gigantin	**Active principle** Plumbagin
Action Local: Irritation CVS depressant	**Action** Local: Irritation CVS depressant	**Action** Local: Irritation CVS depressant
Fatal dose: 6–8 seeds **Fatal period:** 12 hrs to 3 day	**Fatal dose:** Uncertain **Fatal period:** 12 hrs to 3 days	**Fatal dose:** Uncertain **Fatal period:** 12 hrs to 3 days
Clinical features 1. Local: Contact of juice to skin— bruise like painful lesion with marginal small blister called **"Branding"**, the lesion may itch and may ulcerate	**Clinical features** 1. Local: Contact of juice to skin—irritation of skin with blister formation which excoriates later	**Clinical features** 1. Local: Contact of juice to skin-irritation of skin with blister formation which excoriates later

2. Burning pain in mouth/throat, difficulty in speech and deglutition, increase salivation, Abdominal pain, nausea, vomiting, diarrhea, dizziness, dyspnea, dilatation of pupil, flushing of face, cold calmy skin, rapid pulse, fall in BP, with muscular weakness, cramps, tremor, convulsion, collapse, coma

Treatment 1. Local: Wash with soap water, application of bland ointment 2. Stomach wash 3. Demulcent 4. Supportive	**Treatment** 1. Local: Wash with soap water, application of bland ointment 2. Stomach wash 3. Demulcent 4. Supportive	**Treatment** 1. Local: Wash with soap water, application of bland ointment 2. Stomach wash 3. Demulcent 4. Supportive
PM findings: Not specific 1. Local reaction 2. GIT—inflamed, hemorrhagic, crushed seeds may be present	**PM findings:** Not specific 1. Local reaction 2. GIT—inflamed, hemorrhagic, crushed leaves/stem may be present	**PM findings:** Not specific 1. Local reaction 2. GIT—inflamed, hemorrhagic, crushed root may be present

3. Organs—congested, petechial hemorrhage present

3. Organs—congested, petechial hemorrhage present

3. Organs—congested, petechial hemorrhage present

ML aspects
1. Suicidal: Rare
2. Homicidal: Rare
3. Accidental: By mistake, quack medicine
4. Abortifacient
5. Arrow poison—not used
6. Cattle poison—not used
7. False charge: Juice split on the body to cause injury and make a false charge of assault against enemy

ML aspects
1. Suicidal: Rare
2. Homicidal: Rare
3. Accidental: By mistake, quack medicine
4. Abortifacient: By juice
5. Arrow poison—used
6. Cattle poison—used
7. False charge: Juice split on the body to cause injury and make a false charge of assault against enemy

ML aspects
1. Suicidal: Rare
2. Homicidal: Rare
3. Accidental: By mistake, quack medicine
4. Abortifacient
5. Arrow poison—not used
6. Cattle poison—used
7. False charge: Juice split on the body to cause injury and make a false charge of assault against enemy

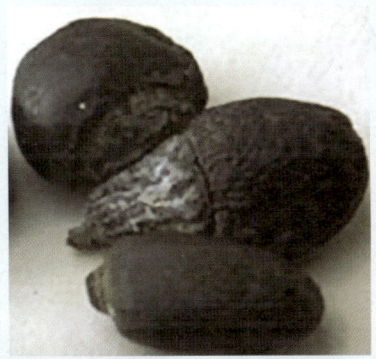

Seeds of semicarpus

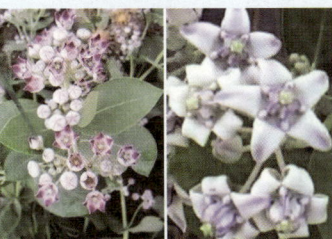

C. gigantae   C. procera

Flowers of calotropis

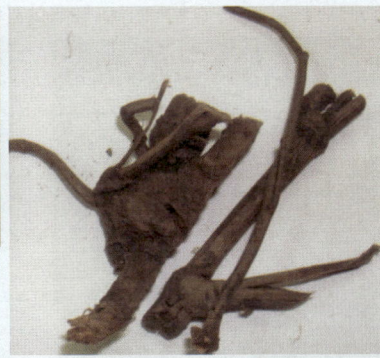

Roots of plumbago

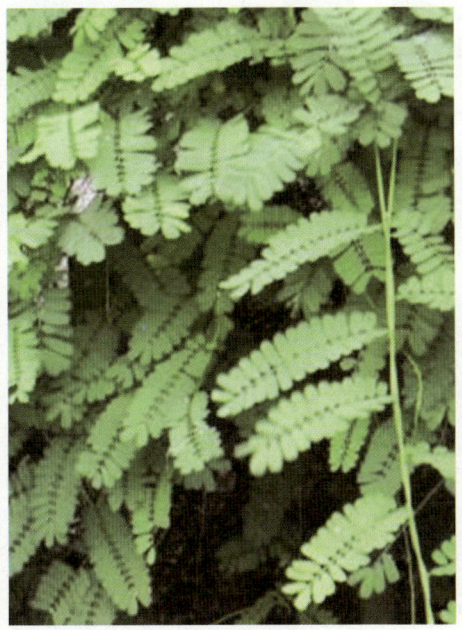

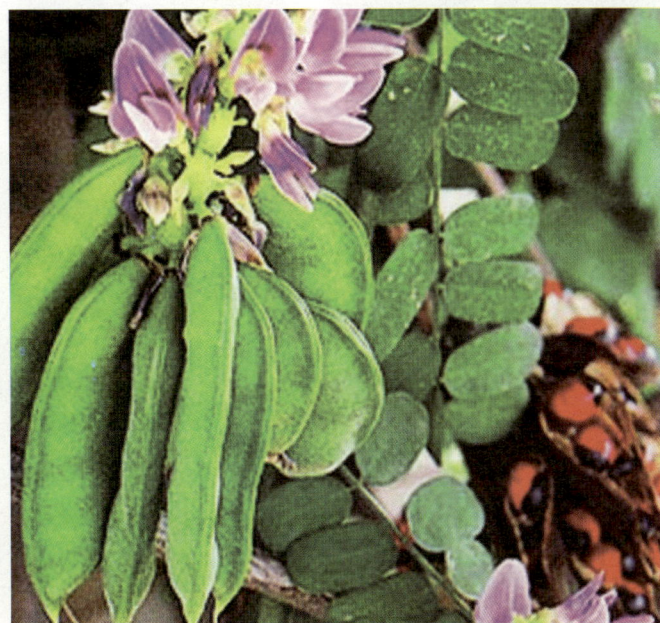

Fig. 8.1: *Abrus precatorius*

Fig. 8.2: Beans of abrus with seeds

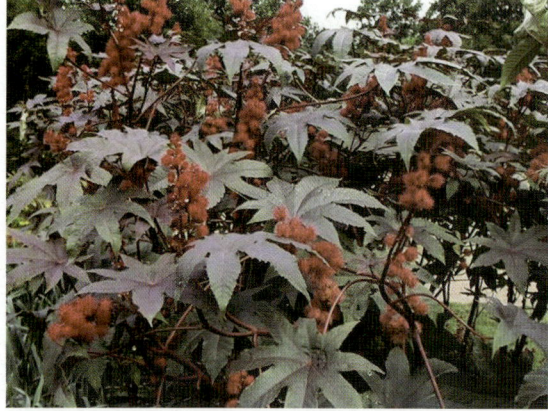

Fig. 8.3: Ricinus

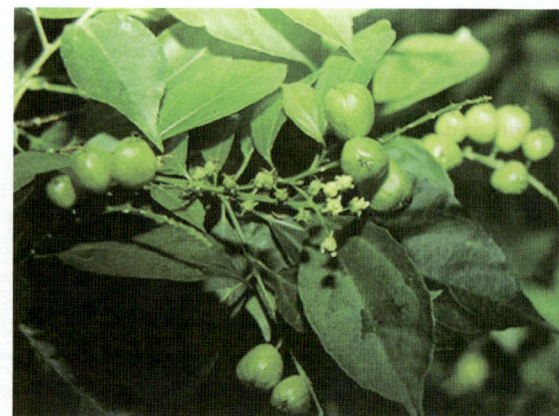

Fig. 8.4: *Croton tiglium*

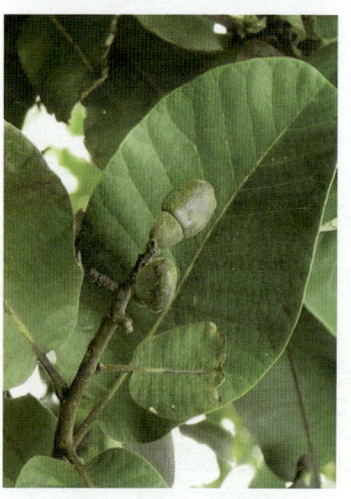

Fig. 8.5: Semicarpus

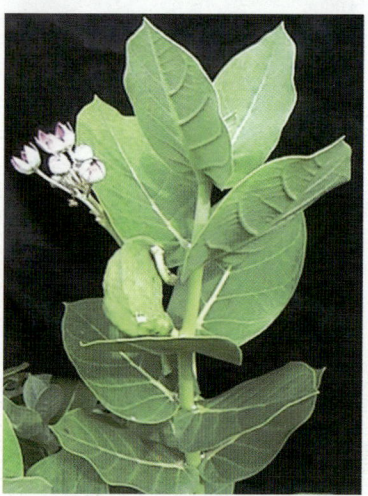

Fig. 8.6: Calotropis

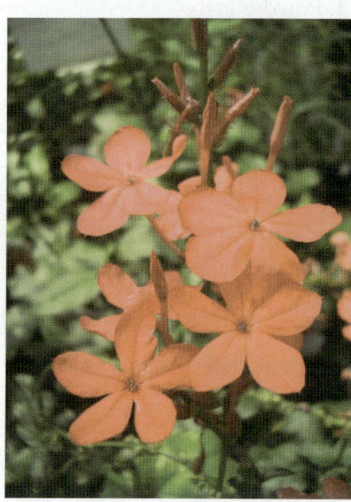

Fig. 8.7: Plumbago

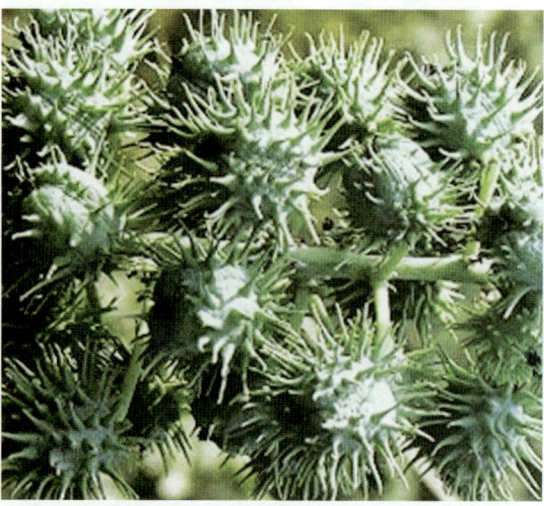

Fig. 8.8: Fruit of ricinus (castor fruit)

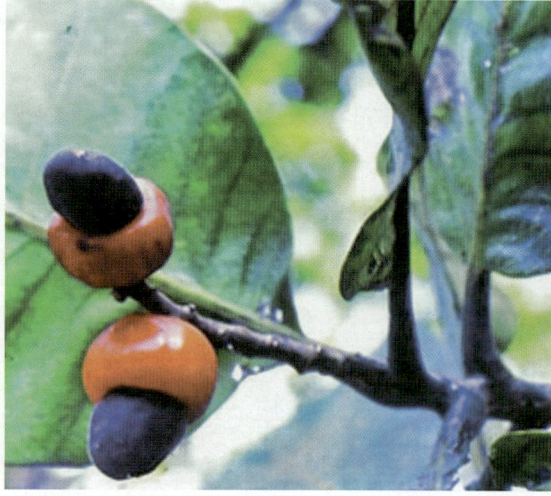

Fig. 8.9: Fruit of semicarpus

Capsicum annum (chilli)

Active principle: Capsicin, capsaicin fruit, seeds and dust causes irritation

Signs and symptoms

Burning, irritation, redness and swelling of mouth/throat, increase salivation, increase perspiration, watering from eyes and nose, abdominal pain, burning sensation during defecation

Death is unusual except in neonates.

Treatment

When swallowed—curd, bulky food and demulcent. Applied to skin/eyes—wash with water, xylocaine ointment

Medicolegal aspects

1. Powder is thrown in the eyes either to snatch money/ articles or to escape arrest after crime
2. It is used to kill unwanted newborn baby
3. It is applied in eyes/nose/anus/vagina/ or injury to extract confession
4. It is applied in the vagina for giving punishment for infidelity
5. **Hyderabadi goli:** It is the paste of chilli powder used to push in the rectum for torture and confession

Ergot (ergotism)

It is present in the dried sclerotium of fungus *Claviceps purpurae*

Active principle

Ergotoxin, ergotamine, ergometrine

Uses

1. It is used as oxytocic agent
2. It also causes vasoconstriction

Fatal dose: 10 gm/10–12 ml

Fatal period: A few days

Acute manifestation: It causes vasocon striction, leads to raised BP and causes dizziness, dimness of vision, vertigo, etc.

- It also causes contraction of smooth muscle
- Respiratory disturbances
- GIT—nausea, vomiting, diarrhea

Chronic manifestation

a. **Convulsive type:** Tingling, numbness, twitching, pain in muscle, cramps, tremors, convulsion
b. **Gangrenous type:** Burning pain in the limbs, inflammation and swelling with alternate heat and cold sensation

Treatment of Ergot Poisoning

- Nitrate for vasoconstriction.
- Gastric lavage with activated charcoal.
- Diazepam/pentobarbital for convulsion.
- Nifedipine, captopril—peripheral ischemia.
- Heparin/dextran for hypercoagulable state.

Medicolegal Aspect of Ergotism

1. **Accidental:** Due to consumption of contaminated food with fungus or when used for prolonged period of time or while use in the treatment of migraine and uterine hemorrhage.

2. Abortifacient.

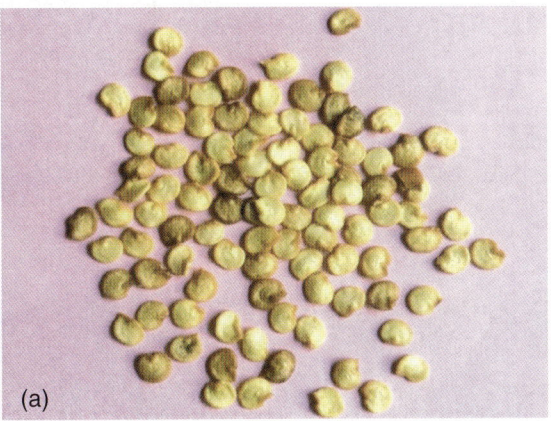
(a)

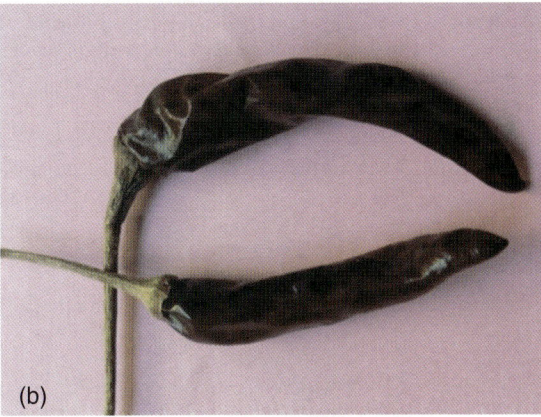
(b)

Figs 8.10a and b: Chilli seeds and fruit

Table 8.1: Other vegetable irritants

Name	1. Aloe	2. Anacardium occidentale	3. Argemone mexicana	4. Chrysanthemum cinerariaefolium
Synonyms:	Aloe vera, Ghritakumari, Gheekumar, Kumarpathu	Cashewnut	Argimone oil	Pyrethrum
General:	Bitter taste	Bitter taste. Active principle present in the pericarp of the fruit	All part poisonous, but maximum concentration is in seeds	Active principle present in the flowers, acrid bitter taste
Active principle:	Dried juice contains glycoside and barbaloin	Cardol	Berberine, protopine, sangunarine	Pyrethrin I and I, Cinerin I and II
Clinical feature:	Abdominal pain, vomiting, diarrhea, inflammation of kidneys increases intestinal movement and causes congestion of pelvic organs	Contact dermatitis with redness and urticaria-like lesion	Consumption of contaminated edible oil with argemone oil causes circulatory collapse, abortion and **epidemic dropsy** and generalize neuropathy	Acrid bitter taste, numbness of tongue/mouth, with nausea, vomiting, diarrhea, headache, restlessness, tremor, muscle weakness and respiratory failure. **Chronic exposure:** person gets sensitizes and there are different allergic manifestation
Treatment:	Symptomatic.	Wash the part with soap water. Symptomatic	Stop consumption of adulterated/contaminated oil. Symptomatic, nursing care and physiotherapy for epidemic dropsy	Prevention of exposure. Symptomatic. Artificial espiration and oxygen inhalation
PM findings:	Nonspecific	Nonspecific	Nonspecific	Nonspecific
ML aspect:	**Abortifacient:** Procure abortion—quackery use	Accidental to workers who collect and process the fruit for extraction of nuts **Abortifacient:** Quack	**Accidental** Contaminated or adulterated edible oil	**Accidental:** Exposure and inhalation of pollen grain leading to allergic reaction. Suicidal—unusual. Homicidal—unusual

	5. Eucalyptus globulus	6. Cytrullus colocynthis	7. Pinus palustris	8. Narcissus
Synonyms:	Nilgiri oil	Bitter apple, colocynth, makal, indrayan, pava, mekka, kayi	Turpentine	Daffodil
General:	Active principle present in the leaves of plant	Active principle present in the fruits of plant	–	Active principle present in the bulb of plant
Active principle:	Cinehole—a volatile oil in stem and leaves	Colocynthin	d and l-pinene	Lycorine
Clinical feature:	Dyspnea, cyanosis, excitement, ataxia, convulsion. Death due to circulatory collapse	Abdominal pain, diarrhea (blood tinged), increase body temperature, circulatory collapse	Abdominal pain, vomiting, diarrhea. When inhaled—RT irritant. Excitement, confusion, coma, oliguria, hematuria	Abdominal pain, nausea, vomiting, tetanic convulsion
Treatment:	Symptomatic. Artificial respiration and oxygen inhalation. Maintenance of circulation	Symptomatic	Stomach wash. Symptomatic	Stomach wash. Symptomatic

(Contd...)

Table 8.1: Other vegetable irritants *(Contd...)*

Name	5. Eucalyptus globulus	6. Cytrullus colocynthis	7. Pinus palustris	8. Narcissus
PM findings:	Nonspecific	Nonspecific GIT—irritation Kidneys— inflammation Organs—congested	Nonspecific	Nonspecific
ML aspect:	**Accidental:** Consumption of oil by mistake **Suicidal:** Uncommon **Homicidal:** Not possible due to the smell	**Accidental:** By mistake. Abortifacient	**Accidental:** By mistake **Suicidal:** Occasionally	**Accidental:** By mistake **Suicidal:** May be used

Table 8.2: Other vegetable irritants

Name	Synonyms	Active principle	Clinical features
1. Mangifera Indica	Mango	Resinous exudate	Irritation, contact dermatitis
2. Nephrolipis Rosaltata	Fern	Filicin	–
3. Poison Oak	Sumac	–	Skin irritation causes rash and dermatitis
4. Aristolocia Indica	–	Aristolocin	Contact dermatitis, respiratory paralysis, hemorrhagic nephritis, GIT irritation
5. Rhus Toxicodendron	Poison Ivy	3-pentadecyl-catechol	contact dermatitis
6. Indian Wintergreen	(Jav)	Methyl salicylate	–
7. Pherulanarthex	(Asafoetida, hing)	–	Digestive stimulant, psychogenic and neurogenic action
8. Eugenia Caryophyllus	(Cloves, lavang)	Tannin, caryophyllin	–
9. Colchicum Leutium	(Hirah tutigu)	Colchicine	–

Animal Irritants

Animal irritants includes snakes, scorpions, bees, wasps, cantharides, spider, etc. which causes venomous bite or stings.

SNAKES (OPHIDIA)

Snakes belongs to class reptilia, order squamata and suborder serpentes. Snakes are found all over the world except in Greenland, Ireland and New Zealand. In the world, there are about 2500 species of snakes, 500 are poisonous to humans. In India, there are about 250 species out of which about 50 species are poisonous. The common poisonous snakes in India are Cobra, Krait, Russell's viper, Saw-scaled viper and Sea snakes. Deaths due to snakebites are mainly accidental in nature.

GENERAL CHARACTERISTICS

1. Snakes have an elongated body and a short tail that is the part behind vent, and has no limbs. Vent is an opening in the rear part of the body for intestine and genitourinary system.
2. The body is covered with scales.
3. On the head, there are 2 eyes, 2 nostrils, but no external ear.
4. Tongue is forked and serves as a sense organ.
5. They are cold blooded creatures with carnivorous habits. They use sharp teeth and strong muscles to catch the prey. The mouth is easily distensible allowing it to swallow even large animals as a whole.
6. Teeth are thin, directed backwards and the upper marginal teeth are modified and are known as fangs. Fangs can be replaced in 3–6 weeks when broken. The fangs are solid in non-poisonous and grooved/canalized in poisonous snakes for transport of venom from the poison glands, i.e. modified parotid salivary glands, to which they are connected through ducts.
7. In poisonous snakes, parotid glands are situated below and behind the eyes, one on each side secreting toxic saliva and acts as poison glands. Fangs of elapids/sea snakes are short, fixed and grooved, and that of vipers are long, movable and canalized.
8. During the process of bite, the glands are pressed and venom is squeezed and channeled through the grooves or canal of the fangs.
9. Some are viviparous (gives birth to young ones in vipers) and some are oviparous (lays eggs, e.g. cobra, pythons, water snakes).

Snakes are classified as

1. Poisonous
2. Nonpoisonous

Classification of Poisonous Snakes
On the Basis of their Families

1. Colubridae: African boomslang, twig snake
2. Elapidae: Cobra and krait (commonly called elapids)
3. Hydrophidae: Sea snakes.

4. Viperidae: Vipers

5. Alractaspididae: Mole vipers or adders.

On the Basis of Venom

1. Elapids—neurotoxic—fangs are 4–6 mm.
2. Vipers—vasculotoxic—fangs are 12–15 mm.
3. Sea snakes—myotoxic—fangs are 2–4 mm.

Venomous snakes: There are about 52 species of venomous snakes in India, of which 4 are important. These are Cobra, Krait, Viper and Sea snakes. Each of these snakes is easily distinguishable, though it is easy to confuse with other non-poisonous snakes.

Common Poisonous Snakes in India

1. Cobra: King/common cobra
2. Krait: Common/banded
3. Viper: Pit/Russell's/Saw-scaled
4. Sea snakes: Banded sea snakes, amphibian sea snakes

Common Non-poisonous Snakes in India

1. Rat snake (Dhaman)
2. Vine snake
3. Bronze back tree snake
4. Banded kukri
5. Sand boa

The non-poisonous snakes, which may resemble poisonous snake are as follows:

Non-poisonous snakes	Poisonous snakes
Rat snake	Common cobra
Common cat	Saw scaled viper
Banded kukri	Banded krait
Sand boa	Russell's viper
Commom wolf	Common krait

Difference Between Poisonous and Non-poisonous Snakes

Table 9.1 shows the differentiating features. *However, there are a few exceptions*

a. **In pit viper, there is a greenish pit between eye and nostril.**

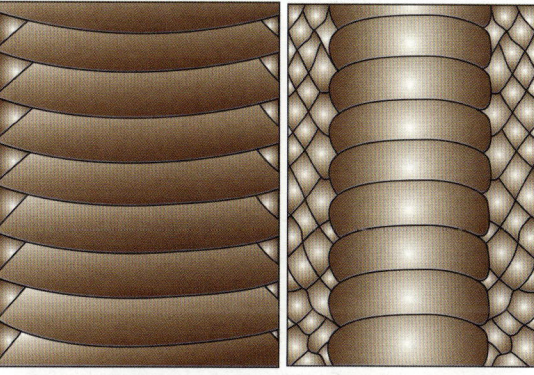

Poisonous   Non-poisonous

Fig. 9.1: Belly scales

Table 9.1: Differences between poisonous and non-poisonous snakes

Features		Poisonous snakes	Non-poisonous snakes
1. Belly scales:	**Size**	Large	Small
	Distribution	Cover entire breadth	Never cover entire breadth
2. Head:	**Size**	Usually small (pit, cobra, krait)	Usually large
	Scales	Usually small except cobras	Usually large
3. Teeth		At least one pair of teeth in upper jaw is modified to form fangs	All teeth are uniformly small, attached to short maxillary bone
4. Fangs		Present and canalized/grooved	Absent
5. Tails		Abruptly tapering tail, rounded	Gradually tapering long tail
6. Habits		Usually nocturnal	May be nocturnal or diurnal
7. Physical features		Stout, dull colour	Slender, bright-coloured
8. Bite marks		Usually two fang marks present	Semicircular set of teeth mark present

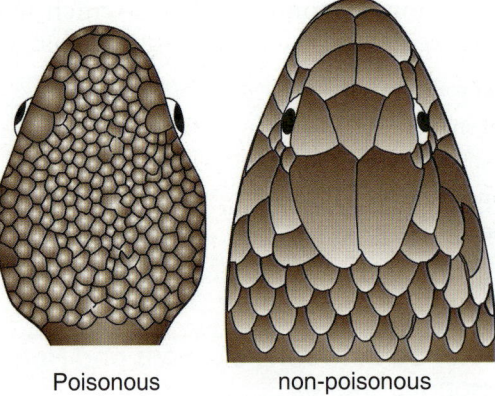

Poisonous   non-poisonous

Fig. 9.2: Head scales

b. In cobra and King-cobra, the third labial is large and touches the eye.

c. In krait, the central row of scales on the back is large, and the 4th infralabial is very large.

Features of Poisonous Snakes in India
(Tables 9.3 and 9.4)

1. **Cobra:** It is usually black, 5–6 feet, has a hood on dorsal side on which there is a single or double spectacle mark or an oval spot surrounded by half circle. **It prefers populated areas.** The third supralabial is big.

2. **King-cobra:** It is 6–18 feet, has a hood without any mark on hood, **prefers forests.**

3. **Common krait:** It is usually steel-black, 3–5 feet. **It prefers area in or near the houses.** The head shields are large, there are four infralabial shields and scales in central row on back are large and hexagonal.

4. **Banded krait:** It is 5–7 feet and has alternate black and yellow bands on the body.

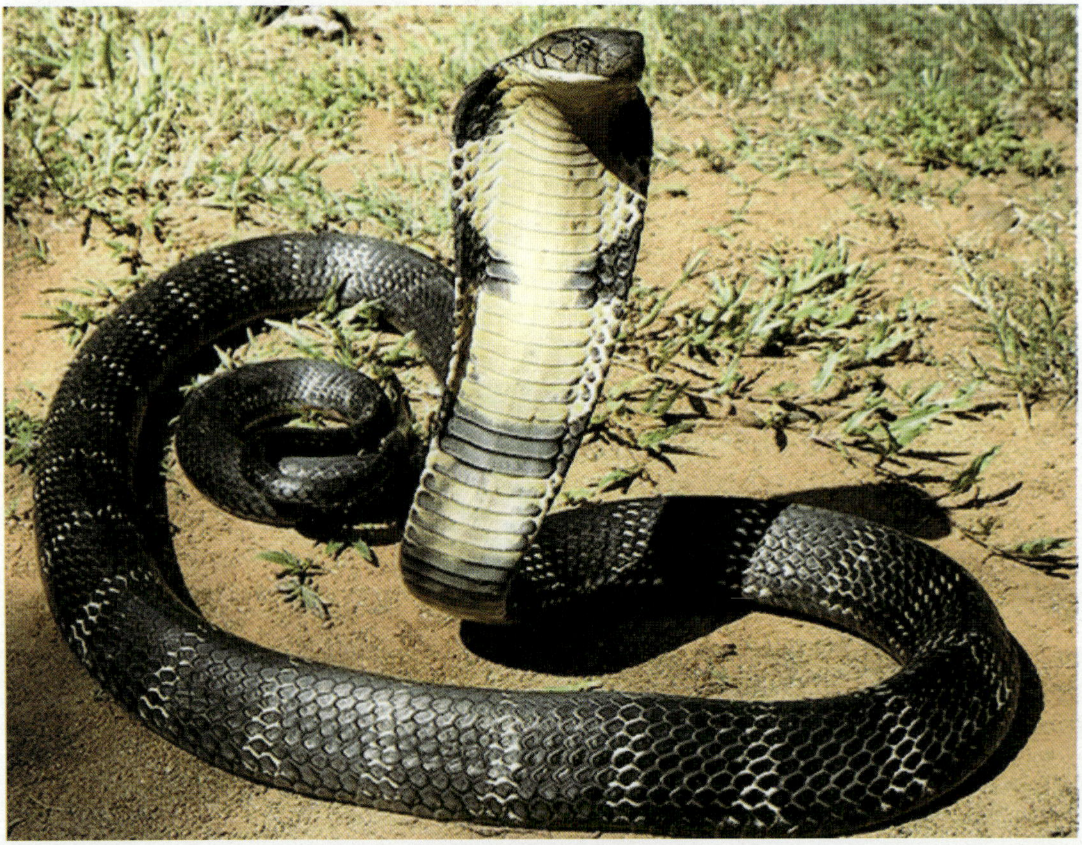

Fig. 9.3: King-cobra without spectacle mark

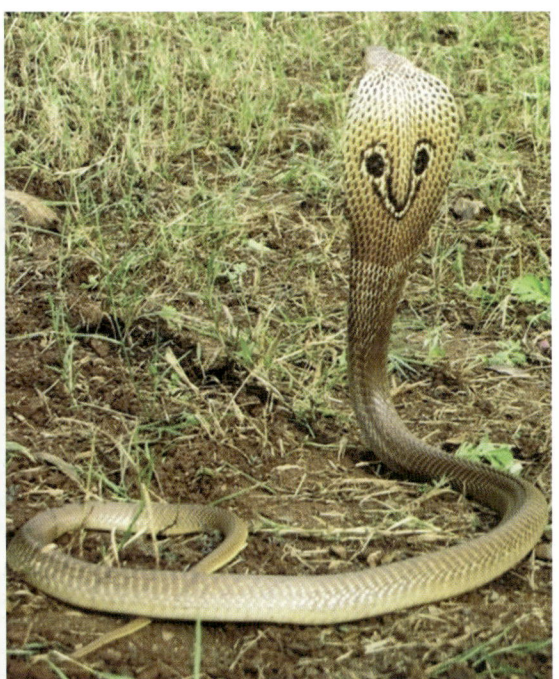

Fig. 9.4: Common cobra with spectacle mark

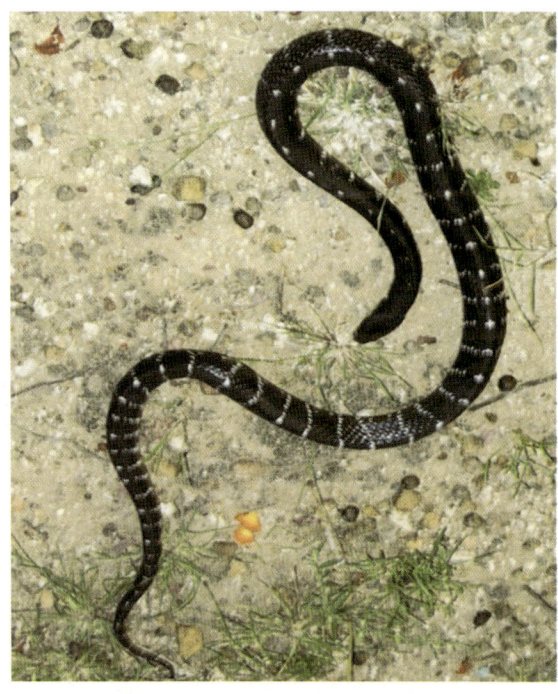

Fig. 9.5: Common krait (*Courtesy*: Shrikant Uike)

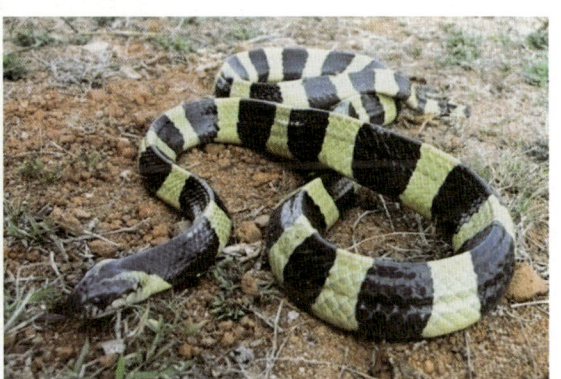

Fig 9.6: Banded krait (*Courtesy*: Shrikant Uike)

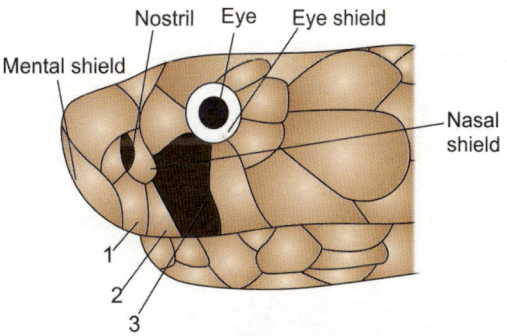

Fig. 9.7: Cobra head scales—large scales and 3rd labial touches the eye and nasal shields

Table 9.2: Differences between cobras and vipers

Features	Cobras	Vipers
1. Body	Long and cylindrical	Short and stout
2. Head	Small with hood seldom broader than body Same width as neck	Large and triangular broader than body Wider than neck
3. Upper jaw	Has 2 fangs and other teeth	Has only 2 poison fangs
4. Fangs	Short, fixed, grooved	Long, movable, canalized
5. Venom	Neurotoxic	Hemotoxic (vasculotoxic)
6. Eyes	Round pupil	Vertical pupil
7. Tail	Round	Tapered
8. Parity	Oviparous	Viviparous

5. **Pit viper:** It is 1–3 feet and has a green pit between eye and nostril. Usually found in hills.

6. **Russell's viper:** It is 4–5 feet long. Head is flat, triangular and has white V-shaped mark pointing forwards.

7. **Saw-scaled viper or echis carinata:** It is 1–1.5 feet usually brown, head is triangular and having a wide mark which resembles an arrow or foot of a bird. The ridges in the middle of each scale are like a saw—hence the name saw-scaled viper.

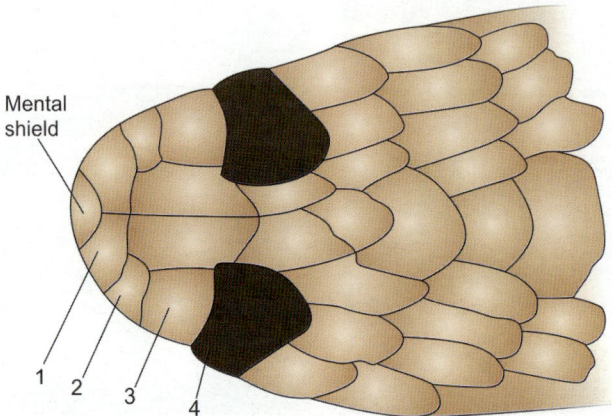

Mental shield

1 2 3 4

Fig. 9.8: Krait head—4th infralabial is largest (view from below)

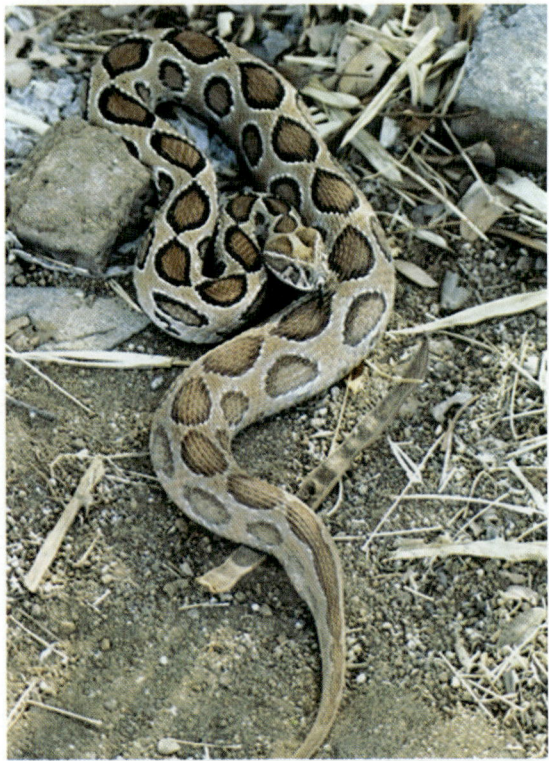

Fig. 9.9: Russell's viper (*Courtesy*: Shrikant Uike)

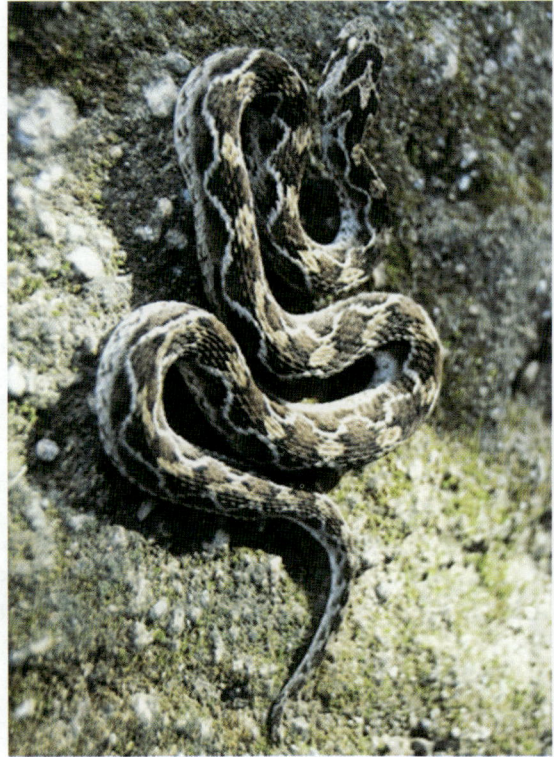

Fig. 9.10: Saw-scaled viper

Table 9.3: Characteristic features of common poisonous snakes in India

Snakes	Common cobra	King-cobra	Common krait	Banded krait
Synonyms	Nag, Gokhurra	NagRaja, Daras	**Maniyar** (Maharashtra), Kawariya (Punj), Chitti (Cal), Kalotaro (Guj)	–
Found in	All over India, Sri Lanka, Burma	Hills and forest of S. India, Odisha, Assam, Himalaya	All over India, and near dwelling house	–
Length	5–6 feet	8–18 feet	3–5 feet	5–7 feet
Colour	Usually black or cream to black to brown	Usually jet black or brownish black, greenish, yellow	Usually steel black with single or double narrow band across their back all over up to tip of tail	Alternate jet black and yellow bands across its back
Head shape and mark	Flat with hood present with one or two dark round spots surrounded by an eclipse c/s 'spectacle mark' on dorsal aspect	Flat with hood present with no 'spectacle mark' on dorsal aspect	Oval with one enlarged central row of hexagonal scales on dorsal aspect	Oval with one enlarged central row of hexagonal scales on dorsal aspect
Head scales	Head scales are large with 3rd supralabial touches the eye and nasal shields	Head scales are large with 3rd supralabial touches the eye and nasal shields	Head scales are small	Head scales are small with black mark on its neck spreading up to the eyes
Pupils	Round	Round	Round	Round
Ventral aspect of mouth	• Ventral aspect of hood bears 3 dark bands on central part and a white band in an area where hood touches the body • Tiny triangular shield between 4th and 5th infralabial shield	• Ventral aspect of hood bears 3 dark bands on central part and a white band in an area where hood touches the body • Tiny triangular shield between 4th and 5th infralabial shield	• Ventral aspect of mouth has only 4 infralabials and 4th infralabial is the largest	• Ventral aspect of mouth has only 4 infralabials and 4th infralabial is the largest
Belly scales	Cover the entire width	Cover the entire width	Cover the entire width	Cover the entire width
Tail	Scales are entirely present proximally but divided in the distal ends	Scales are entirely present proximally but divided in the distal ends	Scales are entirely present and not divided	Scales are entirely present and not divided
Toxin	Neurotoxin	Neurotoxin	Neurotoxin	Neurotoxin
Fatal dose	15 mg	15 mg	1 mg	10 mg
Fatal period	20 mins to 6 hours	20 mins to 6 hours	20 mins to 6 hours	20 mins to 6 hours

Table 9.4: Characteristic features of common poisonous snakes in India

Snakes	Pit viper	Russell's viper	Saw-scaled viper
Synonyms	–	Ghonus (Marathi), Kander (Hindi), Chital (Gujrati), Daboia	Phoorsa
Found in	Hilly area	Throughout India in the plains	–
Length	2–4 feet	4–5 feet, heavy body with narrow neck	1–1.5 feet
Colour	Usually green or **yellow** with pit between eye and nostril	Buff or light brown and pitless with 3 longitudinal regular chain-like pattern or rows on the back	Brownish or brownish grey
Head	Triangular, heavy with deep **depression 'pit'** on each side between eye and nostril.	Triangular, heavy with **white V-shaped mark** with its apex pointing forward	Triangular, heavy with **white mark resembling a bird's foot print or an arrow**
Head scales	Smaller	Smaller	Smaller
Pupils	Vertical	Vertical	Vertical
Body	Flat and broad	Roundish, smooth	Broad and rough having **serrated ridge** and **continuous wavy line along** each **flank** of the back
Other peculiar	–	Snake produces **terrible hissing sound** when about to attack	Snakes produce peculiar **rustling sound while moving**
Belly scales	Cover the entire width	Cover the entire width and broad	Cover the entire width and broad
Tail	Scales are divided throughout	Scales are divided throughout	Scales are divided throughout
Toxin	Vasculotoxic	Vasculotoxic	Vasculotoxic
Fatal dose	100 mg	40 mg	8 mg
Fatal period	2–4 days	2–4 days	2–4 days

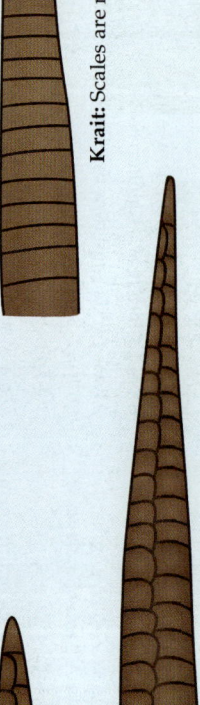

Tail of poisonous snakes

Cobra: Scales are divided distally

Viper: Scales are divided throughout the tail

Krait: Scales are not divided

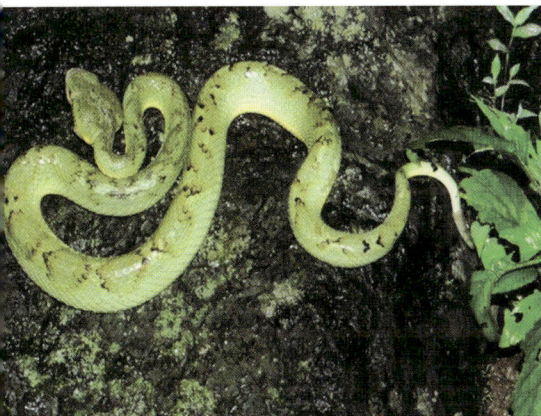

Fig. 9.11: Pit viper

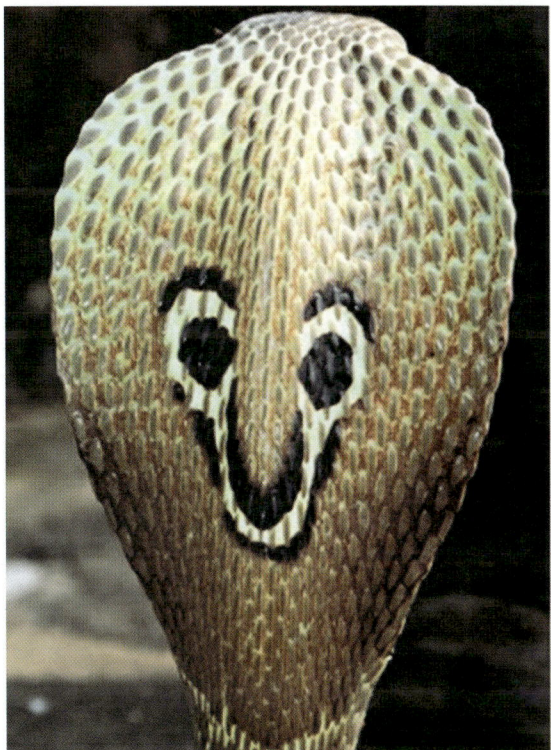

Dorsal aspect
Fig. 9.14

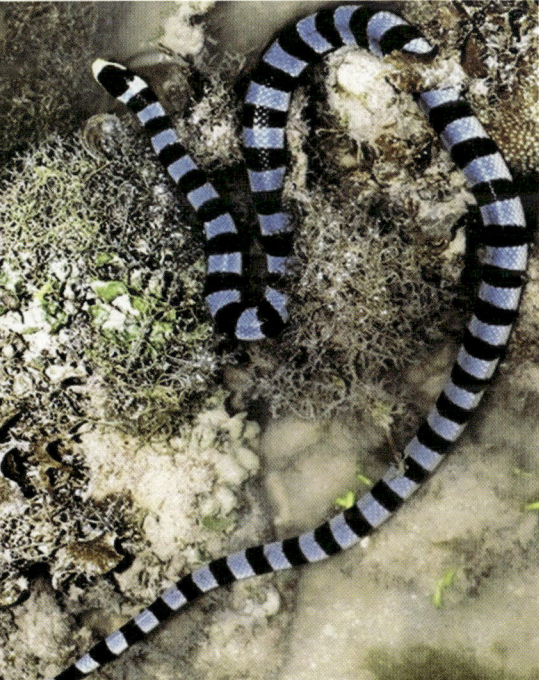

Fig. 9.12: Belcher's sea snake

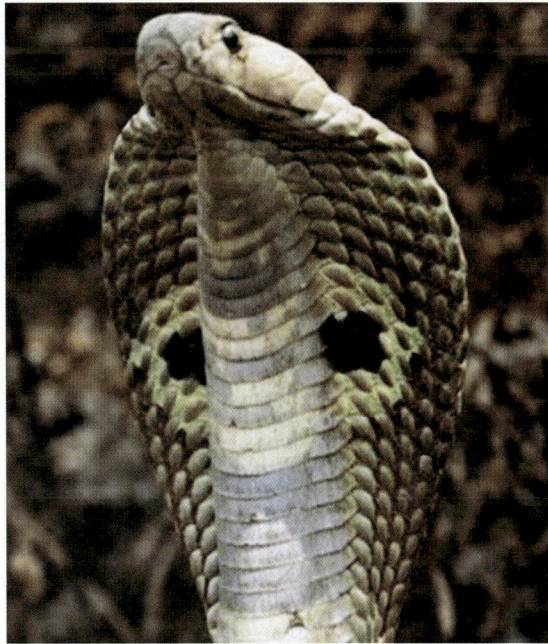

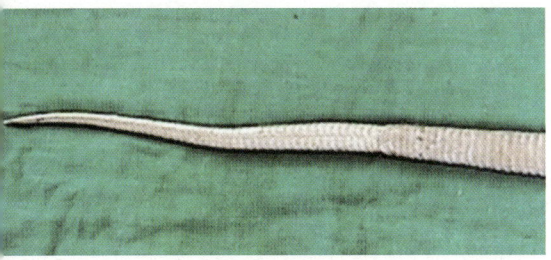

Fig. 9.13: **Poisonous snake:** Viper-Belly scales complete and tail scales are divided throughout

Ventral aspect
Fig. 9.15
Figs 9.14 and 9.15: Hood of common cobra

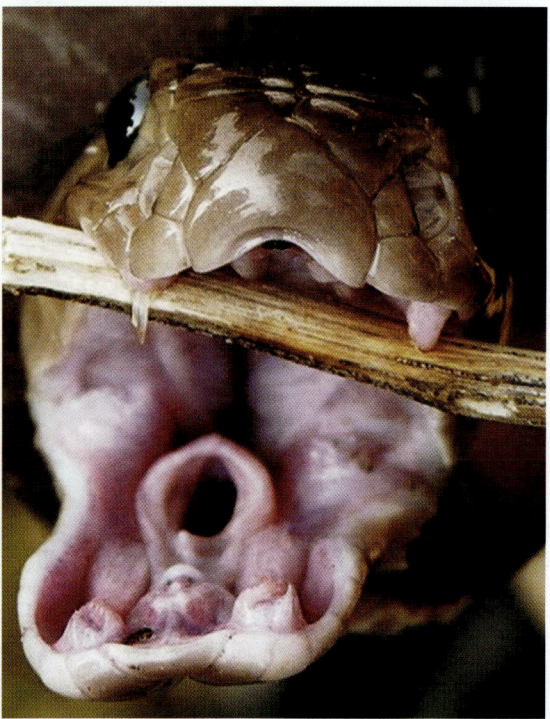

Fig. 9.16: Fangs of cobra

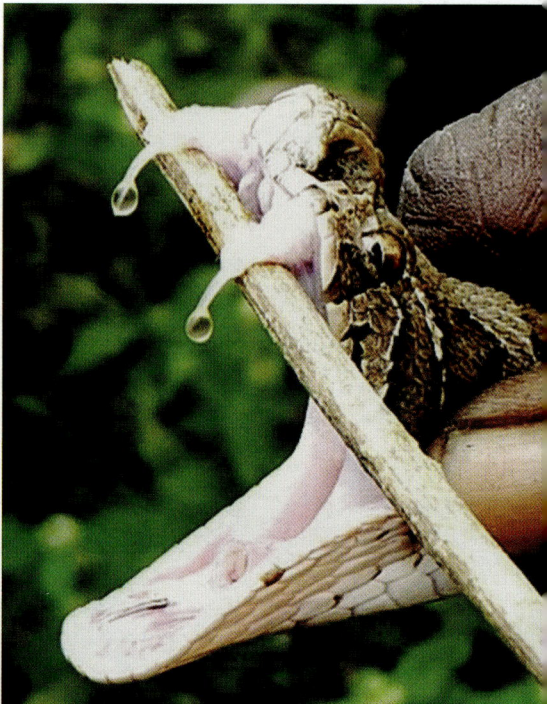

Fig. 9.17: Fangs of viper

SNAKE VENOM

It is the toxic saliva secreted by the specialized salivary glands.

Features

1. **Physical:** Clear, transparent, pale liquid when fresh. It becomes yellowish, opaque, granular powder on drying and remains active for many years.
2. **Chemical:** It is a heterogeneous mixture of proteins in the form of enzymes, peptides and polypeptides.
3. **Enzymes:** The constituents of different snakes venoms are proteinases, hydrolases, transaminase, hyaluronidase, phospholipase A, B, C and D, ribonuclease, deoxyribonuclease, phosphomonoesterase, phosphodiesterases, 5-nucleotidase, ATPase, alkaline phosphatase, acid phosphatase, cholinesterases, coagulases, agglutinins, fibrinolysin, hemolysin, etc.
4. **Types of venoms and action**
   - **Elapids:** Neurotoxin—it blocks the neuromuscular junction (curare-like action) and thus decreases the output of acetylcholine.
   - **Vipers:** Hemolytic and hemotoxic. It causes intravascular hemolysis and depression of coagulation mechanism and leads to hemorrhage and necrosis.
   - **Sea snake:** Myotoxic. It leads to muscle pain, myoglobinuria and hyperkalemia
5. **The action of different constituents of snake venom is as follows**
   - **Proteolytic enzymes:** Cause digestion and destruction of tissue proteins.
   - **Hyaluronidase:** Helps to spread venom
   - **Phospholipase:** Causes hemolysis.
   - **Hemolysin:** Causes lysis of RBC.
   - **Leukolysin:** Causes lysis of WBC.
   - **Cytolysin:** Damage of internal viscera.
   - **Rhabdomyolysin:** Necrosis of muscles.
   - **Proteases:** Dissolution of blood vessels.
   - **Fibrinolysin:** Breakdown of fibrin and causes lysis of clot.

6. Fatal dose, fatal period and amount of venom injected per bite:

Snakes	Fatal dose (of dried venom)	Amount injected per bite
Cobra	12 mg	200–350 mg
Krait	6 mg	20–22 mg
Russell's viper	15 mg	150–200 mg
Saw-scaled viper	8 mg	25 mg

Fatal period

Colubridae: 20 mins to 6 hrs.

Viperidae: 2 to 4 days.

Absorption: The snake venom on ingestion is non-poisonous since it can be digested. Poisoning occurs due to direct snakebite, injection of venom or absorption through abraded skin or mucous membrane.

CLINICAL FEATURES OF NON-POISONOUS SNAKES BITE

- Fear and apprehension; sweating.
- Feeble pulse, hypotension, syncope, rapid and shallow breathing.
- Bite area may show multiple teeth marks.

DIAGNOSIS OF SNAKEBITE POISONING (IN OPHITOXEMIA)

Diagnosis depends on

1. **Fang marks:** Usually two fang marks are seen in the form of punctured wound, separated from each other by about 1 to 4 cm.
2. **Identification of snakes:** Refer Tables 9.3 and 9.4.
3. **Laboratory methods:** Lab diagnosis is poor but are useful for monitoring, prognosis and determining stages of intervention:

Signs and symptoms of poisonous snakes bite

1. **Psychological trauma:** Fright is the most common symptom following snakebite due to enhanced systemic absorption of venom. It develops almost rapidly and may produce psychological shock and cause sudden death. Fear may cause transient pallor, sweating and vomiting

2. **Local manifestations** are present in the form of one or more fang (bite) marks seen as punctured wound. Local features are more prominent in vipers as compared to elapids
   a. **Elapids:** They are mild in the form of **burning with triple response** (i.e. redness, swelling, and inflammation) at the site of bite. In Krait, the bite may be unnoticed as it occurs usually at night. The patent wakes up with vomiting and pain in abdomen (predominantly ANS involvement)
   b. **Vipers: Intense pain with radiation** and tenderness followed by **edema, swelling, irritation, cellulitis, cyanosis, oozing of blood and formation of blisters** containing sera-sanguinous or rarely serous fluid. There is tingling, numbness over tongue/mouth and scalp and paresthesia around the wound. Local area of bite may become devascularized with features of necrosis/gangrene. Secondary infection like tetanus and gas gangrene may also develop
   c. **Sea snakes:** The prick is initially painful but is soon painless and takes 2 hours to produce signs

3. **Systemic manifestation:** Systemic manifestation depends upon the type of venom predominantly present like neurotoxic (cobras and kraits), hemorrhagic (vipers) and myotoxic (sea snakes). Regional lymphadenopathy has been reported as an early and reliable sign of systemic poisoning
   a. **Elapids:** Neurotoxic features are similar to *d*-tubocurarine leading to flaccidity of muscles. However, **Cobra** venom is almost 15–40 times more potent than tubocurarine. There is vomiting, blurred vision, headache, dizziness, giddiness, drowsiness, vertigo, lethargy and flushing of face. There will be drooping of head and eyelids (ptosis), difficulty in speech and deglutition with salivation and frothing from mouth. This is followed by respiratory paralysis, muscle weakness and pain, staggering, spreading paralysis (ascending from lower limbs), convulsions and death. With **Krait** bite, the s/s is less rapid and there is no convulsion, nausea and frothing but there is more drowsiness
   b. **Vipers:** Bleeding from multiple sites including gums, nose, GIT (haematemesis, malena), urinary tract, injection sites, skin (multiple petechiae and purpura), and internal organs particularly kidneys. There is intravascular hemolysis leading to hemoglobinuria and hypotension. Even SAH, SDH and EDH have been reported. **Renal failure** is the major cause of death in viper bites
   c. **Sea snakes:** Myalgia, vomiting, collapse, muscular pain, muscle stiffness, myoglobinuria (due to muscle necrosis), hyperkalemia (increased K^+) and increased serum transaminase levels

Table 9.5: Difference in clinical manifestation of colubrine bite and viperine bite

Features	Colubrine bite (cobra)	Viperine bite (viper)
1. Onset of sign and symptoms	Within 10–20 mins	Within second to 10 min
2. Feeling of intoxication	Marked	Not marked
3. Speech and deglutition	Lost	No effect
4. Involvement of tongue/larynx	Paralyzed	No effect
5. Salivation	Drooling of saliva from mouth	Absent
6. Drooping of eyelids (ptosis)	Present	Not observed
7. Pupils	Normal	Dilated, Not reacting to light
8. Gait	Staggering	Not so, but s/o general paralysis
9. Blood coagulability	Not affected	Completely deranged
10. Hemorrhagic features	Not present or less marked	Most important feature
11. Death	Due to respiratory paralysis	Pulmonary thrombosis or toxic action on heart, blood, kidneys.
12. Development of gangrene	Early, wet type	Slow, dry type

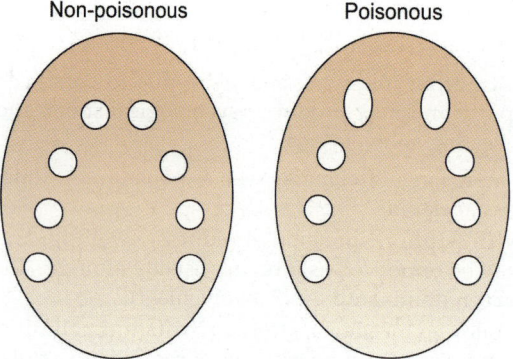

Non-poisonous   Poisonous

Fig. 9.18: Fang marks of snakes

a. Blood changes: Include anemia, leukocytosis and thrombocytopenia and hypofibrinogenemia.

b. Peripheral smear: Shows evidence of hemolysis, particularly in viperine bites.

c. Deranged coagulant activity: Manifested by prolonged clotting time and prothrombin time.

d. Immunodiagnosis: Consist of:

  i. ELISA: To identify the species based on antigens in the venom. These tests are expensive and not freely available and hence are of limited value.

  ii. Radioimmunoassay (RIA).

  iii. Immunodiffusion.

  iv. Countercurrent immuno-electrophoresis.

4. Metabolic changes: Like hyperkalemia and hypoxemia with respiratory acidosis, especially with neuroparalysis.

5. Urine changes: Reveals hematuria, proteinuria, hemoglobinuria or myoglobinuria.

6. CSF: Hemorrhage has been documented in certain cases.

TREATMENT

In non-poisonous snakes

a. Allay the fear and anxiety.

b. Console the patients that not all snakes are poisonous.

In poisonous snakes, the treatment includes

a. Field management

b. Hospital management

A. FIELD MANAGEMENT

1. To allay fear and anxiety: The first step in the snakebite treatment is to allay fear and anxiety, which is the commonest cause of mortality in snakebite. Every patient should be reassured that every snake is not poisonous and that the poisonous snakebite can be treated. The patient should be taken to the hospital at the earliest for hospital management.

2. **Washing the area of bite:** Bite should not be washed as traces of venom that are left on the skin can be used to identify the snakes (where such facilities are available) and type of anti-venom that should be used.

But some prefer to clean the bite area with soap and water/saline or washing with $KMnO_4$ solution (it neutralizes the poison). Some recommended saline cleaning and dressing and some prefer to keep it open.

3. **Avoid incision and sucking:** There is no benefit in cutting or sucking the bite as the venom is deeply injected and or absorbed. Rather avoid incising or cooling bite site, as neurotoxin may be rapidly absorbed through it.

4. **Pressure immobilization technique:** Immobilization is the most effective first aid. It greatly restricts absorption and circulation of these venoms (usually in elapids/sea snakes bites) which tends to cause more limited local tissue effects than viper bites. It prevents spread of venom and relieves pain.

To minimize the movement of the venom around the body until the victim reaches hospital, **apply firm bandage/broad** tourniquet **proximal to the site of bite** (if on extremity, preferably on a single bone). The pressure of torniquet should be **tight enough to occlude the lymphatics,** but not venous drainage. The tourniquet should be released for 20–30 sec. every 20–30 min. to avoid gangrene.

But, in viper bites, application of tourniquets are at risk as the procoagulant enzymes present in viper venom cause the blood to clot. When such torniquet is released, the clot will rapidly enter the circulation and cause embolism and death. Moreover confining or restricting the toxin in a small area creates a greater risk of serious local damage.

B. HOSPITAL MANAGEMENT

1. Specific Therapy: Antivenom Serum or Antivenene

Preparation: It is prepared by injecting the snake venom into horse and extracting the antibodies in the serum. **Antivenoms or Antivenins** may be **monovalent** (species specific, not available in India) or **polyvalent** (effective against cobra, krait, pitless viper). This serum is freeze dried (lyophilized) and is available as granular powder. It is reconstituted by adding 10 ml of distilled water or saline/dextrose. (This solution should be clear.) The serum remains potent for about 10 years.

Indications: Antisnake venom (ASV) should be used cautiously because of its hypersensitivity reactions, but should be given irrespective of the sensitivity.

1. Serious manifestation of envenomation like coma, hypotension, shock, bleeding, DIC, ARF, neurotoxicity, rhabdomyolysis and ECG changes.

2. In absence of these systemic manifestations, swelling involving more than half the affected limb, extensive bruising or blistering and progression of local lesions within 30–60 minutes.

Dose: Firstly, sensitivity test is done (if time and condition of the patient permits) by giving 0.1 ml reconstituted serum intradermally on one forearm. Control with 0.1 ml saline in opposite forearm.

- **If a person is sensitive,** i.e. +ve test (appearance of erythema or wheal >10 mm within 30 minutes) then desensitize with 0.01 ml of 1 : 100 solution and increase the concentration gradually at intervals of 15 minutes, till 1.0 ml SC can be given 2 hourly; **under cover of adrenaline, antihistaminic, and corticosteriods.**

- **If not sensitive,** 20 ml of the serum is given IV and repeated if required. (Some recommended, the serum should be given 20 ml IV, 20 ml IM and 20 ml at the site of bite.) Local injection is useful in vipers to avoid local gangrene.

Types

a. Polyvalent Antisnake Venom Serum (**ASV Serum**—prepared in Haffkine's Institute, Bombay) is given 20 ml IV prepared by dissolving powdered serum in distilled water, administered at the earliest, but may be helpful even after 6–7 days after bite.

b. Polyvalent antivenene (prepared at Kasauli) may be used as a substitute, if ASV serum is not available or patient is very sensitive.

Despite widespread use of Antivenom, there are virtually no clinical trials to determine the ideal dose.

Conventionally: 100 ml ASV (10 bottles) dissolved in DNS/normal saline in IV drip for 1–2 hours. Then after 6 hours, whole blood clotting time is done. If clotting time is more than 20 min, then 50 ml ASV is repeated; and if less than 20 minutes, then there no need of further dose.

2. Supportive Treatment

For Absorbed Venom

a. **In elapids:** 0.6 mg atropine and 0.5 mg neostigmine.

In paralytic cases—adrenaline SC and calcium chloride IM.

b. **In vipers:** 30–40 thousand units heparin. 300–600 gm fibrinogen.

  i. In case of bleeding—blood transfusion: replacement with fresh whole blood.

  ii. In respiratory failure—mechanical ventilation/artificial respiration.

  iii. Acute renal failure—conservative managements or hemodialysis.

  iv. In DIC—heparin.

  v. Antibiotics to prevent post-bite infection

  vi. Tetanus toxoid, antihistaminics, barbiturates, steroids, analgesics.

  vii. IV immunoglobins (IgG)—use of IgG with ASV eliminates the need of repeat ASV. It also improves coagulopathy.

PM FINDINGS

a. Colubrine Snakebite

- Two puncture marks of fangs: ½ inch deep with oozing of serum and blister and necrosis at the site of bite.

- Blood is fluid with dark red color.

- Froth in mouth/nostrils.

- Signs of asphyxia present.

- Histology: Nervous tissue shows changes in Nissl's granules, fragmentation and swelling of nuclei. Cells of medulla show acute granular degeneration.

b. Viperine Snakebite

- Two puncture marks of fangs: 1 inch deep with oozing of fluid blood and swelling, inflammation, discolouration, extravasation of blood or cellulites. On cut section underlying soft tissue edema, hemorrhage and oozing of fluid blood present (marked local features).

- Blood is fluid with dark red color.

- Evidence of hemorrhage in GIT, RT, UT and petechial hemorrhage in pleura, pericardium, *lungs, and kidneys. Hemorrhage present* over endocardium, IV septum, papillary muscle.

- Visceral organs are congested.

MEDICOLEGAL ASPECTS

1. **Accidental:** Snakebite is usually accidental. Annually about 2 lakh people are bitten by snakes and about 20,000 die. It is also seen in snake charmers.

2. **Suicidal:** Rarely except by Cleopatra.

3. **Homicidal:** Rarely and mostly by indirect method or for giving punishment in ancient period.

4. Cattle poisoning by placing snakes and banana in an earthen pot and irritating snakes by firing it. The cobra bites the banana. Fruit is then taken out and smeared into a rag to be injected into rectum of the animal by bamboo stick.

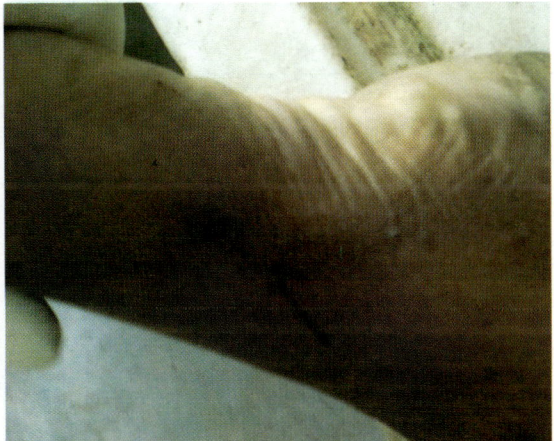

Fig. 9.19: Cobra bite mark

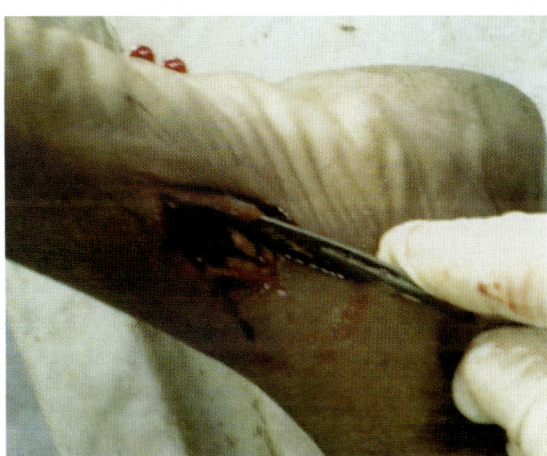

Fig. 9.20: Hemorrhage on cut section

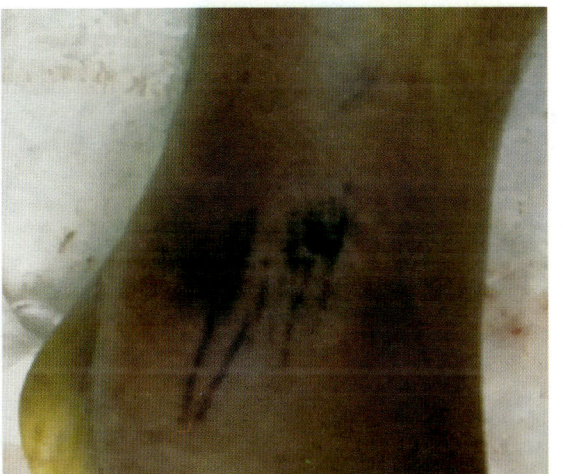

Fig. 9.21: Viper bite marks

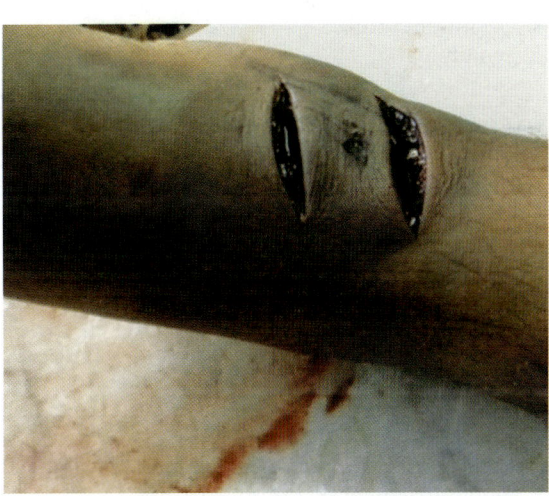

Fig. 9.22: Extensive hemorrhage on cut section

Cantharides (Spanish fly—not seen in India)	*Scorpions*
Cantharide is locally irritating and also a nephrotoxic agent. It is an insect about 1.5 cm long, shining greenish in appearance	Scorpions are long, fleshy, five segmented, eight legged, and have a tail. The end part of the tail has two poison glands and a sting. The agitated scorpion presses its sting onto the body of victim injecting the venom and sometimes leaves the broken tip of the sting in the tissue. Colour varies from light yellow to black
Uses 1. As counterirritant and in other medicinal preparation 2. Aphrodisiac	–
Active principle—cantheridin	Active principle—scorpion venom toxalbumin (a proteinous substance)
Action: Locally irritant, remotely—nephrotoxic	**Action:** Locally irritant, remotely—neurotoxic and hematotoxic actions

Fatal dose: 30 mg cantheridin **Fatal dose:** 12–24 hrs	**Fatal dose:** Uncertain **Fatal period:** Uncertain
Clinical features External application causes burning pain, redness and vesiculation When ingested—burning pain in throat, abdominal pain, vomiting Urine—scanty containing blood, albumin. Painful swelling of penis, blood tinged mucus stool and straining during motion, followed by renal failure, CV collapse, convulsion, coma, death	**Clinical features** Since only a small quantity of the venom is injected—mortality is negligible Local manifestations—more severe than snakes-pain, edema and reddening Systemic manifestations—nausea, vomiting, restlessness, fever, convulsions, coma and cyanosis
Treatment 1. Restriction of fat as it dissolves cantheridin and helps absorption 2. Stomach wash 3. Plenty of water to drink 4. Demulcent drinks 5. Symptomatic	**Treatment** 1. Immobilization and application of tourniquet proximal to bite 2. Wash the wound with water or $KMnO_4$ 3. Local infiltration of anesthetics to lessen pain 4. Antivenin 5. IV calcium gluconate to control swelling 6. IV glucose, saline and hydrocortisone
PM findings • Suggestive of irritation in mouth/esophagus/stomach • Stomach: Wall—swollen • Mucosa—hemorrhagic • Contains—particles of exoskeleton of insect • Visceral organs—congested with haemorrhagic spots present • Urinary bladder—reddish urine • Mucosa—hemorrhagic • Kidney—hemorrhagic	**PM findings** • **Local:** At site of scorpion bite—swelling, edema, underlying tissue haemorrhagic • Visceral organs congested
Medicolegal aspects 1. **Accidental:** During medicinal use for counterirritant or for aphrodisiac use 2. **Suicidal/Homicidal:** Rare 3. **Abortifacient** 4. **Aphrodisiac:** To increases sexual desire	**Medicolegal aspects** 1. Poisoning is accidental 2. Spraying DDT kills scorpions

1. Bees	*2. Wasps, hornet*
It causes manifestation by stinging	It causes manifestation by stinging
Venom 1. Biogenic amines: Histamine, 5-hydroxytryptamine, acetylcholine 2. Enzymes: Phospholipase A, hyaluronidase, cardiotoxin 3. Toxic peptides: Mellitin, apamin, mast cell degranulating peptides	**Venom** 1. Biogenic amines: Histamine, 5-hydroxytryptamin, acetylcholine 2. Enzymes: Phospholipase A, hyaluronidase, cardiotoxin 3. Toxic peptides/other: Kinin/antigen-5, acid phosphatase

Clinical features
Local: Stinging causes local pain, redness, swelling
Systemic effect: S/o collapse with sweating, fall of BP, nausea, vomiting, bronchospasm, tingling sensation, flushing, dizziness, syncope, urticaria, glottis edema, angioedema, renal failure, haemolysis with hematoglobinuria

Treatment	Treatment
1. Wash the bite site with bicarbonate solution	1. Wash the bite site with vinegar
2. Epinephrine HCl: 0.3 mg SC	2. Epinephrine HCl: 0.3 mg SC
3. Ca Gluconate: 1–2 gm IV	3. Ca gluconate: 1–2 gm IV
4. Glycocorticoids IM	4. Glycocorticoids IM
5. Artificial respiration + O_2 inhalation	5. Artificial respiration + O_2 inhalation
6. Antihistaminic cream locally	6. Antihistaminic cream locally
ML aspect: It is almost always accidental	**ML aspect:** It is almost always accidental

3. Black spider	*4. Brown spider*	*5. Red ants*
Black spider bite is toxic	Bite inject haemolysin and norepinephrine	Red ants bite injects alkaloid, solenopsin A (has haemolytic and phytotoxic actions)
Clinical manifestation Local: At the site of bite, pain and cramps which extends upward Systemic: Increase BP, nausea, vomiting, respiratory difficulty when acts on CNS and nerve endings of the diaphragm	**Clinical manifestation** Local: At the site of bite, painful ulceration Systemic: Nausea, vomiting, fever, haematuria, albuminuria, arthralgia	**Clinical manifestation** Local: Urticarial lesion followed by pustulation Systemic: Increased BP, retrosternal pain, respiratory difficulty
Treatment 1. Sedatives 2. Ca gluconate 3. Neostigmine + atropine sulphate (0.5 mg each) 4. Curariform drug	**Treatment** 1. Symptomatic	**Treatment** 1. Adrenaline 2. Antihistaminic
ML aspect: Accidental	**ML aspect:** Accidental	**ML aspect:** Accidental

6. Centipedes and millipedes
They secrete phenol, quinone and cyanogens from base of their feet which may produce ulcers

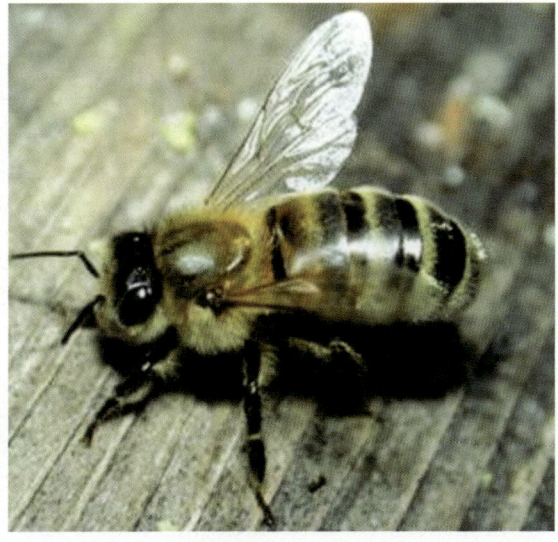

Fig. 9.23: Honeybee

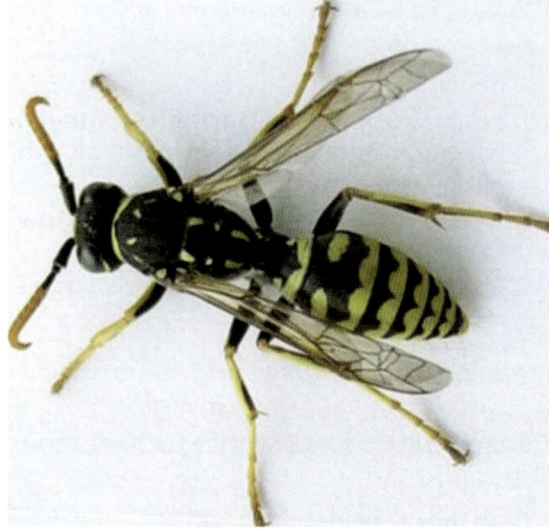

Fig. 9.24: Wasps

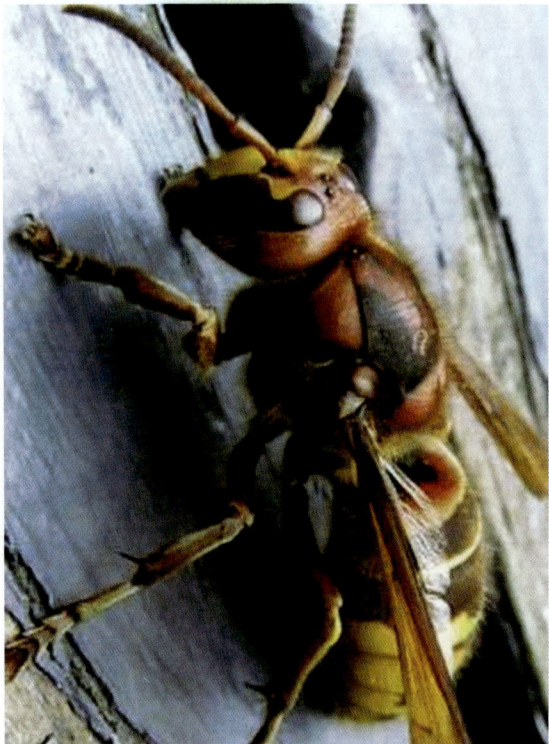

Fig. 9.25: Giant Indian hornet

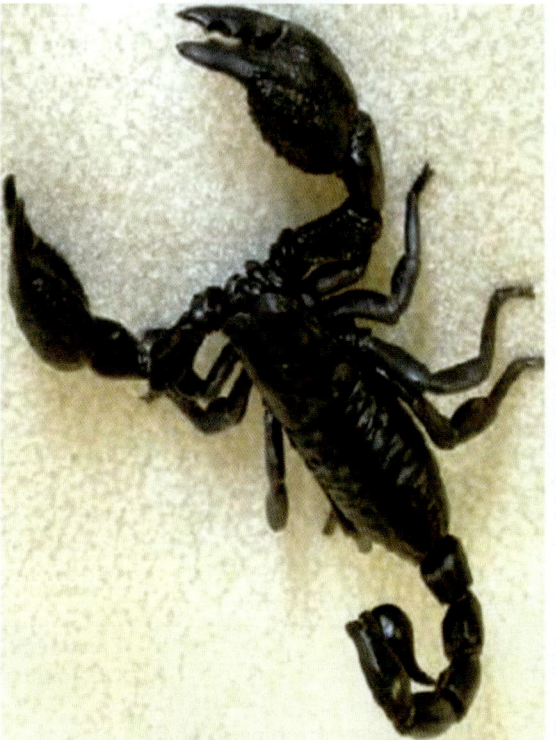

Fig. 9.26: Black scorpion

VENOMOUS AQUATIC ANIMALS

Some of the venomous aquatic animals are
a. Vertebrates: Sea snakes, venomous fishes.
b. Invertebrates: Shells, mussels, squids, crustaceans, jelly fish.

Poisoning by venomous aquatic animals occurs by way of
a. Biting: Sea fish.
b. Stinging: Spines of various venomous fishes: Stingray, horn sharks, cat fish, scorpion fish, weever fish.
c. Surface contact: Jelly fish, sea urchins, blood worm, bristle worm.
d. Consumed as food: Shells, mussels, squids, crustaceans.

Poisoning by biting/stinging of venomous fish (Table 9.6)

Treatment in Cases of Stinging of Venomous Fishes

1. To relieve pain—analgesic.
2. Symptomatic treatment.
3. Prevents secondary infection.
4. To attenuate the venom, hot compression with MgSO$_4$ solution or plain hot water is useful.
5. Local: Antihistaminic cream.

Poisoning by surface contact
Poisoning occurs due to injection of the venom by stinging cells of the invertebrates when they come into contact with the skin of person.

1. Jelly fish like Portuguese man of war/sea anaemone: Venom contains 5-HT, urocanyl-choline.
2. Molluses or mussels (conch shells, squid, octopus) have developed venom apparatus which cause punctures on the skin and inject venom.
3. Sea urchins: Venomous spines covering their body surface.
4. Bristle worm
5. Blood worm: Bites and inject toxic substances.

Table 9.6: Venomous fishes

V. fishes	Sting/spines	Venom gland	Local manifestation	Systemic manifestation
1. **Stingray:**	Sting is located in the dorsal aspect of tail. The sting/spine has furrows	Venom is secreted from ventro-lateral glandular tissue and causes vasoconstriction and inhibits auricular and ventricular contraction and dilatation	**Bite:** Intense, sharp, shooting, spasmodic or throbbing pain. Area is swollen and necrosis of marginal tissue	**Systemic:** Nausea, vomiting, faintness, vertigo, drowsiness, sweating, fall of BP, arrhythmia and muscular paralysis (flaccid/spastic)
2. **Horn-sharks:**	There are 2 dorsal spines at anterior margins of two dorsal fins. The spines are grooved	Near the base of spines, there are glandular cell which secretes venoms	**Sting:** Immediate, intense, stabbing pain with swelling, redness	Death due to shock
3. **Cat fish:**	Have 3 stings, one dorsal in front of anterior dorsal fin and 2 pectoral stings one in each side in front of pectoral fins	Venomous glands are axillary glands for pectoral stings and glandular structure at base of dorsal sting. The venom of cat fish consists of both neurotoxic and haemotoxic agents	**Sting:** Intense pain may lead to primary shock leading to death. Secondary infection occurs and takes time to heal	**Systemic:** Respiratory distress
4. **Scorpion fish:**	Have 12 dorsal spines, 3 anal spines and 2 pelvic spines with associated venom glands	Venoms consist of neurotoxic, haemotoxic and cardiotoxic agents	**Stinging:** Intense pain + swelling, warm, bluish area surrounding red zone	**Systemic:** Nausea, vomiting, nervous disturbances, convulsion, delirium, fever, pain in joints, respiratory distress and cardiac failure • Lymphadenitis and lymphangitis
5. **Zebra fish and stone fish:**	Have 13 dorsal spines, 3 anal spines and 2 pelvic spines with associated venom glands	–	**Stinging:** Intense pain with swelling	**Systemic:** Nausea, vomiting, nervous disturbances, convulsion, delirium, fever, pain in joints, respiratory distress and cardiac failure
6. **Weever fish:**	Have 5–7 dorsal spines and 2 opercular spines with associated venom glands	The venom stimulates sensory motor cortex and is also cardiotoxic	**Stinging:** Extreme pain with tingling and numbness. Area is firstly ischaemic and then becomes red and swollen	**Systemic:** Nausea, vomiting headache, chill, fever, palpitation, bradycardia, cardiac failure, respiratory distress, ankylosis, convulsion, delirium • Aphonia, psychic depression **Complications:** Ankylosis, peripheral neuritis and muscular atrophy

Clinical manifestation: In poisoning by surface contact.

Local: Pain, swelling, redness.

Systemic: Nausea, vomiting, muscular cramps, paralysis, convulsion, collapse, coma, respiratory distress and death.

Treatment in Case of Surface Contact

1. Washing with mineral oil or alcohol or alkaline solution.
2. Analgesic.
3. Symptomatic.

Poisoning by Consumption of Poisonous Aquatic Animals as Food

1. California mussel (which eats planktons having deadly toxins): May cause sensory and motor disturbances like tingling, numbness, muscular weakness and paralysis.
2. Some shells, shrimps and crabs: May cause chronic arsenic poisoning.
3. Puffer fish: Cause tetra-dotoxin poisoning leading to vomiting, retching, lethargy, muscular weakness, fall of BP and respiratory distress.

Treatment in Case of Eating/Consumption as Food

Symptomatic.

ML ASPECT OF POISONING BY AQUATIC ANIMALS

1. Accidental.
2. Poisoning occurs in divers.

10

Somniferous Poison: Opium and Its Alkaloids

Somniferous poison/drugs: These are the sleep inducing drugs obtained or derived from the *Papaver somniferum* plant. It includes opium and their alkaloids. Opium has a peculiar smell and bitter taste. It is obtained by giving incision to the unripe fruit (poppy capsule) of *Papaver somniferum* (poppy plant). It is the milky exude which on exposed to air becomes dark brown or black crude opium commonly called **"Afim"**.

Plant: *Papaver somniferum* is a herb growing up to a length of 1 meter. Flowers are large purple white or white in color. Each plants bear 5–10 fruits (poppy capsules) containing numerous small poppy seeds. The plant is a native of Turkey and is cultivated worldwide under Government control. In India, it is cultivated and distributed in Ghaziabad, Uttar Pradesh under Government supervision and also in Rajasthan and Madhya Pradesh. Opium has 20 alkaloids of which morphine is most important. Ripe poppy capsule and poppy seeds are not toxic. A dried poppy capsule contains a little narcotine.

Types of opiates and active principle: It has alkaloids classified as:

1. **Natural:** It has two groups:
   a. Phenanthrene: Morphine, codeine and thebaine.
   b. Benzyl isoquinolene: Papaverine, noscapine/narcotine and narcine.

2. **Semisynthetic opiates:** Diacetyl morphine (heroin), dehydromorphine, benzyl morphine, oxymorphone, hydromorphone, N-allyl-normorphine (nalorphine), hydrocodeine bitartrate, dehydrocodeine bitartrate.

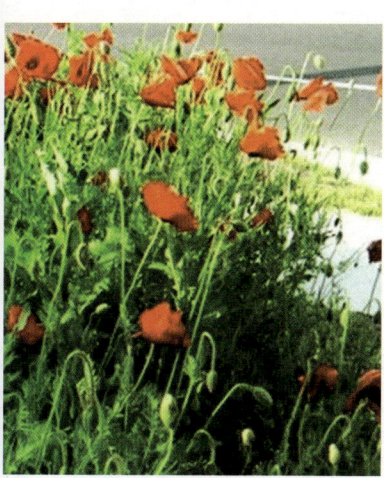

Fig. 10.1: Poppy plant

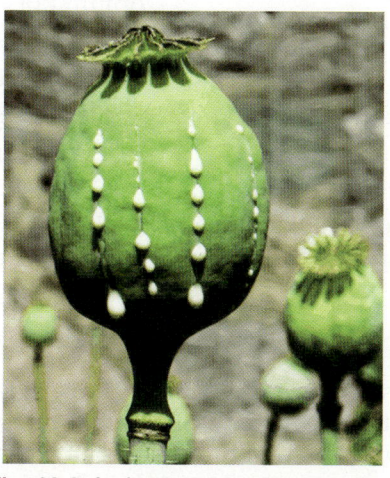

Fig. 10.2: Incised unripe poppy capsules

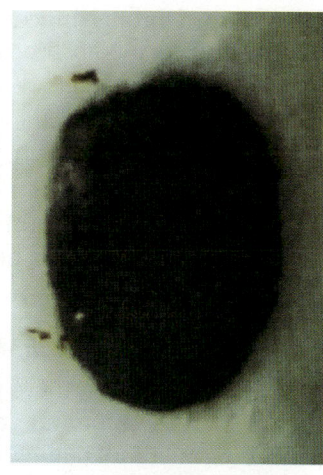

Fig. 10.3: Afim-crude

3. Synthetic opiates: Pethidine, hydroxy-pethidine, methadone, isomethadone, nor-methadone, α-methadol, acetyl-methadol.

Uses

1. Morphine and codeine have maximum use as analgesic and cough depressant respectively.
2. Poppy seeds (khas-khas) are used in different food preparations.
3. Heroin is used as cough suppressant and is a drug of addiction.
4. Pethidine is used as analgesics. A single dose of pethidine may make an individual addict.
5. Morphine being respiratory depressant, is contraindicated in head injury and is a drug of addition.
6. Apomorphine, prepared from morphine is used as an emetic.

Mechanism of Action

It causes CNS depression and narcosis (analgesic + hypnosis). It depresses all centers (in cortex and medulla—respiratory and cough) except vomiting center, occulomotor center and sweating (vagus).

Fatal dose: Opium—2 gm, morphine—100–200 mg, codeine—500 mg, heroin—50 mg, pethidine—1 gm, methadon—100 mg.

Fatal period: 6–12 hours.

Absorption, Fate, and Excretion

It is absorbed through mucous membrane of GIT. When smoked, it is absorbed through lungs.

Metabolised in liver.

Excreted through kidneys, bile, milk, saliva and also through stomach and intestine.

Signs and symptoms: Poisoning occurs due to ingestion of opium or its alkaloids or injection of morphine. There are 3 stages of opium poisoning:

Stage I: Stage of Excitation and Euphoria

There is excitement, increased sense of well-being, increased mental activity, flushing of face and sometimes hallucinations. In children-marked feature is convulsions.

This stage is short-lived and may not be there, if large dose is taken. But soon there is restlessness, anxiety, dizziness, nausea and dysphoria.

Stage II: Stage of Depression or Stupor

Headache, giddiness, drowsiness, dizziness, disorientation, ataxia, lack of interest/concentration, uneasy feeling, contracted pupils, cyanosed face and itching all over the body.

Stage III: Stage of Narcosis/Coma

Muscles relaxed, reflexes are lost, pinpoint pupils (and dilated only after prolonged coma, severe anoxia), sleep, coma, death.

There is hypotension, Cheyne-Stokes breathing, sweating, hypothermia (due to reduction in oxygen consumption, low metabolic activity and failure of heart regulating mechanism), cyanosis and froth at mouth and nose with progressive respiratory depression.

Pulse is slow, and skin is moist, cold, clammy, and pale. Face is flushed, conjunctiva suffused.

There is constipation due to constriction of smooth muscles of the sphincter. Emptying of stomach is delayed. There is oliguria, hyperglycemia, glycosuria and renal failure.

Pulse, perception, pain and conscious are depressed.

DIAGNOSIS OF OPIUM POISONING

The triad of following features strongly suggests opium poisoning:

- **Coma,**
- **Pin point pupils,**
- **Depressed respiration**, along with
- **Typical opium smell (raw flesh)**
- Cyanosis
- Froth at nose and mouth
- Cheyne-Stokes breathing
- Slow pulse
- Moist cold skin and hypothermia.

Differential diagnosis: Uremia, diabetic coma, cerebral malaria/encephalitis/meningitis, epileptic coma, hysterical coma, cerebrovascular accidents (IC hemorrhage with compression of the brain), heat stroke, Poisoning due to carbolic acid, carbon monoxide, barbiturates and alcohol.

Treatment

1. Stomach wash with 1 : 5000 dilution of $KMnO_4$. 200 ml of the solution is left in the stomach after last wash to neutralize morphine, which is resecreted in the stomach after absorption even if morphine is given parenterally.
2. Enema and purgatives: $MgSO_4$: 20 gm.
3. Antidote: **Naloxone:** 0.2–0.5 mg IV every 5 minutes till person becomes conscious and pupils dilate. Newer antidote is nalmefene: 0.1 mg IV followed by 0.5 mg IV. (Nalorphine or atropine is not used nowaday due to their terminal depressive action on respiration.) Methadone in chronic poisoning. (Levo-alpha-acetyl methadol (LAAM) is superior.)
4. Safeguarding respiration:
   • Bronchial suction to make airway free from obstruction.
   • Artificial respiration and O_2 inhalation
   • Endotracheal intubation: It increases the lumen width to ensure free air passage.
5. Stimulants: Methyl amphetamine HCl— 10–20 mg, acts as stimulant to different system. Coramine as cardiorespiratory stimulant.
6. Supportive: Antibiotic to prevent pulmonary infection.

Correction of fluid and electrolyte imbalance.

Benzodiazepines for convulsion.

Postmortem Appearance

External

Face congested with deep cyanosis over fingertips, lips and ear lobules.

• Black postmortem lividity.
• Froth at mouth and nostrils.
• Smell of opium (raw flesh) present.

Features of drug addiction—injection marks with pigmented and scar formation and tattooing.

Internal

Stomach: Content give characteristic smell of opium or show unabsorbed lump of opium.

Respiratory tract: Froth present.

Lungs: Congested, edematous with petechial hemorrhage over surface.

Brain: Congested, edematous with petechial hemorrhage on cut section.

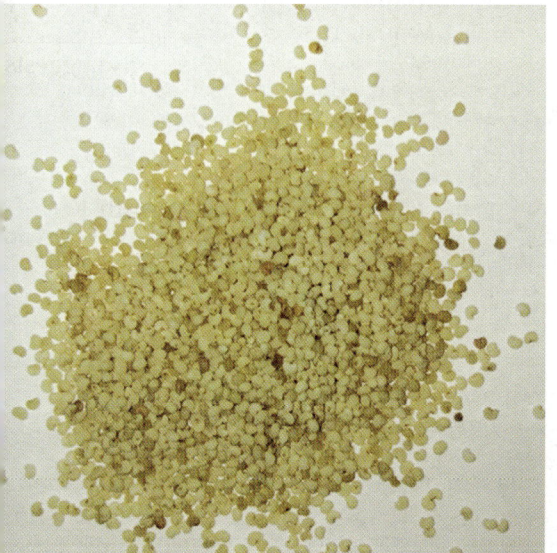 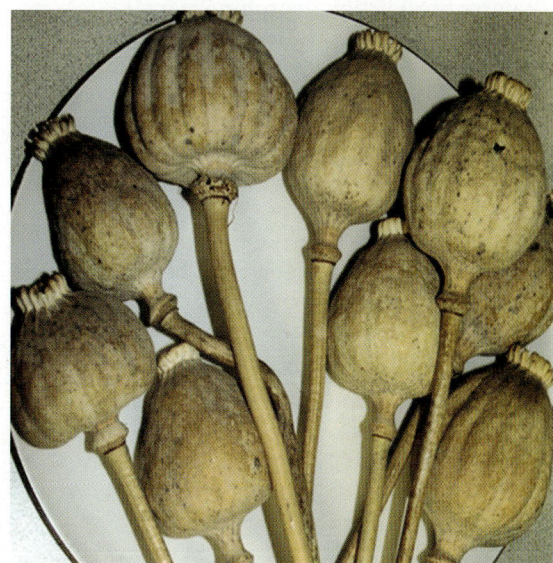

Fig. 10.4: Poppy seeds and dry poppy capsules

- **Blood:** Dark and fluid.
- Visceral organs congested.

Medicolegal Aspects

1. Suicidal: It is a popular suicidal agents leading to painless death.
2. Homicidal: Not used due to its bitter taste, characteristic smell, and delayed death.
3. Accidental: Due to overdose in addicts and in children; and due to therapeutic misadventure.
4. Aphrodisiac: Morphine is used as aphrodisiac agents but it diminishes the performance.

5. Addicts can consume high dose of morphine/opium. There is moral degradation, lack of judgement and may lead to commit any crime in order to get the drug out of desperation.

Chemical test: Marquis test

Blotting paper soaked with test material. Put one drop of mixture of 3 ml of conc. H_2SO_4 + 3 drops of formalin.

If the test material contains opium or morphine, then there is a change of color first to purple, then violet and finally blue.

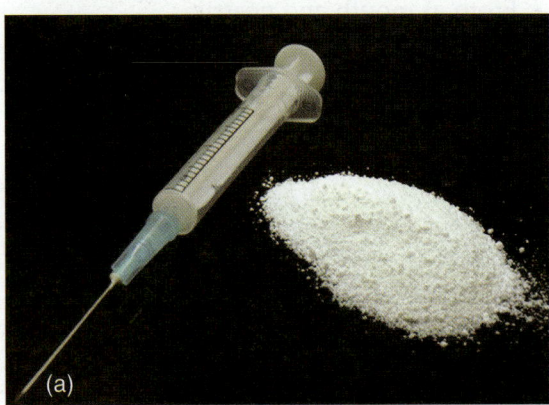
(a)

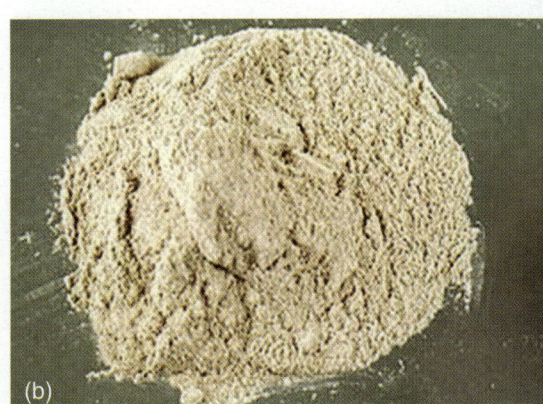
(b)

Fig. 10.5: Heroin/brown sugar

Opium/morphine addiction	Withdrawl symptoms in opium addict
Features of addiction (morphine mania)	**Features of withdrawl**
1. Irritability, fatigability, lack of interest/ concentration, loss of weight and appetite, constipation, furred tongue, impotence/ frigidity	1. Weeping, running nose, sweating, scratching, restlessness
2. Mental depression, **moral degradation**, loss of self respect and morality and a desire to procure drug by any means	2. Pain in legs, shivering, goose skin appearance
	3. Vomiting, diarrhea, abdominal pain, muscle spasm, tremor, hypertension, anxiety, drug seeking behavior
3. For parentral use (skin popping in SC use and main lining in IV use): There will be **pigmentation and scar formation** at the site of injection often masked by **artificial tattooing**	4. Insomnia, hot and cold flushes and weight loss
4. **Toxic dementia** may develop	5. Dangers: There may be debility, injury, intercurrent infection
Treatment of opium addiction	**Treatment of withdrawal symptoms**
1. Gradual withdrawal of drug	1. Chlorpromazine 50–100 mg or pentobarbitone
2. Substitution therapy with methadone 30–40 mg/day and then gradually tapered off	2. Low dose of morphine or methadone
	3. Physical restrains to protect from accident and injury
3. β-Adrenergic blocker like propranolol (80 mg) is quite effective in anxiety and craving	4. Maintenance of food, nutrition and vitamins
	5. Nursing care

4. Maintenance of food, nutrition and vitamins
5. Nursing care
6. Physical restrain
7. Psychiatric counseling

6. Antibiotic in some cases

Other opiates

Codeine (methyl morphine): (Natural)
It is popularly used as cough depressant. It is also used as an analgesic. It is less toxic than morphine and is less miotic, less constipating and more nauseating. In toxic doses, it excites medulla and spinal cord and causes convulsion and delirium

Pethidine and methadone (synthetic opiates)
Pethidine is good analgesic, narcotic and sedative and causes mydriasis and dryness of skin. It liberates histamine and mast cells. It has direct inhibitive action on heart muscles

Brown sugar: It is crude heroin **(semisynthetic)**
Heroin (diacetyl morphine)
It is semisynthetic opiate derived from morphine
It is 2–3 times more toxic than morphine. It is also a narcotic. It causes more euphoria and no vomiting. Addiction occurs easily and more quickly than other narcotic drugs
It is 'downer' or depressant drug that affects the brain's pleasure system and interferes with the brain ability to perceive pain. It is a white to dark brown colored powder

Nalorphine (N-allyl-normorphine): Semisynthetic opiate
It causes analgesic, respiratory depression, dysphoria, and hallucination. It was popularly used as an antidote to morphine but because of its depressive action and other side effects, it is not used nowadays

11

Inebriant Poison: Alcohols

Inebriants are the drugs producing excitement. Inebriant means to cause drunkenness or to intoxicate. It includes alcohols and their derivatives, anaesthetic drugs, and fuels like kerosene and petrol.

These are the poisons, which are characterized by two sets of symptoms

1. Excitement
2. Narcosis—It is the combination of hypnosis (sleep) + analgesia.

Definition of alcohol: It is an organic hydroxy compound obtained by replacing one or more hydrogen atoms from aliphatic hydrocarbons by hydroxyl group (–OH). Absolute alcohol is 99.8% concentrated.

Spirit: Means any liquor containing alcohol and obtained by distillation (whether denatured or not)

Liquor: Term used for any liquid containing alcohols obtained by any method (distillation or not) and includes spirits, denatured spirit, wine, beer, toddy, etc.

Rectified spirit: It is the spirit subjected to rectification (process whereby liquor is purified or refined) for making it potable (Fig. 11.1)

Denatured spirit: It is the spirit subjected to a process for the purpose of rendering unfit for human consumption, e.g. French polish, varnish (Fig. 11.1)

Methylated spirit: Rectified spirit with 5–10% wood naphtha, i.e. impure methyl alcohol. It contains 90–95% ethanol + 5–10% methanol

Surgical spirit: 95% ethanol + 5% methanol + oil of wintergreen (sweetish flavor for easy detection and pleasant use)

Beverages are drinks used for their flavor or stimulating effect, e.g. tea, coffee, aerated water, wines, etc. These may be alcoholic or non-alcoholic

Toddy is liquor not a spirit. It means fermented or unfermented juice extracted from palm tree, e.g. coconut, barb, date, etc. **Neera** is unfermented juice extracted from any palm tree

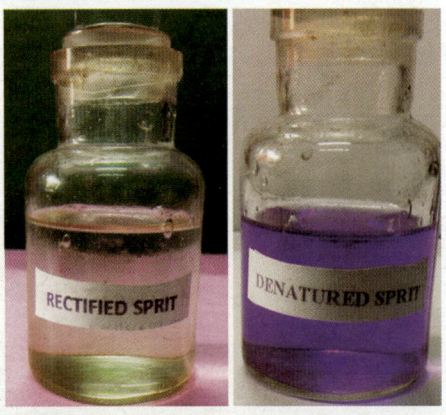

Fig. 11.1: Rectified/denatured spirit

Types of methylated spirit

1. Mineralized (light pink color)—90% ethanol + 10% wood naphtha.
2. Industrial (colorless)—95% ethanol + 5% methyl alcohol.

Arrack is an Eastern name for any country liquor

- Distilled from rice/sugar or jiggery, cashew nut, coco palm, and mohua flowers.
- Fortified with powerful knock out agents like potassium bromide, chloral hydrate, Datura and bhang.

Different names: Andra Pradesh—Gudamba; Maharashtra—Khopri; Gujarat—Lattha; Feni—Goa, Tequila—Mexico; Sake—Japan.

Alcohol is obtained by enzymatic fermentation of:

- Carbohydrates—sugars and starch;
- Raw materials—cereals, corn, barley, etc;
- Jaggery;
- Molasses;
- Potatoes; and
- Fruits—grapes.

Beverages	Origin	Alcohol % by volume	Proof %
Rum	West Indies	42.8	75
Whisky	Scotland	42.8	75
Brandy	–	42.8	75
Gin	Holland	42.8/40.0/ 37.2	65–75
Beer	Brazil	2–10.0	3.5–17.5
Country liquor		11.4–45.7	20–80

Vodka is the purest form of beverages and does not contain any congeners. It is virtually odorless.

One peg: Large peg = 60 ml and small peg = 30 ml.

Types of drink		
Soft	04–08% alc	Beer
Moderate	10–20% alc	Wines, champagne
Hard	40–55% alc	Whisky, brandy, gin, rum

Proof spirit: (57.10%) defines such strength of alcohol which when poured onto gunpowder allowed it to burn, since the remaining 42.90% of water did not prevent it. It indicates a mixture containing 57.10% by volume (or 49.28% by weight) of absolute alcohol.

Proof strength of a liquid is obtained by dividing the alcohol percent in volume by 0.571, e.g. wine—10% alcohol. Therefore, proof spirit = 10/0.571.

Similarly % of alcohol in liquid is obtained by multiplying the proof strength by 0.571, e.g. brandy 75° proof = 75 × 0.571= 42.8% by volume.

ETHYL ALCOHOL: C_2H_5OH

Properties: Colorless, sweetish smell, sweet-fiery (piercing) taste, soluble in water.

Uses

1. Beverages/drink: It is used as a drink for pleasure to reduce tension and to satisfy thirst.
2. Solvent: For aftershaves, colognes, mouthwash, perfumes (15–80%).
3. Preservatives: Rectified spirit is used as preservatives of viscera for chemical analysis.
4. In industries and laboratories.
5. Medicinal uses:
   a. Surgical spirit is used as an antiseptic.
   b. Several multivitamins and cough syrups contains varying amount of alcohols—2–20%.
   c. Antidote for methanol and ethylene glycol poisoning.
   d. Ethanol sponging is an effective remedy for hyperthermia.
   e. It is also used in trigeminal neuralgia.

Action

CNS—excitation followed by depression. It removes the restraints on primitive behaviour.

Fatal dose: For non-addicts: 150 ml at a time/very rapidly in one setting.

Fatal period: Death within 24 hrs.

Absorption, Distribution, and Excretion

Absorbs rapidly from intestine and rate is more than glucose.

Distributed: Alcohol is distributed in intracellular and extracellular fluid of the tissue. 'Walked off'—exercise sharply fall of alcohol supply to the brain.

Fate/excretion: 90% alcohol is oxidized in liver and rest is excreted as it is in urine and exhaled air.

Absorption of Alcohol

Depends on

1. Amount of food: Empty—absorbs rapidly.
2. Quality of food: Fat and protein—delays absorption.

3. Concentration:

a. Higher concentration is absorbed rapidly due to irritation and inflammation of gastric mucosa.

b. But in chronic user, it is not rapidly absorbed as higher concentration destroys the mucosa.

4. Presence of CO_2: Increases absorption by increasing the absorption surface.

5. Condition of stomach wall: Gastrectomy, chronic gastritis—increases the absorption.

6. Quantity and rate of drinking.

7. Weight of person.

8. Development of tolerance.

Metabolism

Ethyl alcohol → acetaldehyde → acetic acid → CO_2+H_2O

Oxidation yields 7 cal of energy/gm and causes reduction of intake of other food by alcoholic (vitamin and nutrients), leading to degenerative changes in liver.

Methyl alcohol → formaldehyde → formic acid (highly toxic)

Rate of oxidation of methyl alcohol is very slow, about 15% of ethanol.

Blood alcohol level reduces by about 10 mg% per hrs and about 7 ml is washed out per hour in this way.

Concentration of alcohol in blood reaches a maximum (peak) in about 1 to 1½ hrs after ingestion. However, it is present in the blood within 30 min and urine within 60 min.

Level of alcohol in mg/100 ml of blood	Minimum consumed volume of 75% proof spirit in ml
50 (0.05%)	69.5 ml
100 (0.1%)	139.0
200 (0.2%)	278.0
300 (0.3%)	417.0
400 (0.4%)	556.0
500 (0.5%)	695.0

Acute poisoning: Result from consumption of any preparation containing alcohol either in small doses at short interval or one big dose.

Clinical Features and Stages

I. Stage of excitement: 0.05% to 0.1% blood alcohol (>0.1% not fit to drive a vehicle)

- Inhibits the higher centers, which controls judgment and behaviour leading to unrestrained and unabstained character of a person.
- There is loss of restraints of code of conduct (habit, duty, behaviour).
- The person becomes excited and talkative.
- Skin—flushed, warm (increased temperature).
- Conjunctiva—reddened or congested.
- Pupils—dilated, sluggish reacting to light/accommodation.
- Smell of alcohol present in breath.
- Pulse increases, increased HR/BP.

II. Stage of in-coordination (0.1 to 0.3%)
There is in-coordination of

- Thought—recent memory impaired
- Speech—slurred, incoherent
- Action (incoordination of muscle)—staggering gait, and skill movement impaired and reaction time increased.
- Eyes—suffused,
- Vision—blurred, double,
- Pupil—dilated, sluggishly reacting to light,
- Mouth—dry, and
- Tongue—furred.

III. Stage of narcosis (0.3% to 0.5%)
Deep sleep responds to strong stimuli

- Pulse—rapid, temperature—subnormal,
- **Pupil—constricted,**
- **Macewen's sign** present (pinching of skin of neck/face leads to dilation of pupil).
- A fine lateral **nystagmus**—oscillatory movement of eyeball (alcoholic gaze nystagmus—AGN). Alcohol causes nystagmus by two mechanisms.
  1. Firstly by acting on vestibular system, it causes positional alcoholic nystagmus (PAN), when the person is lying supine with head turned either left or right.
  2. Secondly by inhibiting smooth pursuit system due to alcohol effect on ocular

movement via neural mechanism results in horizontal gaze nystagmus (HGN).

IV. Stage of medullary paralysis (>0.5%):

a. Slow, stertorous respiration

b. Cold calmly cyanotic skin,

c. Dilated pupil, abolished reflexes, very weak pulse.

Treatment—acute alcoholic	Treatment—chronic alcoholic
1. 25% dextrose drip	1. Gradual withdrawal of alcohol
2. Inj B₁ (thiamine) 100 mg IM stat followed by once daily till the patient becomes conscious. Then, switch to oral Benalgis (B-complex)	2. **Antabuse: Disulfiram**— it blocks metabolism at acetaldehyde level, gets accumulated and causes untoward symptoms **Dose:** 0.75 gm × 2 days; 0.5 gm × 3–5 days; 0.25 gm × week: 0.125 gm—follow-up dose
3. **Proton pump inhibitor:** Inj pantoprazole/ rabeprazole/ ranitidine	3. **Citrated calcium carbimide (CCC):** Temposil—50 mg— OD
4. Sucralfate—if GIT bleeding	4. Chlorpromazine— 50 mg
5. IV fluids maintenance	5. Diet
6. Respiration is safeguarded by artificial respiration and O₂ inhalation	6. Supportive

Chronic poisoning: Result from continued uses of alcohol and is characterized by **physical, moral and mental deterioration.**

Physical: Lack of personal hygiene, loss of appetite, gastroenteritis, wasting, peripheral neuropathy, fatty changes in liver and heart, impotence and sterility.

Moral: Wide sociological abnormal.

Mental: By dementia, loss of memory, impaired judgement.

Thus, there is GIT disturbance, liver damage with jaundice, ascitis, peripheral neuritis, tremor, insomnia, loss of memory, intermittent infection.

Complication resulting from chronic alcoholism (alcohol withdrawal syndrome)

1. **Delirium tremens:** It is a psychotic condition in chronic alcoholic associated with tremors and hallucination. It is characterized by tremor, convulsions, insomnia, loss of memory, confusion, disorientation, and failure to recognize known things, hallucination and agitated behaviour

   Causes
   i Sudden increase of dose
   ii. Sudden withdrawal
   iii. Injury/infection
   iv. Shock from injury
   v. Exposure to cold

   Treatment
   i. Largactil—100 mg orally
   ii. Meprobamate—2.4 gm daily
   iii. Sedation—phenobarbitone, paraldehyde or chlorpromazine injection is given
   iv. 5% dextrose IV drip, vitamins
   v. Symptomatic

2. **Korsakoff's psychosis:** It is a psychological and neurogenic deranged condition occurring in some alcoholics. It is characterized by hallucinogens, disorientation, multiple neuritis and muscular degeneration, i.e. weakness, wasting and unsteady gait, retrograde amnesia—loss of recent memory.

3. **Acute hallucinosis:** Auditory hallucinogens, delusion of persecution.

4. **Alcoholic confusional insanity:** It is one of the withdrawal problems in chronic alcoholic with disorientation of time and place, hallucinations, delusions and mania/attack.

PM Findings

- Clothes are dirty, torn, soiled with vomitus and earth particle.
  - There may be minor and major external injuries. Visceral organs—congested.
  - Stomach contents—smell of alcohol with mucosa congested, hemorrhagic at places.
  - Lungs and brain are congested and edematous;
- Liver—cirrhotic, fatty.
  - Other signs of hazards of alcohol may be present.

Material Preserved

1. Routine viscera—in saturated solution of common salt. (Rectified spirit—not to be used.)
2. Blood—in sodium fluoride/oxalate.
3. Urine—without any preservatives.

Medicolegal Aspects

1. Alcohol causes death mostly due to the hazards associated with its use.
2. Accidental death—due to inhalation of vomitus or due to adulterated drinks or due to consumption of synergistic drug along with alcohol.
3. Suicide—alcohol is commonly used with other poison to commit suicide. Poisons were also taken under the influence of alcohol.
4. Homicide—for this the poison is mixed with alcohol to mask taste and smell. The person was killed by inflicting fatal injury or by pushing from height or by drowning after making him unconscious/intoxicate by giving alcohol.
5. It is said to be aphrodisiac agents, it increases sex desire but decreases the capacity of sex performance.
6. Used to strengthen the nerve before committing a crime.
7. It may lead to desire to commit a criminal act.

Hazards Associated with Alcohols

1. Vehicular accidents.
2. Fall from height.
3. Electrocution/drowning/burns
4. Choking-café coronary
5. Cooking gas poisoning
6. Death
7. **Saturday night paralysis**—by compression of circumflex nerve. In intoxicated state, the person rests his armpit on the back of his chair. When intoxication is over he suffers from temporary paralysis of his arm.

CHEMICAL TEST

Apply 50 ml of potassium dichromate to filter paper in neck of test tube containing urine.

Heat the test tube for 1 min.

If alcohol is present, color of filter paper changes from orange to green.

DETERMINATION OF BLOOD/ URINE ALCOHOL

1. **Kozelka hine/cavett method**—aeration/distillation method:

$$\text{Alcohol} \xrightarrow[\text{Oxidized}]{\substack{\text{Potassium dichromate or} \\ H_2SO_4}} \text{acetic acid}$$

Each ml of 0.05 N dichromate solution that is reduced in the process is equivalent to 0.575 mg of alcohol.

2. **Gas chromatography**

3. **Alcohol dehydrogenase method**

4. **Breathalyzer**—estimation of blood alcohol concentration (BAC) on breath analyzer is legally admissible as per the section of MV Act, 1988.

Widmark formula—It is used to estimate alcohol absorbed in the body by

- a = CPR , therefore C = a/PR
- R is the constant, for male = 0.68, for female = 0.54,
- C is the blood alcohol concentration (gm/kg), and
- A is the total amount of alcohol in gm absorbed in the body.
- For urine, a = 3/4 qpr, where q is the concentration of alcohol in urine (gm/L)
- **Example:** 70 kg male has consumed 120 ml of 25% proof liquor. What will be the blood alcohol level?
- a = CPR, but proof spirit and density of alcohol (ml/kg) consumed should be considered for calculation.

Therefore,
C = a × proof spirit × density of alcohol/PR
= 120 × 0.428 × 0.8/70 × 0.68 = 86 mg%

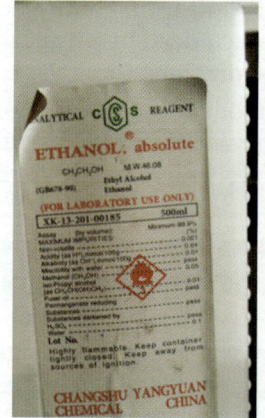
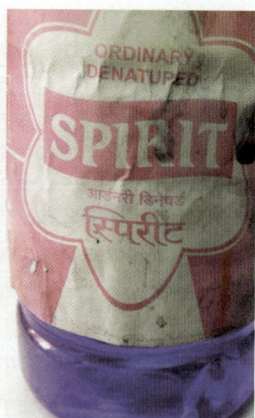

Fig. 11.2: Ethanol and spirit

Methyl alcohol: CH_3OH	Isopropyl alcohol: C_3H_7OH
Synthesized from coke and water. It is a volatile, colorless, flammable liquid with distinct odor similar to ethanol, but highly toxic and unfit for human consumption (Wood naphtha/spirit)	It is a colorless flammable liquid with a strong odor, used in disinfecting pads/hand sanitizers It is 3 times more toxic than methyl alcohol, which is more toxic than ethyl alcohol
Uses 1. Used as industrial solvents 2. With ethanol, used as antiseptic spirit 3. Methylated spirit = Mixture of ethanol + methanol	**Uses** 1. Used as industrial solvents 2. Used as gasoline additive 3. Alternative to formaldehyde as tissue preservatives
Fatal dose: 60–140 ml **Fatal period:** 24–36 hrs	**Fatal dose:** >100 mg% in blood **Fatal period:** A few hours
Action: CNS depression.	**Action:** Cerebral depressant and renal damage as it oxidizes to acetone.
Absorption, distribution, excretion Same as ethanol.	**Absorption, metabolism, excretion** Absorption through mucosa of GIT/RT. Metabolism in liver. A part of it is converted to acetone. Excreted through urine as such or acetone, and small amount through breath.
Clinical features **GIT:** Nausea, vomiting, abdominal pain, dehydration, low BP, collapse, smell present **CNS:** Headache, dizziness, vertigo, muscular pain/weakness, cramp, restlessness, convulsion, coma **Ocular:** Blurring of vision, pupil-dilated and fixed, conjunctiva—congested, blindness **RS:** Dyspnea, death due to respiratory failure	**Clinical features** It causes cerebral depression and drunkenness Nausea, vomiting, abdominal pain, dehydration, low BP, smell present, headache, dizziness • With loss or sluggishness of reflexes • Pupils are constricted in coma • S/o renal damage
Treatment Patient must be hospitalized and kept under close observation 1. Stomach wash with $NaHCO_3$ 2. O_2 inhalation + artificial respiration 3. Eyes—covered and protected 4. Combat acidosis by IV $NaHCO_3$ infusion (2 gm in 250 ml water every 2 hrs) prevents retinal damage and other symptoms. Potassium chloride infusion for hypokalemia due to alkali therapy 5. Circulation should be maintained by amphetamine, fluid or noradrenaline 6. Dehydration—electrolyte balance + sodium bicarbonate given 2 gm orally every 4 hrly 7. Renal failure correction	**Treatment** Stomach wash 1. Symptomatic 2. Protection of the kidneys: • Hemodialysis • Dialysis if renal failure 3. Oxygen therapy to excrete acetone from lungs 4. Fluid replacement if dehydration

Specific antidote of methyl alcohol poisoning

1. Ethanol 100 mg/dl in blood saturates alcohol dehydrogenase and retards methanol metabolism and thereby reduces the rate of generation of toxic metabolite. Ethanol 10% in water is given through nasogastric tube in a loading dose of 0.7 ml/kg followed by 0.15 ml/kg/hr drip
2. Fomepizole is a specific inhibitor of alcohol dehydrogenase, is given in 15 mg/kg IV followed by 10 mg/kg 12 hrly till serum methanol falls below 20 mg/dl

Methyl alcohol	Isopropyl alcohol
PM findings	**PM findings**
• S/o asphyxia with cyanosis and marked PM staining.	• Nothing specific
• Frothing from mouth with presence of smell.	• Visceral organs—congested
• Stomach/intestine—mucosa congested, alcoholic smell present	• Liver/kidneys—congested, edematous
• Lungs/brain—congested and edematous	• Renal degeneration
• Liver—fatty changes	
• Kidney—tubular degeneration	
ML aspects	**ML aspects**
1. Accidental: Most of cases are accidental due to adulteration of alcoholic drink with methylated spirit	1. Accidental—mostly by way of external medicinal use
2. Suicidal and homicidal uses may occur but are not common	2. Suicidal—due to easy availability as it is the main ingredient in many cleaning products

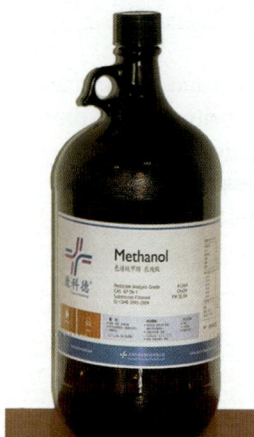 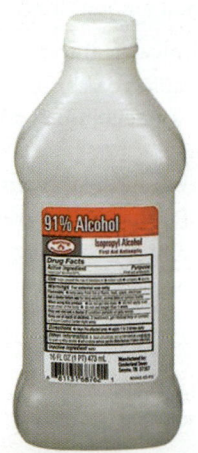
Fig. 11.3: Methanol and isopropyl alcohol

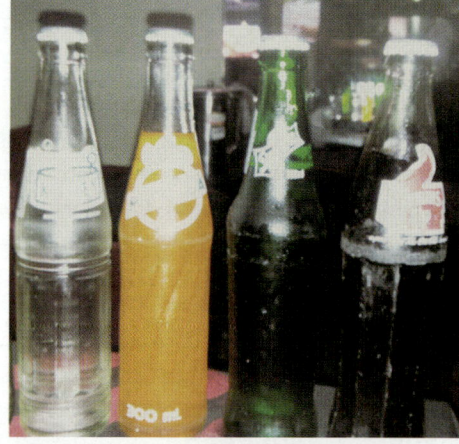
Fig. 11.4: Non-alcoholic beverages

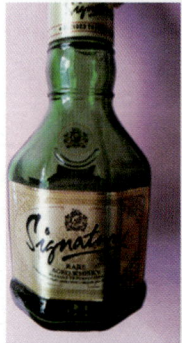 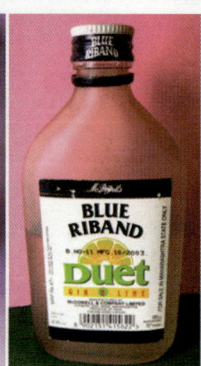 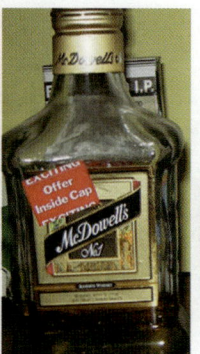 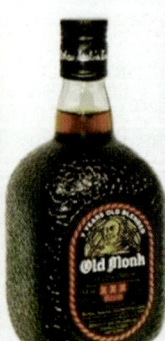 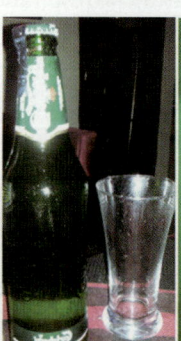 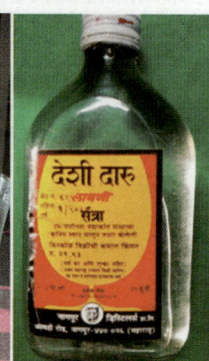
Fig. 11.5: Different types of alcoholic beverages

EXAMINATION OF ALCOHOLIC PERSON

Medical man is often required to examine a person and certify whether the person is under the influence of alcohol or not. So it is examined as per the following proforma:

Examination of Alcoholic

To

The Investigating Officer

PS ....

Ref: Your letter No. ...., dated ....

1. Name: .... Age: ..... Sex: ......

    Address: ....
    ....

2. **Identification marks** (two)

3. **Consent**

    Under Section 53(1) of CrPC: Examination of accused can be carried out by a medical practitioner at the request of police even without his consent and by use of force if necessary.

    Brought by PC: .... No.: .... PS ....
    Date and time of examination: ....
    Place of examination: ....
    Examination in presence of: ....

4. **History** of consumption of alcohol/ medication:

    - Type, duration
    - Consumption of any mouth washes
    - History of diabetes
    - Past history of: Head injury

5. **General behaviour:** Whether polite, excited, hilarious, talkative, carefree, sleepy, cooperative, indifferent, antagonistic, combating, insulting, etc.

    (Polite = Polished; Excited = Agitated, roused emotionally; Hilarious = Very Funny; Talkative = Repeated talk; Carefree; Sleepy; Cooperative; Indifferent = Not very good, uninteresting; Antagonistic = One who straggles with other; Combating = Opposing)

6. **Memory:** Recent event

    - Whether having orientation of time/ place/person.

- Ask a few personal questions and then ask the same at the end of examination.
- Ask about some article/object in the examination room like number of tube light/tables, etc. and then ask the same in the last.

7. **Mental alertness:** Ask simple sums of addition or subtraction and see how much time person will take.

    How quickly the person responds to you and your question during examination.

8. Temp

9. Pulse

10. Resp

11. BP

12. **Skin:** Dry, moist, flushed, pale

13. **Smell of alcohol in breath**

14. **Eye:** Normal, watery, congested, suffused.
    Pupils: Normal, dilated, constricted.
    Reaction to light: Normal, poor.

15. **Gait**

    Balance: Sure, fair, swaying, wobbling, sagging knee, falling other.
    Walk: Sure, fair, swaying, uncertain, staggering to reel.
    Turning: Sure, fair, swaying, uncertain, staggering to reel.
    (Sure = Safe; Fair = Clear; Swaying = Incline from side to side; Wobbling = To move unsteadily from side to side; Sagging knee = To bend; Uncertain = Lacking confidence)

16. **Speech:** Whether fair, slurred, stuttering, confused, incoherent, other.

    (Slurred = Blurred; Stuttering = To speak, say or pronounce with spasmodic repetition of words, especially initial; Confused = Disordered; Incoherent = Loose)

17. **Muscular coordination**

    Finger nose test: Sure, uncertain.
    Picking up coins: Sure, slow, uncertain, unable.

    Unbuttoning and buttoning of shirt.

18. **Handwriting and copying of sentence:** Missing of letters; not in straight line

19. Reflexes: Knee and ankle: Delayed and sluggish.

20. Systemic examination

RS

CVS

P/A

21. Investigation

Blood: Spirit must not be used

Preservatives: 10 mg sod fluoride + 30 mg Potassium oxalate per 10 ml of blood

Urine: 100 ml

Preservatives: 30 mg phenyl mercuric nitrate for 10 ml urine or 5 ml conc. HCl for 200–500 ml urine.

Note: The sample are preserved, sealed and handed over to police on duty at the earliest for chemical analysis.

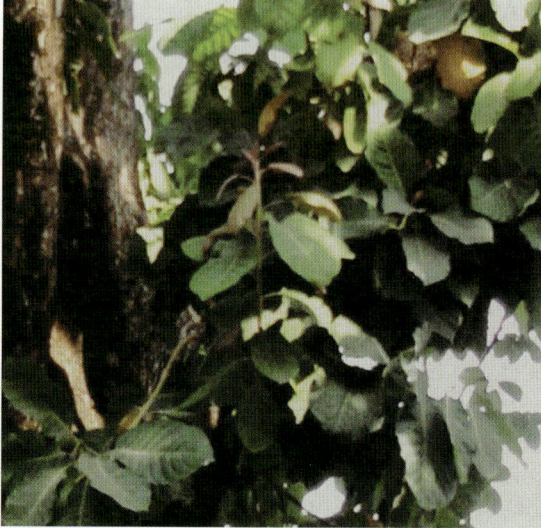

Fig. 11.6: Mohua plant and seeds

Opinion

1. The above person has not consumed alcohol.

2. The above person has consumed alcohol but is not under its influence.

3. The above person has consumed alcohol and is under its influence.

Place .... Signature ....

Date ....

Name of doctor ....

Time ....

Designation ....

Seal ....

But, the opinion whether the person is under or not under the influence of alcohol is purely based on the clinical examination. The signs and symptoms of alcoholism are based on the personal tolerance to alcohol and various other factors. The same amount of alcohol consumed or same BAC (blood alcohol concentration) in two individuals give different clinical manifestation; one may be under influence and other may not be under influence of alcohol. Chemical analysis of the blood in this examination reveals only the amount or concentration of alcohol.

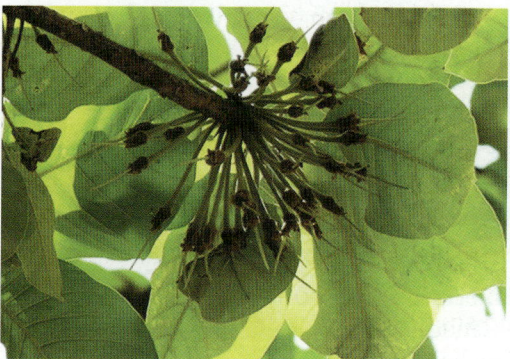

Fig. 11.7: Mohua flower

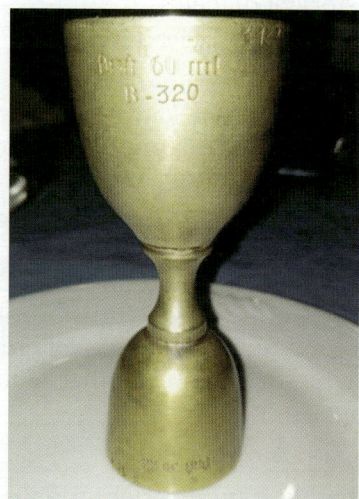

Fig. 11.8: Large and small pegs—measurement

Alcoholic anonymous: It is an association (without having a formed body and place) of people who have given up alcohol. The addicts, who desire to give up alcohol, narrate their bad experiences to other alcoholics through meetings, symposiums, letters, press, etc.

Alcoholic intoxication: It is a state occurring in a person due to consumption of alcohol in a quantity sufficient to loose control of his faculty to such an extent that he is unable to perform his activities.

Drunkenness: It is a condition which results from excessive intake of alcohol and the person concerned is so much under its influence that:

1. He loses control over his mental faculties.
2. He is unable to perform his duties in which he is engaged at a particular time.
3. He may be a source of danger to himself or others.

Features at Different State of Alcohol Consumption

Slight: Flushed face, dilated pupils, euphoric, loss of restraints.

Under the influence: Flushed face, dilated and sluggish pupils, loss of restraints, increase in reaction time, stagger in sudden turning.

Drunk: In addition to the above symptoms, there is staggering gait with reeling and lurching while making sudden turn.

Bombay Prohibition Act

It is the Act (operated in Maharashtra/Gujarat) in relation to drinking, drunkenness, pleas in relation to drinking of nonprohibited preparation and possession of intoxicant. Some important sections of BP Act are as follows:

Sec. 65 and 66(1): Provide penalty for illegal import, export, manufacture, sale, and purchase of an intoxicant without proper license, permit or authorization.

Sec. 62(2): If blood alcohol concentration is not less than 0.05% (50 mg%), then accused person is supposed to prove the cause.

Sec. 84: Provides penalty for being found drunk or drinking in a common drinking place/house or being present for the purpose of drinking. Punishment of ₹ 500.

Sec. 85: Provides punishment for being drunk and disorderly in any public place, street, thoroughfare. Punishment for imprisonment of 1–3 month with or without fine of ₹ 500.

Sec. 129(A): A prohibition officer who has reasonable ground for believing that the person has consumed an intoxicant, is authorised to get such a person medically examined and his blood test for quantitative estimation of alcohol.

Rule 3 of BP Act: Deals with clinical examination and certification of a person by RMP in alleged consumption case.

Rule 4: Provides for the manner of collection of blood and forwarding to CA.

Rule 5: Deals with certificate of test in relation to blood sample examined by the chemical examiner.

Rule 117: Prohibition officer authorized to search any person, article or premises believed to provide evidence of possession of in-toxication.

Rule 121(1): Opens any package and examines any goods and stop and search any vehicle.

Rule 123(1): Seize and detain any articles likely to contain intoxicant.

Rule 123(2): Forward the article to nearest police station for CA.

Sec 117 of motor vehicle Act: Offence to drive/attempt to drive a motor vehicle with any quarter of alcohol in blood.

Blood alcohol concentration (BAC)	
BAC	*Different stages*
0.05%	Changes in special test
0.10%	Stimulation
0.15%	Incoordination
0.2–0.3%	Confusion
0.4%	Stupor
0.5%	Coma
0.6%	Death

If the BAC is 0.1% and above, then person is usually considered to be under the influence.

Formaldehyde	*Kerosene*	*Naphthalene*
40% formaldehyde is formalin. It is colorless, pungent irritating odor	It is a clear liquid formed from hydrocarbons obtained from the fractional distillation of petroleum between 150 and 275°C	**Properties:** White scaly powder which volatiles at room temperature
Uses 1. Preservation of tissue for histopathology 2. Embalming fluid	**Uses** 1. Used as fuels/and solvent in paints, pesticides 2. For preserving yellow phosphorus	**Uses** 1. Moth repellent—as mothballs 2. Deodorant cakes
Action Locally—GIT irritation, and precipitation of protein After absorption it causes systemic acidosis	**Action** Locally—irritation of GIT Systemic—nephrotoxic, neurotoxic, respiratory depression	**Action** The metabolites alpha and beta naphthol and naphthaquinone are powerful hemolytic agents, especially in individual with G6PD deficiency
Absorption, fate, and excretion Absorption through mucosa of GIT/RT After absorption it is changed to formic acid (like in methyl alcohol)	**Absorption, fate, and excretion** Kerosene is poorly absorbed from GIT but there is often aspiration into respiratory tract especially, if child vomits	**Absorption, fate, and excretion** Absorbed through mucosa of GIT. It is metabolized in liver and distributed to visceral organs and excreted in urine
Fatal dose: 30–90 ml	**Fatal dose:** 30 ml	**Fatal dose:** 2–5 gm
Fatal period: Within 24 hrs	**Fatal period:** Not fixed	**Fatal period:** Uncertain
Clinical features GIT—nausea, vomiting, diarrhea, abdominal pain, followed by death due to shock In diluted form, after absorption it produces systemic acidosis and other features like in methyl alcohol poisoning When vapor is inhaled—it causes bronchitis, pneumonitis	**Clinical features** Nausea, vomiting, diarrhea, abdominal pain, smell of kerosene in breath, headache, giddiness, dizziness, confusion, convulsion, coma, death Respiratory failure, glycosuria, proteinuria, pneumonitis, pulmonary edema	**Clinical features** General—nausea, vomiting, abdominal pain, fever, confusion, convulsion Hemolytic manifestation—pallor, weakness, jaundice, cyanosis, and dark urine (hemoglobinuria) with increase WBC count, fragmented RBC, anisopoikilocytosis, Heinz bodies Chronic exposure leads to aplastic anemia, hepatic neurosis and jaundice
Treatment 1. Stomach wash: 0.1% ammonia solution and sodium bicarbonate solution 2. Demulcent 3. Antidote: Sodium bicarbonate IV infusion	**Treatment** 1. Stomach wash: Sodium bicarbonate with precaution to avoid aspiration 2. Artificial respiration and O_2 inhalation 3. Liquid paraffin—250 mg oral 4. Symptomatic: Steroids, pantoprazole, IV fluids, antibiotics	**Treatment** 1. Stomach wash and emesis 2. Avoid demulcent 3. Treat hemolysis with blood transfusion, packed/red cell transfusion or exchange transfusion

PM findings

Stomach: Mucosa—inflamed; Wall—hard and leathery; Content—formalin smell present

Adjacent organs: Also becomes hard and inflamed due to the transudation of formalin through stomach

Lungs/brain: Congested, edematous

Liver/kidneys: Shows fatty degeneration

ML aspects

1. Suicidal: Rarely
2. Homicidal: Not occur
3. Accidental: Mostly

PM findings

On opening the body cavities— smell of kerosene present.

Stomach: Mucosa—inflamed; Wall—soft; Content—kerosene smell present

Organs: Congested

Kidneys: Degenerative changes

Lungs: Congested, edematous, pneumonitis

ML aspects

1. Suicidal: Some cases are recorded
2. Homicidal: Not occur
3. Accidental: Mostly in children

PM findings

Not specific

Stomach: Mucosa—inflamed; Wall—soft; Content—naphthalene particle with peculiar smell present

Organs: Congested

Kidneys: Hemorrhagic on cut section

Lungs: Congested, edematous

ML aspects

1. Suicidal: Rarely
2. Homicidal: Not occur
3. Accidental: Mostly in children

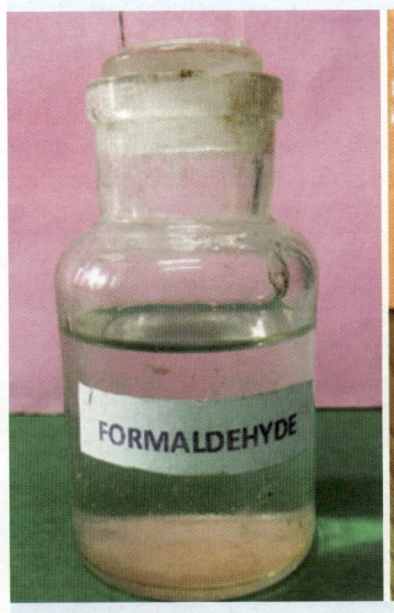

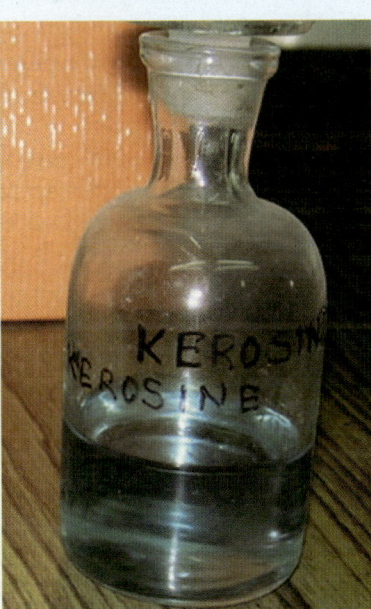

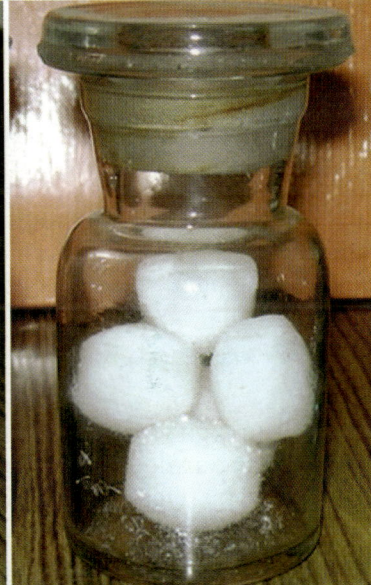

12

Deliriant Poisons: Datura, Cannabis and Cocaine

Deliriants are the substance, which causes delirium, means great excitement and ecstasy. The poisons in this group are characterized by well marked stage of delirium. Delirium is an acutely disordered state of mind involving incoherent speech, hallucination and frenzied excitement, occurring in intoxication, fever, metabolic states, etc. Important examples are datura, cannabis, and cocaine. However, cocaine is actually CNS stimulant, but it is commonly used to include it among the deliriants.

DATURA

Common Name

Jimson weed, thorn apple, stinkweed.

Family: Solanaceae.

Plant: Characteristics

Datura stramonium—grows in Himalayan altitudes.

Datura fustuosa—grows on plains all over India.

There are two varieties of *Datura fustuosa*—niger (with purple flowers), and alba (with white flowers) (Figs 12.1 and 12.2).

Toxic part: All parts of the plant are toxic, but maximum concentration is in the seeds present in the fruit commonly called 'Thorn Apple', which is spherical in shaped having multiple spikes on the surface and containing about 400–500 seeds. The white or purple color flowers are tubular in shape.

Datura seeds: Odorless, bitter taste, yellowish brown, larger and thicker than chilly, kidney shaped, rough surface, have two ridges on their convex surface, on dissection embryos are curved outward near hilum (Fig. 12.3).

Seeds: These are similar to chilly (capsicum) seeds, but are very bitter to taste. Points of differences are shown in Table 12.1.

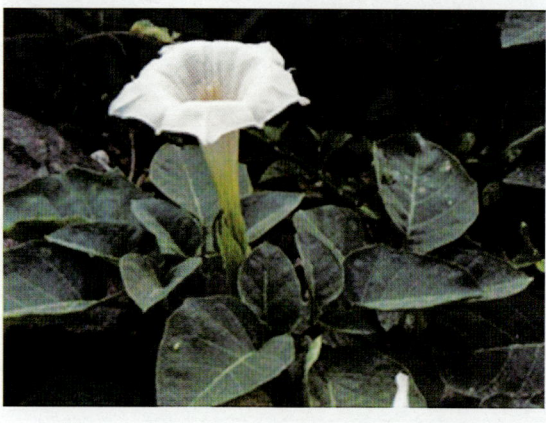

Fig. 12.1: *Datura fustuosa*—white flower

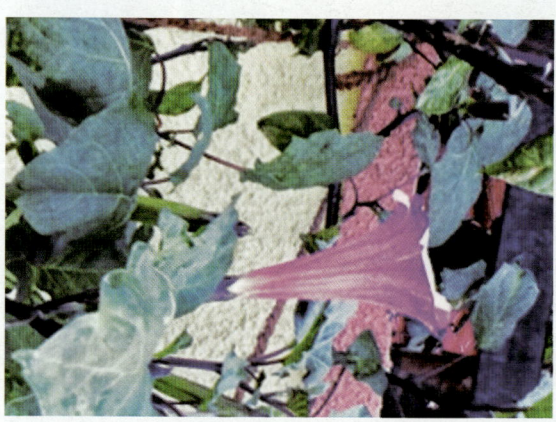

Fig. 12.2: *Datura fustuosa*—purple flower

Table 12.1: Difference between seeds of Datura and capsicum (chilly)

Points	Datura	Chilly
1. Odor	Odorless	Pungent
2. Taste	Bitter Irritating	Burning
3. Color	Yellowish/ brown	Pale yellow
4. Size	Larger	Smaller
5. Thickness	Thick	Thin
6. Shape	Kidney	Round
7. Surface	Rough	Smooth
8. Ridge on convex surface	Two ridges	No ridge
9. On cut section	Embryo curved outward	Embryo curved inward

Capsicum seeds: Pungent irritating smell, burning irritating taste, pale yellow, smaller and thinner, roundish, smooth surface, no double ridges on the margins, on dissection embryos are curved inward near hilum (Fig. 12.4).

Active Principles

- Hyoscine (scopolamine)
- Hyoscyamine
- Atropine.

Uses

1. Atropine as one of the active principle is used as medicine in:
   a. Antidote for organophosphates and carbamates poisoning.
   b. Pre-anesthetic medication.
   c. Mydriatic.
   d. Antispasmodic.
2. Datura seeds powder is used as kicking agent in the alcohol.
3. The seeds are also used in preparing *sui* (needle) from *Abrus precatorius* seeds.

Fatal Dose

Atropine—50–60 mg, hyoscine—10 mg.
   Seeds—75–100 seeds, for stupying uses—40–50 seeds.

Fatal Period

24 hrs.

Absorption, Metabolism, and Excretion

- It is absorbed through mucosa of GIT/RT.
- Metabolized in liver (atropine is destroyed by enzyme atropinase).
- Excreted through urine.
- Atropine is retained for long periods in dead bodies.

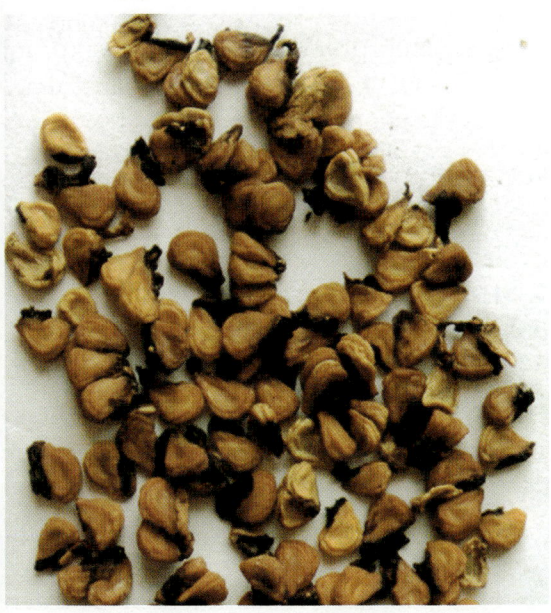

Fig. 12.3: Datura seeds

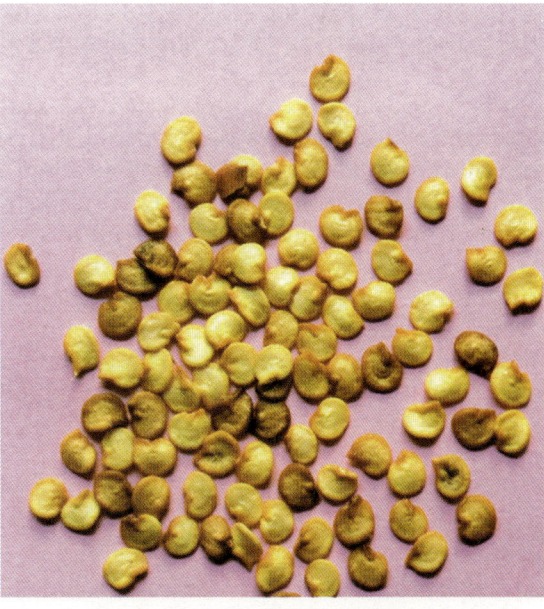

Fig. 12.4: Capsicum seeds

Action

- It blocks the ACh receptor and thus produces sympathomimetic or parasympatholytic action.
- CNS—it first stimulates and then depresses.

Clinical Manifestation

The alkaloids of datura stimulate the higher centers of the brain and then the motor centers. Thus, they inhibit secretion, dilate the cutaneous blood vessels, dilate the pupils and stimulate the heat regulating center. The initial stimulation is followed by depression and paralysis of the vital centers in the medulla.

The symptoms are classically described as classic phrase—**dry as a bone, red as a beet, blind as a bat, hot as a hare, and mad as a wet hen.**

There is bitter taste in mouth, difficulty in speech/deglutition, vomiting, abdominal pain. Body temperature is raised and **skin is dry** and hot due to inhibition of sweat secretion and stimulation of heat regulating centers **(hot as a hare)**. Face is flushed due to dilatation of cutaneous blood vessels **(red as a beet)**. Conjunctiva congested, pupils are dilated, insensitivity to light, blurring/double vision **(blind as a bat)**. Pulse is rapid, respiration is hurried. This is followed by giddiness, staggering gait, incoordination of muscle.

The mind is affected, first restless and confused, later becomes delirious, talkative and mutters indistinct words **(mad as a hen)**. This is followed by mania, convulsion, delirium and hallucination (visual/auditory). The person tries to run away from the bed, picks up bed sheets, grasp imaginary object, draws imaginary threads from tip of finger and threads imaginary needles. This excitation phase is followed by depressive phase, where the person is in deep sleep/coma, respiratory depression and death.

Thus, the main features can better be summarized under 9 Ds mistaken for drunkenness:

1. Dryness of mouth/throat, nausea, vomiting.
2. Difficulty in talking.
3. Dysphagia.
4. Dilated pupils, diplopia.
5. Dry, hot skin.
6. Drunken gait (ataxia).
7. Delirium, with confusion, agitation, and hallucinations.
8. Drowsiness leading to coma.
9. Dysuria (urinary retention).

Death is due to respiratory failure or cardiac arrhythmias.

Thus, the clinical picture is like anti-cholinergic poisoning.

Treatment

1. Stomach wash
2. Purgatives
3. Antidotes:
   a. Physostigmine—0.5 mg IV/IM, 1–2 hrly, relives both cerebral and peripheral symptoms (usually preferred). OR
   b. Neostigmine (2.5 mg IV every 3 hourly), or pilocarpine nitrate (6–15 mg SC) relives only peripheral symptoms. OR
   c. Morphine—15 mg SC, but not given due to its depressant action on brain.
4. Symptomatic:
   a. Inj chlorpromazine (50–100 mg) or inj diazepam, if patient is violent.
   b. Cold sponging.

Postmortem Findings

- Not specific.
- Signs of asphyxia.
- **Stomach:** Broken seeds of datura.
- Visceral organs are congested.
- Datura resists putrefaction and found even in decomposed bodies.

Medicolegal Aspect

1. **Accidental:** While using for other purposes, mistaken with capsicum seeds usually by children, adulterated country liquor/toddy (mixed with datura seeds powder, chloral hydrate for kicking effect).

2. **Suicidal:** Mostly reported from rural areas.

3. **Homicidal:** Extremely rare.

4. **Stupefaction:** Prior to robbery, kidnapping or rape. The seeds are crushed and mixed with food, tea, drink, paan, prasad and given to unwary travellers by co-passengers. When given it produces confusion, agitation, disorientation, and loss of consciousness, thereby facilitating robbery or rape (Figs 12.5 to 12.7).

Children may be easily kidnapped by giving them candy or sweet mixed with datura. They follow all the instructions of the person (who gave these sweet) to follow him. Likewise, women have been abducted, robbed or raped.

5. **Aphrodisiac agent:** To increase sexual desire.

Chemical Test

If a drop of stomach content (having Datura) is put in rabbit's eye, then there is dilatation of pupil.

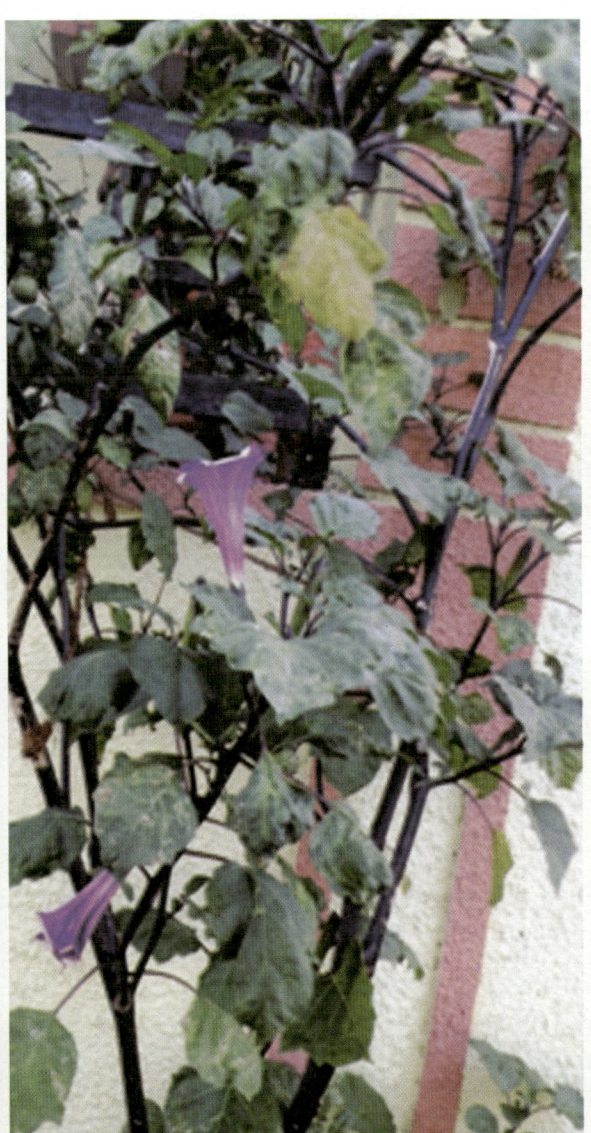

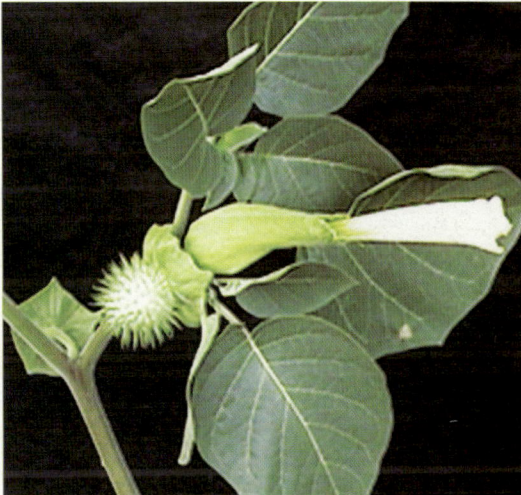

Fig. 12.6: *Datura fustuosa*—alba variety

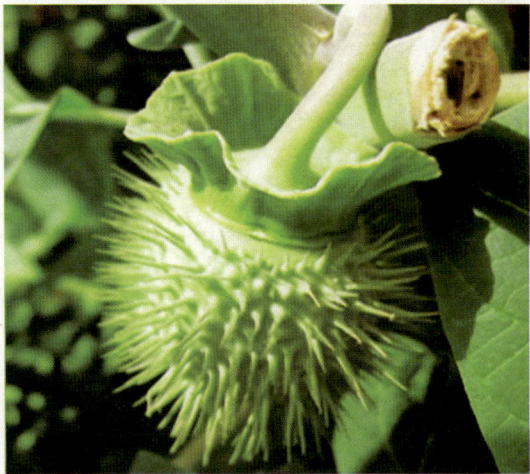

Fig. 12.5: *Datura fustuosa*—niger variety

Fig. 12.7: Thorn apple—Datura fruit (alba)

Cannabis	*Cocaine (Erythroxylum)*
Common name: Indian hemp	**Common names:** Coke, snow, cadillac, white lady
Family: Cannabaceae	**Family:** Erythroxylaceae

Plant: Characteristics

Cannabis sativa is having two varieties

C. indica—grows all over India.

C. mexicana—grows in Mexico.

The term cannabis refers to the flowering and fruiting tops of Cannabis plant. Cannabis is a tall weed growing up to 15 feet in height and it is a dioecious plant, i.e. the sexes are separated. But its cultivation and marketing is under strict legislation and control under government.

Toxic part: All part is toxic. It is a drug of dependence and consumed in different preparation containing different concentration of **active principle,** namely **Tetrahydrocannabinol (THC)**

Plant: Characteristics

Cocaine is an alkaloid, extracted from the leaves of the coca tree, namely ***Erythroxylum coca*** and *E. novograna-tense*. They grow in mountains of South America, Indonesia, and India.

Cocaine is the strongest **drug of psychological** dependence but also causes strong **physical dependence** that makes it a notorious drug of addiction. The synthetic variety of the drug is non-addicting but has acute toxic effects. Cocaine is usually abused by nasal insufflations (snorting or sniffing), but it can also be smoked, ingested, or injected intravenously

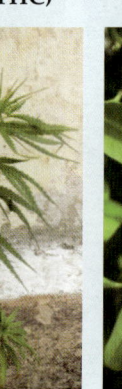

Fig. 12.8: Cannabis plant

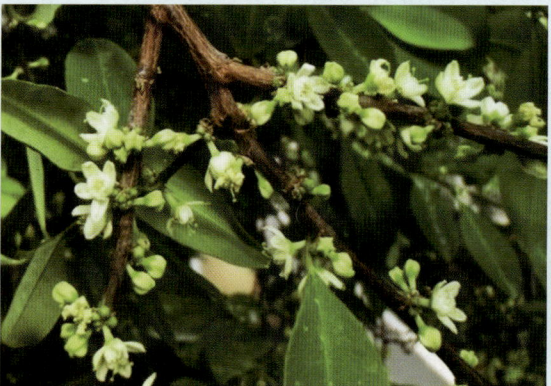

Fig. 12.9: *Erythroxylum coca* (cocaine plant)

Cannabis is a drug of abuse, being particularly popular among sanyasis and sadhus, Western musicians and painters, and college going youth, however, physical dependence is not common

Cocaine is usually abused by the upper classes of society to enhance self-image or improve professional performance

Common preparations of cannabis and concentration of THC in brackets

1. **Bhang:** (Siddi/patti) prepared from dried leaves and stem (2–5% THC)
2. **Majun:** Sweetmeat preparation of bhang
3. **Ganja:** Prepared from flowering tops of female plant (5–10%)
4. **Charas/hashish:** It is resinous exudate from stem and leaves. It is dark green or brown-colored powder (25–40%)

Cocaine: Cocaine can be **synthesised** in the laboratory, and is often sold as **crack**, which is a smokable form obtained by combining cocaine hydrochloride with baking soda and water, followed by heating and drying

Cocaine occurs as white, shiny crystalline odorless substance with a bitter, numbing taste. It is sparingly soluble in water

Ganja is smoked either as it is or mixed with tobacco in a pipe/hookah/chilam or in the form of cigarette. The cigarette preparation of ganja is called '**Reefer**'. When ganja is smoked in a pipe, then it is called **Marijuana** (marihuana, mary jane, pot, weed, grass)

There is a characteristic **odor** like that of a **burnt rope** to all cannabis preparations, especially to the smokable forms

Cannabis	Cocaine
Uses At present, cannabis is a banned drug in India and most parts of the world 1. **Antiemetic** against nausea and vomiting induced by anticancer drugs 2. Possible role in the treatment of convulsions, anxiety, pain, and inflammation	**Uses** 1. Medicinally used as local **anesthetic agent** in minor surgery/procedures 2. **Brompton's cocktail:** It contains cocaine, morphine, chlorpromazine, and alcohol. It was previously popular as a pain reliever in terminal cancer 3. Used as a snuff to reduce appetite and feeling of fatigue 4. Used as aphrodisiac and as a pleasant intoxicant

Fatal dose: Very high, fatality is uncommon
    Charas—2 gm; Ganja—8 gm
    Bhang—10 gm/kg body weight
Fatal period: 12 hours to a few days
	Fatal dose
	    Oral—1.5 gm
	    Injection—1 gm (hypodermic injection 40 mg)
	    Fatal period: A few min to 2 hrs

Absorption, fate, and excretion
    Absorbed through mucosa of GIT and also through RT when smoked
    Metabolized in liver
    Excreted through urine, feces, bile
	Absorption, fate, and excretion
	    Absorbed through mucosa of GIT/RT/nose (when used as snuff)
	    Metabolized in liver
	    Excreted through urine

Action 1. It is a **hallucinogen** causes excitement followed by sleep 2. CNS—stimulant	**Action** 1. It is a strong **amino-oxidase inhibitor** and potentiator of effects of adrenaline or noradrenaline 2. CNS—stimulant and local anesthetic

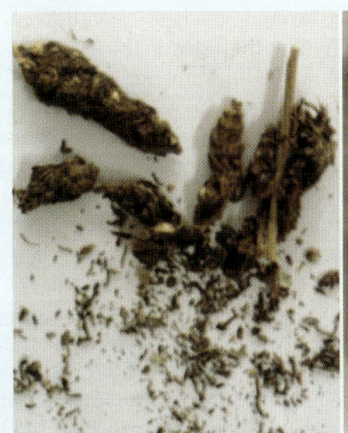

Fig. 12.10: Ganja

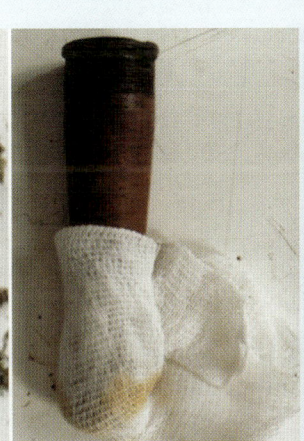

Fig. 12.11: Chilam

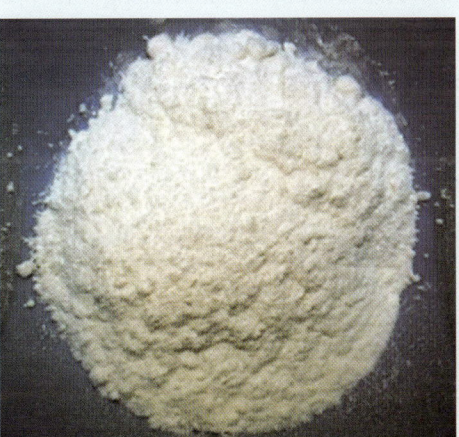

Fig. 12.12: Cocaine powder

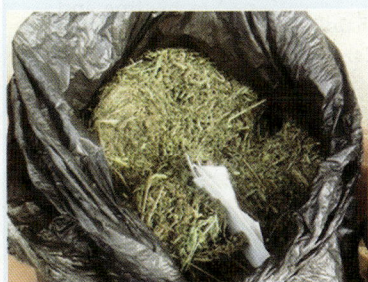

Fig. 12.13: Bhang

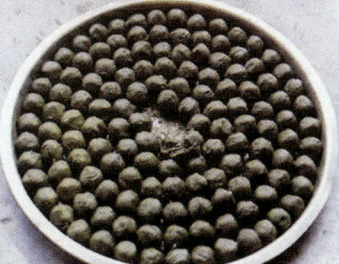

Fig. 12.14: Majun

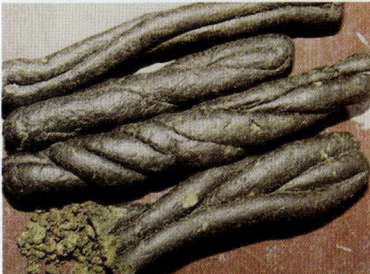

Fig. 12.15: Charas

Clinal features: Cannabis

Generally considered, cannabis is not very toxic and fatal. It is a hallucinogen. In acute poisoning, it causes excitement followed by sleep. The overall signs and symptoms depends on:

1. Personality of the subject
2. Whether accustomed or not
3. Environment at the time of consumption
4. Route of administration, inhalation is associated with more pronounced effects than ingestion

Acute poisoning: The manifestations are grouped into two stages

a. Stage I: Stage of excitement/euphoria and release of inhibition

- Sense of well-being, excitement, euphoria, talkativeness, **uncontrollable laugh,** marked increase in appetite specially sweet, craving for sleep, purposeless muscular movement and **visual hallucination and ideas** (sees nude beautiful women dancing before him, playing music, and singing amorous songs)
- **Motor incoordination,** tachycardia, conjunctival congestion, miosis
- There may be vomiting along with **disorientation** of time, place and person and gradually patient passes to next stage

b. Stage II: Stage of narcosis

- It is characterized by giddiness, confusion and ataxia. The person is in **dreamy state,** with frightful hallucination and delirium. Sometimes there is development of homicidal tendency or thanatophobia
- There is **tingling and numbness** of skin or generalized anesthesia and becomes deeply narcotized
- Characteristic **(burnt rope) odor,** if the drug has been used for smoking. Intravenous use can cause headache, vertigo, dyspnea, diplopia, hypotension, and renal failure
- Usually recovery occurs after a deep sleep, and death if occur, is due to respiratory failure

Clinical features: Cocaine

Acute poisoning

Initially there is a sense of well-being, euphoria with excitement, restlessness, increases reflexes **with increase in the BP, heart rate, and respiratory rate.**

There may be sudden rise of temperature with rigor **(cocaine fever),** dryness of mouth, dysphagia, tingling and numbness of tongue/mouth.

Pupils—dilated, pulse—weak, irregular, BP—fall, Respiration—shallow, gasping with profuse sweating, and cold calmy skin

There may be hallucination, muscle twitching, tremor, and convulsion, followed by loss of reflexes, collapse, coma and death

Body packer: The smuggler smuggled **contraband drugs (mostly cocaine/ heroin and amphetamines, hashish and marijuana),** across international border in specially devised packages in the carrier's rectum, vagina or alimentary canal. Typically the drug is wrapped in several layers of latex by using condoms, gloves or even toy balloons. **Up to 214 packages have been found in a single "mule"** means 'potli or sack containing packages'. The packages, which are round or oval of 1–2 cm in diameter, usually contain 3–7 gms of narcotics

The smugglers are termed "packer", "swallowers" or "stuffers". On arrival at their destination, they check into their hideout, self-administer cathartics, and defecate the ingested packets of cocaine. Sometimes rectal suppositories or disposable enemas are used. Sometimes the packing may **burst,** leading to overdose, collapse and acute poisoning (cacaine **body packers syndrome/minipacker syndrome)**

Diagnosis of an asymptomatic body packer can be accomplished with the help of an abdominal **X-ray, ultrasound, or CT scan.** The last two methods should be resorted to only if X-ray is unclear. In some cases, fecal examination over a period of a few days may be necessary. **Water soluble iodinated contrast material** has been given orally to confirm or exclude body packages

---

Chronic cannabis poisoning: Seen in person who consumed for long period with the development of strong psychological dependence

- There is **general loss of weight/appetite,** weakness, emaciation, tremor, impotence
- There is **mental and moral deterioration/ degradation,** insanity and sometimes person turns violent and may **'run amok',** who go on killing person who comes in his way to either surrender or killing himself ultimately. The person suffers from some **hallucination or delusion** of

Chronic cocaine poisoning: Cocainism/cocainomania— Immediately upon intake, there is euphoria (rush), followed about an hour or so later by rebound depression (crash). To get rid of the unpleasant effects of the later, the individual feels compelled to take the drug again, and the vicious cycle continues until physical, financial, or drug resources are exhausted

Features

- There is **loss of weight/ appetite,** weakness, tremors, impotence, insomnia, and emaciation

persecution/infidelity, due to which the patient is overpowered by an irresistible impulse to destroy life and property

- **Amotivational syndrome:** Chronic abusers of cannabis gradually become lethargic, apathetic with lack of interest and concentration
- **Hashish insanity:** Chronic, heavy abuse of cannabis causes paranoid psychosis with violent behaviour, culminating in homicide or suicide (running amok)
- **Increased susceptibility to** pharyngitis, bronchitis, asthma, and gynecomastia (in males)

- There is **mental and moral degradation.** There is degeneration of CNS with development of dementia and may get involved in crimes
- **Psychosis:** There is **tactile hallucination** with feeling of insects crawling on the skin, or of sand lying under the skin **(cocaine bugs, Magnan's syndrome).** The person may suffer from dreadful hallucination and delusion of persecution and melancholia
- **Sexual perversion** in males and erotic tension/nymphomania in females is a characteristic feature of chronic cocaine takers
- There is **blackish pigmentation of tongue and teeth,** perhaps due to the action of saliva and lime on cocaine when **taken orally,** and ulceration/**perforation of nasal septum when cocaine is sniffed**

Treatment of acute poisoning Cannabis

1. Stomach wash with warm water, in case the drug has been ingested, and purgatives
2. Artificial respiration
3. Antidotes—no specific antidotes
4. Supportive:
   - Strong tea/coffee by oral or per rectum
   - Haloperidol or other antipsychotic for psychosis
   - Maintenance of nutrition and
   - Hypodermic injection of strychnine

Death occurs due to hazards like:
a. Inhalation of vomitus
b. Accidents—injury, electrocution, drowning, etc. when the person takes cannabis

Treatment of acute poisoning—cocaine

1. Stomach wash with activated charcoal when ingested
2. Antidote: Amyl nitrite inhalation
3. Artificial respiration and O_2 inhalation
4. Symptomatic/supportive:
   - Benzodiazepines or barbiturates for restlessness and convulsions
   - Haloperidol or other antipsychotic for psychosis, and
   - Ice bath for hyperthermia
5. For cardiac irritability:
   a. Vagal stimulant—acetylcholine HCl 1 mg IV or carbachol 0.25 mg IV
   b. Inhibit cholinesterase enzyme—100 mg procainamide IV
   c. Slow injection of dilute phenoxybenzamine 10 mg has antiadrenaline action
   d. Propranolol for hypertension; death due to respiratory failure or cardiac arrest

Treatment in bodypacker syndrome (cocaine)

1. Asymptomatic patients: It should be treated by **whole bowel irrigation with polythylene glycol** solution. However, polythylene glycol can dissolve the heroin from a package, rupturing it and increasing absorption of heroin. Hence, **low-volume phosphosoda enemas or high-volume saline enemas** are given when all packages pass into the colon from the stomach. Food ingestion must not be permitted until all packages have moved into the colon. **Metoclopramide 10 mg,** 8 hourly, may be administered to encourage gastric emptying. It may be advisable to **empty the rectum first by a bisacodyl suppository**

2. Symptomatic patients: It must be managed with specific drugs, activated charcoal, and whole bowel irrigation. Intestinal perforation or obstruction by packets requires surgical intervention

Treatment of chronic poisoning

Gradual withdrawal of the drug
Diazepam for anxiety
Antipsychotics for psychosis; Psychotherapy

Treatment of chronic poisoning

Gradual withdrawal of the drug
Psychotherapy

PM findings
Not specific
Suggestive of asphyxia

PM findings
Acute poisoning: Nothing specific
Suggestive of asphyxia and cardiac dilatation
Cerebral and pulmonary edema
Generalized visceral congestion
Chronic poisoning: Evidence of nasal erosions,
ulceration, or perforation (in "snorters"). Nasal
swabs must be taken for chemical analysis

Medicolegal aspects
1. Accidental: Mostly due to overindulgence. It is
   a drug of addiction commonly used by sadhus
   and pujaris
2. Suicidal: Rare
3. Homicidal: Rare
4. Stupefying: Used prior to robbery, kidnapping or
   rape
5. The person committing a crime under this
   condition will not be held responsible for the act
   under Section 84 IPC
6. Abrupt stoppage after habitual use can result in
   a mild withdrawal reaction characterized by
   restlessness, insomnia, anorexia, and nausea

Medicolegal aspects
1. Suicidal: Not used
2. Homicidal: Not popular
3. Accidental: Due to overdose from its intradermal/
   urethral or other uses as a drug of abuse/addiction
   (causes both **psychological** and **physical
   dependence**)
4. Aphrodisiac: Increases the duration of sex
   performance when used locally by causing
   desensitization of the glans penis
5. To improve professional performance

13

Cerebral Depressant

Cerebral depressant are the drugs which causes CNS depression. These are sleep inducing drugs like sedative and hypnotic. It includes barbiturates, benzodiazepines, bromide, chloral hydrate, paraldehyde, etc.

Barbiturates

It is the derivative of barbituric acid (malonylurea)

Uses: Medicinal uses in:
1. Psychiatric disorder
2. Epilepsy/seizure disorder (grand mal)
3. Strychnine poisoning
4. For induction and maintenance of general anesthesia (when given IV)
5. IV thiopentone—used as truth serum in narcoanalysis

Classification: According to duration of action
a. Long acting barbiturates (6–12 hrs): Mephobarbitone, phenobarbitone
b. Intermediate acting (3–6 hrs): Amobarbitone, aprobarbitone, butobarbitone
c. Short acting (<3 hrs): Hexobarbitone, pentobarbitone
d. Ultrashort acting (<15–20m): Thiopentone sodium

Benzodiazepines

–

Uses: Medicinal uses in:
1. Insomnia
2. Epilepsy/seizure disorder
3. Anxiety disorders
4. Also used as sedatives and hypnotics displacing the barbiturates

Classification
A. Major tranquilizers:
 1. Phenothiazine derivatives
  • Chlorpromazine (largactil)
  • Thioridazine (thioryl)
 2. Butophenone derivatives: Haloperidol, carbamazepine, tegritol
B. Minor tranquilizers:
 1. Benzodiazepine derivatives:
  • Benzodiazepines: Diazepam, lorazepam
  • Alprazolam
 2. Chlordiazepoxide (librium)

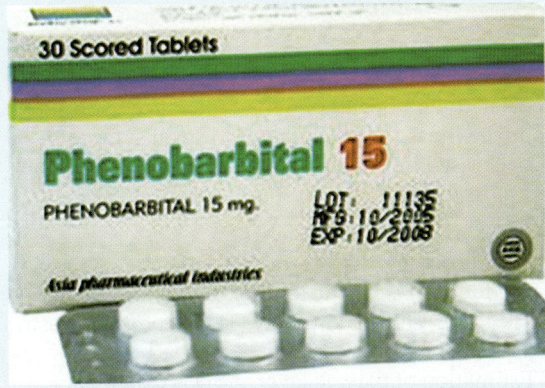

Fig. 13.1: Phenobarbitone

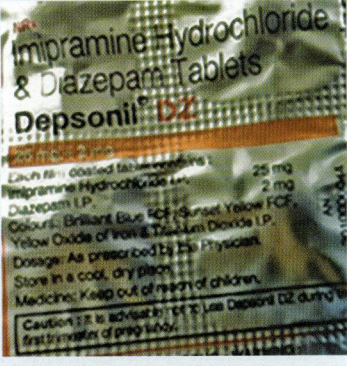

Fig. 13.2: Diazepam and alprazolam tablets

Barbiturates	Benzodiazepines
Fatal dose: 4–5 gm **Fatal period:** 1–2 days	**Fatal dose:** 5–10 gm/variable **Fatal period:** 1–2 days
Absorption, fate, and excretion Absorption: Through GIT Distribution: Equally in all tissues as also in red cells and plasma Metabolism: Detoxified in liver by oxidation and dealkylation Excreted: Slowly in urine up to a week. The rate of excretion reduces in presence of liver and renal disease	**Absorption, fate, and excretion** Absorption: Through GIT Distributed: In all tissue Metabolism: Metabolized extensively in liver by different microsomal enzyme systems Excreted: Through urine
Action 1. CNS depressant, main site being midbrain 2. Sedative, hypnotic, anticonvulsant and anesthetic action 3. Synergistic action of barbiturates with • Sedatives/hypnotics/tranquilizers • Anticonvulsants • Antipyretic, analgesics, antihistaminic • Alcohol Alcohol + barbiturates: Causes dangerous coma Chlorpromazine + barbiturates: Potentiates the effect Their effect depends on type, dose, combination, absorption and weight of the patient	**Action** 1. CNS depressant: Act by stimulating the gamma-aminobutyric acid-B (GABA-B) receptors, thereby opening the chloride ion channel resulting in the increased conduction of chloride ion across the nerve cell membrane. This lowers the potential difference between the interior and exterior of the cell, blocking the ability of the cell to conduct nerve impulses
Clinical features With therapeutic doses, it results in sleep and sometimes confusion so that the person takes more drugs **(barbiturate automatism)** **Acute poisoning** • Headache, confusion • Giddiness, flaccid limbs, areflexia • Ataxia, slurred speech, stupor • Diplopia and pupils shows **alternate constriction and dilatation**, nystagmus • Later face is congested, respiration is slow, BP fall, and skin is cold, with blister/bullae on skin **(barbiturate blister)** • There is oliguria, albuminuria and coma	**Clinical features** With therapeutic doses, it results in sleep and feels relaxed **Acute poisoning** • Nausea, headache • Giddiness, dizziness • Ataxia, weakness • Diplopia, nystagmus • Followed by amnesia, vertigo, slurred speech, lethargy, coma with fall of BP and respiration • Sometimes there may be restlessness, agitation and hallucination
Chronic poisoning Lack of interest and concentration, vertigo, tremor, ataxia, hallucination and barbiturate blisters. Abrupt stoppage is associated with withdrawal symptoms characterized by anorexia, insomnia, headache, tremor, cramps, seizures, and delerium	**Chronic poisoning** It is due to chronic user of benzodiazepines and is associated with development of tolerance. Abrupt stoppage is associated with withdrawal symptoms characterised by anxiety, insomnia, headache, tremor, and paresthesia
Diagnosis: Barbiturates 1. Gas chromatography (GC) can be used to analyse urine level of barbiturate 2. Thin layer chromatography (TLC)—of urine, gastric aspirate or other residue 3. High pressure liquid chromatography is also useful	**Diagnosis:** Benzodiazepines (BD) 1. Gas chromatography—mass spectrometry can be used to analyse urine level of BD 2. Thin layer chromatography (TLC)—of urine, gastric aspirate or other residue 3. Estimation of plasma level of BD is usually not necessary

Treatment
1. Maintain respiration by: Foot end raised, suction of airway, artificial respiration and O₂ inhalation, tracheostomy or endotracheal intubation
2. Maintain circulation: Methyl amphetamine HCl –10 mg dose, IV infusion of noradrenaline 2 mg IV drip, IV fluid and electrolyte; coramine 5–10 ml IV drip
3. Antidote: Not specific
4. **Forced alkaline diuresis** (with soda bicarb –1 mg/kg IV with or without mannitol/ frusemide) **and dialysis**
5. Stomach wash with activated charcoal (if patient is not in coma)
6. Emesis and purgatives
7. Symptomatic:
   Cerebral stimulants: **Bemigrid 50 mg IV, daptazol 15 mg IV, antibiotic**

Treatment
1. Maintain respiration by: Suction of airway, artificial respiration and O₂ inhalation, tracheostomy or endotracheal intubation
2. Correction of hypotension with dopamine or levarterenol
3. **Antidote: Flumazenil**—it is quite effective in reversing the coma. Dose: 1 mg slow IV or series of smaller doses beginning with 0.2 mg and increasing by 0.1 to 0.2 mg every min until total dose of 3.5 mg is reached
4. IV fluids
5. Stomach wash with activated charcoal (if <6–12 hrs)
6. Emesis and purgatives
7. Symptomatic:
   In chronic poisoning: Phenobarbitone is used. However, replacement of short half life BD (alprazolam) with long half life BD (clonazepam) is recommended before tapering and final discontinuation of BD. For acute somatic symptoms in withdrawal of BD, propranolol is used

PM findings
- Suggestive of asphyxia, cyanosis
- Froth at mouth/nostril
- Visceral organs—congested
- Lungs and brain are congested and edematous with punctate hemorrhages
- Bronchopneumonia
- Stomach—parts of tablet may be present, mucosa may be congested, erosion present
- **Barbiturate blisters**—on the buttocks, inner and posterior aspect of thigh and forearms

PM findings
- Suggestive of asphyxia
- Froth at mouth/nostril
- Visceral organs—congested
- Lungs and brain are congested and edematous
- Stomach—parts of tablet may be present, mucosa may be congested

ML aspects
1. Suicidal—ideal, mostly used
2. Homicidal—rare
3. Accidental—due to overdose/or automatism, abuse, due to drug addiction. (Marilyn Monroe was addicted to alcohol and barbiturate and was found dead at home following an overdose of barbiturate

ML aspects
1. In spite of having wide safety margin, death has been reported even in unexpectedly low dose of BD
2. It is used deliberately to induce amnesia in order to accomplish an illegal or immoral act **(Date rape)**
3. Accidental—due to overdose or abuse

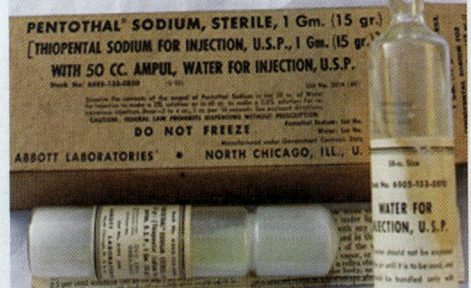

Fig. 13.3: Thiopentone sodium injection

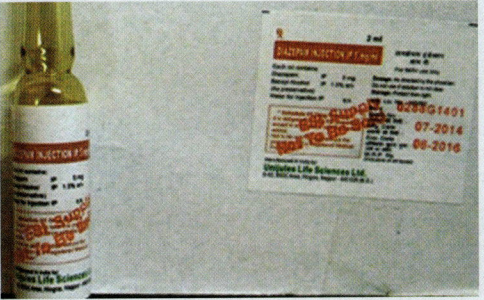

Fig. 13.4: Diazepam injection

Bromides	Chloral hydrate	Paraldehyde
Salts of Na/K or calcium/ lithium: Sodium bromide is a high melting, white crystalline solid resembling NaCl	It is a white, crystalline powder, freely soluble in water, bitter to taste, and has pungent odor. It is a synthetic product	Synthetic drug It is a colorless, volatile liquid with an ethereal odor
Uses 1. For insomnia, epilepsy 2. Disinfectant for swimming pool in conjunction with chlorine	**Use** For kicking effect in alcohol	**Use** As an effective anticonvulsant
Absorption, fate, and excretion Absorbed through S/L intestine. Metabolized in liver and distributed in tissue Excreted mostly through urine, sweat and other body secretions	**Absorption, fate, and excretion** Absorbed through mucosa of GIT, usually stomach Metabolized in liver where it is converted to trichloroethanol and then to trichloroacetaldehyde and trichloroacetic acid Excreted mostly through urine, either free or combined with glucuronic acid	**Absorption, fate, and excretion** Absorbed through mucosa of stomach/intestine **Metabolism:** Oxidised in liver to acetaldehyde and acetic acid. Excreted mostly through kidneys and lungs without alteration
Action **Cerebral depressant:** It replaces chlorides and depresses nervous systems both sensory and motor function	**Action** Cerebral depressant Somniferous Sedatives It enhances the GABA receptor complex	**Action** Cerebral depressant Somniferous Sedatives and basal anesthetics
Fatal dose: 30–45 gm **Fatal period:** 6–8 hrs	**Fatal dose:** 5–10 gm **Fatal period:** 8–12 hrs	**Fatal dose:** 100 ml **Fatal period:** Within a few hrs
Clinical features Nausea, vomiting, abdominal pain. Headache, confusion. Fall of BP, temperature and respiration—depressed, pulse— slow, weak Vertigo, weakness, skin rash, paralysis, coma	**Clinical features** Nausea, vomiting, headache, confusion, giddiness, drowsiness. BP—low, and temperature is low, respiration—depressed, pulse— slow, weak, irregular. Cardiac arrhythmia, muscle relaxed, albuminuria, deep sleep, coma	**Clinical features** Nausea, vomiting, headache, confusion, giddiness, drowsiness BP—low, temperature is low, respiration—depressed, pulse—weak Etheral smell in breath Coma

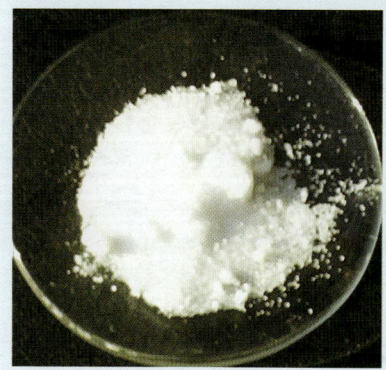
Fig. 13.5: Sodium bromide powder

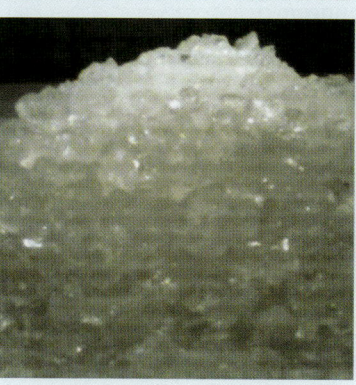
Fig. 13.6: Chloral hydrate crystal

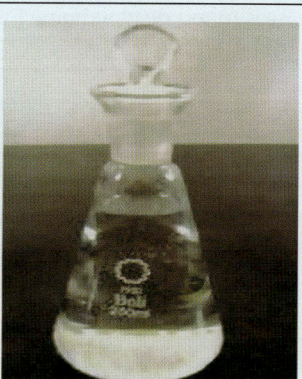
Fig. 13.7: Paraldehyde liquid

Treatment	Treatment	Treatment
1. Stomach wash	1. Stomach wash	1. Stomach/colonic wash
2. Antidotes: NaCl by mouth or in drip	2. Antidotes: Naloxone or flumazenil produce dramatic improvement	2. Antidotes: Not specific
3. Symptomatic	3. Caffeine etsy dibenzoate IV repeated after 15 mins and 1 hr	3. Artificial respiration
	4. Artificial respiration	4. Respiratory stimulant
	5. For liver protection—glucose	5. Calcium gluconate IV
	6. To protect heart—strophanthine 0.3 mg	
PM finding	**PM findings**	**PM findings**
Nothing specific	• Suggestive of asphyxia	• Suggestive of asphyxia
	• Liver damage in chronic cases	• Organs—congested
	• Renal damage	• Lungs—congested, edematous.
		• Smell of paraldehyde on opening the body cavities
ML aspects	**ML aspects**	**ML aspect**
1. Suicidal: Rare	1. Suicidal: Occurs as it is used for knockout drop. It is a habit forming drug	Accidental: Overdose due to addiction. It is a habit forming drug
2. Homicidal: Rare	2. Homicidal: Not possible due to smell/taste	
3. Accidental: Mostly, chronic poisoning when used for insomnia, epilepsy and nervous breakdown (cumulative poison due to gradual accumulation)	3. Accidental: Due to overdose, chronic use due to addiction and gradual accumulation	

14

Cerebral Stimulant

Cerebral stimulants are the drugs which causes CNS stimulation. It includes cocaine, camphor, caffeine, theophylline and theobromine.

CEREBRAL STIMULANTS

Examples

1. Cocaine and its synthetic derivatives like procaine, butacaine, lidocaine, tetracaine and dibucaine. They are used as local and spinal anesthetic agents. The synthetic substitutes of cocaine like Nuvacaine, Nupercaine and Xylocaine are used as local anesthetics.

2. Camphor.

3. Caffeine, theophylline, theobromine.

Cocaine is already discussed in the previous chapter.

PROCAINE

It is a synthetic product almost one-third as toxic as cocaine.

Uses: As local infiltration anesthesia or spinal anesthesia.

Absorption, Fate, and Excretion

Toxic symptoms occur when it is given intra-thecally or when it enters the circulation directly by wrong pushing into a vein or infiltration into a vascular area.

It is partly hydrolyzed by esterase while in circulation and partly by liver to PABA (which is excreted through urine) and diethylamino-ethanol.

Properties and Action

Same as Cocaine

Clinical features: Same as cocaine when it gets into circulation.

In case of spinal use, there may be post-anesthetic myelitis with symptoms of cord degeneration with pulmonary edema and pneumonitis.

Treatment

Prophylactic premedication with barbiturate and ephedrine is necessary before using as spinal anesthesia.

1. For circulatory collapse—noradrenaline drip.
2. For respiration—oxygen inhalation and artificial respiration.

PM findings: Same as cocaine.

ML Aspect

Accidental: From therapeutic use.

BUTACAINE, LIDOCAINE, TETRACAINE, AND DIBUCAINE

These are the synthetic derivative of cocaine. Butacaine and lidocaine are almost two times as toxic as cocaine. Tetracaine and dibucaine are four times as toxic as cocaine.

Action, clinical features, treatment, PM findings and ML

Aspect: Same as cocaine.

Camphor	*Amphetamine*
1. Camphor is naturally obtained from stem/bark of cinnamomum camphora 2. Synthetically, it is produced from turpentine oil	Chemically, amphetamine is phenylpropanolamine. Amphetamine was first synthesized in 1887, but began to be therapeutically used only since the 1930s. Because of its abuse potential, its therapeutic administration is greatly restricted today
Uses 1. Pain reliever in various ayurvedic medicines. Also used in nasal congestion and cold 2. Deodorant 3. Mosquito/cockroaches repellents 4. In worshipping (*pooja*)	**Uses** 1. Abuse—to enhance the performance or to stay awake 2. Narcolepsy 3. Attention deficit disorder 4. Hypotension (mephentermine as IV solution)
Absorption, fate, and excretion • Absorbed from GIT • It is partly oxidized and partly conjugated with glycuronic acid. Excreted mostly through the kidneys (urine) and small amount through lungs	**Absorption, fate, and excretion** • Absorbed from GIT • Excreted mostly through the kidneys and small amount through lungs
Fatal dose: 15 gm **Fatal period:** 24 hrs	**Fatal dose:** 250 mg (addicts can tolerate larger doses) **Fatal period:** Uncertain
Action 1. CNS—stimulant 2. GIT—irritant	**Action** Amphetamines enhance the synaptic concentration of dopamine and norepinephrine, either by direct release from storage vesicles or by inhibition of re-uptake 1. CNS and CVS—powerful stimulants

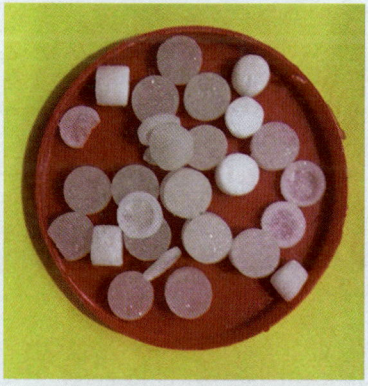

Fig. 14.1: Camphor cakes

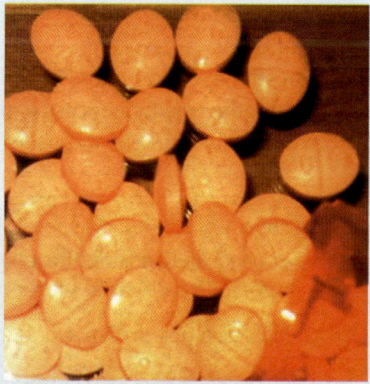

Fig. 14.2: Amphetamine 30 mg tablet

Clinical features *Acute poisoning occurs in two phases* **1. Convulsive phase** **2. Depressive phase** • Abdominal pain, vomiting, diarrhea, circulatory collapse, excitement, anxiety, epileptiform, convulsion, delirium, rise in BT, cyanosis • There may be hallucination and delusion followed by depression, collapse and coma	**Clinical features** **Acute poisoning:** Acute overdose with amphetamines is uncommon in India • Restlessness, insomnia, tremor, sweating, dry mucous membranes, nausea, mydriasis • Hyperactivity, confusion, hypertension, tachycardia, tachypnea, vomiting, hallucinations • Delirium, hyperpyrexia, convulsions, arrhythmias

Camphor	Amphetamine
Chronic poisoning	**Chronic poisoning**
There are neurological symptoms with convulsion	**1. Amphetamine psychosis**
	2. Gilles de la Tourette's syndrome
Treatment	**Treatment**
In acute poisoning	*In acute poisoning*
1. Bromides/paraldehyde/diazepam or inhalation of ether vapor (for convulsion)	1. Stomach wash and emesis
2. Stomach wash	2. Acidic diuresis (controversial)
During depressive phase	3. Benzodiazepines or antipsychotics for agitation and convulsions
1. Caffeine	4. IV Sodium nitroprusside for hypertension
2. Pressure agents	5. Ice bath or cold sponging for hyperthermia
3. IV fluids—maintenance of circulation	6. Supportive measures
4. Dialysis of blood for rapid elimination of camphor	**In chronic poisoning:** Chlorpromazine or haloperidol for amphetamine psychosis; and haloperidol for Gilles de la Tourette's syndrome
In chronic poisoning—precaution against exposure. Death is due to respiratory failure or CV collapse/cardiac failure	
PM findings	**PM findings**
S/o asphyxia	Not specific
Organs—congested	S/o asphyxia
Stomach—congested, smell present	Organs—congested
ML aspects	**ML significance**
1. Suicide—rare	1. Suicide: Due to bizarre behaviour
2. Homicidal—not occur	2. Homicide: Due to bizarre behaviour
3. Accidental—mostly, in children due to	3. Accidental deaths may occur in **abuser** when combined with alcohol and other CNS depressant
i. Mistaken with other medicine/castor oil	
ii. Chronic exposure in workers and users	4. Aphrodisiac

Amphetamine abuse

1. Formerly, it was used (abused) by those who were compelled **to stay awake at nights periodically,** e.g. truck drivers, night shift industrial workers, medical students, etc.

2. Abused by athletes as a performance enhancer

3. Today "designer drugs" are abused in **rave parties, for dancing all night long** by youngsters

Chronic amphetamine poisoning

1. Amphetamine psychosis

Stereotype—obsessed with repetitive activities involving grooming, rearranging, cleaning, etc.

Paranoid behaviour—characterized by suspicion, hostility, and anxiety

Delusions of persecution

Hallucinations—usually visual

2. Gilles de la Tourette's syndrome: Characterized by tic, eye blinking, jaw jerks, humming, etc.

Caffeine (trimethyl xanthine)	Theophylline	Theobromine
Caffeine is extracted from the leaves of tea and coffee beans	It is 1, 3-dimethyl xanthine. It is available from tea leaves and is also synthesized	It is 3, 7-dimethyl xanthine. It is available from the seeds of Theobroma cacao
Absorption, fate, and excretion 1. Absorbed through GIT 2. It is demethylated and further metabolized in liver 3. Excreted through kidneys, partly as methylated xanthine and partly as xanthine	**Absorption, fate, and excretion** Same as caffeine	**Absorption, fate, and excretion** Same as caffeine
Action It stimulates brain and spinal cord	**Action** Same as caffeine	**Action** Same as caffeine
Fatal dose/period: Not certain	**Fatal dose/period:** Not certain	**Fatal dose/period:** Not certain
Clinical features 1. Headache, anxiety, insomnia, vertigo, tremor, convulsion, delirium 2. Due to adrenocortical stimulation, there is a rise in serum catecholamines and increase excretion of 11-hydroxycorticosteriod	**Clinical features** Same as caffeine Theophylline causes hematuria	**Clinical features** Same as caffeine It is irritant to stomach and also causes palpitation
Treatment 1. Sedatives/tranquilizers: Barbiturates, bromides, paraldehyde or diazepam to counter cerebral/spinal stimulation 2. Artificial respiration and O_2 inhalation 3. Symptomatic	**Treatment** Same as caffeine	**Treatment** Same as caffeine
PM findings • Nothing specific • Suggestive of asphyxia	**PM findings** • Suggestive of asphyxia • Cloudy swelling of kidneys	**PM finding** Same as caffeine
ML aspects 1. Suicidal: Rare 2. Homicidal: Not common 3. Accidental: Mostly mistaken with other drugs or overdose or idiosyncratic	**ML aspect** Same as caffeine	**ML aspect** Same as caffeine

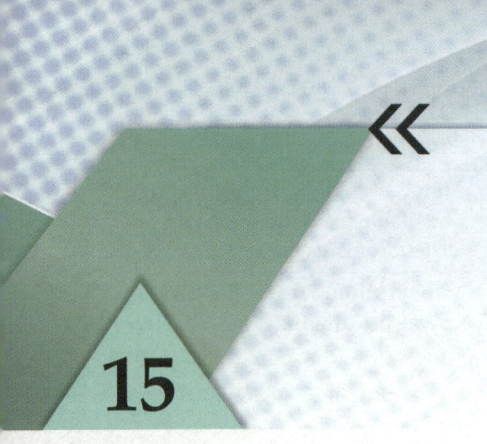

15

Hallucinogens

Hallucinogens are the drugs which causes hallucinations. Hallucination is a false sense of perception. It includes lysergic acid diethylamide, phencyclidine, mescaline.

Lysergic acid diethylamide (LSD)	Phencyclidine
LSD is the most powerful hallucinogen known to man. It was popular among the hippies in the West in the 1960s. It is usually impregnated in stamp sized paper **(LSD blotter)** which is liked or consumed	Phencyclidine is a popular drug of abuse in the West. A common mode of intake involves sprinkling the drug on parsley or marijuana leaves, and then smoking it. It is sometimes used as an adulterant in expensive drugs of abuse such as cocaine
Common name Acid, microdot, purple haze, white lightning, etc.	**Common name** Angel dust, PCP, peace pill, hog, rocket fuel, etc.
Physical appearance Crystalline substance, which is colourless, odourless, tasteless, and water-soluble. It is effective in extremely small doses (micrograms)	**Physical appearance** White crystalline powder
Sources 1. *Rivea corymbosa* (a mexican plant) of family Convolvulaceae 2. Morning glory plant (contains a compound very similar to LSD) 3. Ergot: Synthesized from lysergic acid, a derivative of ergot	**Source** 1. Commercial—drug addicts
Clinical features Mydriasis, tachycardia, tremor, ataxia Hallucinations Panic attacks, psychotic reactions, flashback phenomena, mania Convulsions, focal cerebral deficits, coma. Hyperthermia, bleeding disorders	**Clinical features** Pencyclidine is usually smoked, sniffed, or injected (IV, SC) Nystagmus, miosis, ataxia, tremor, dysarthria, tachycardia, hypertension. Lethargy, catatonia, coma. Acute psychosis with delusions and hallucinations. Agitation, violent tendency, bizarre behaviour
Treatment 1. Quiet, secluded environment 2. Antipsychotics 3. Benzodiazepines 4. Supportive measures 5. Psychiatric follow-up	**Treatment** 1. Stomach wash is usually not applicable, since the drug is rarely taken orally 2. Acid diuresis 3. Supportive care 4. Psychiatric follow-up

ML significance
Suicidal and accidental deaths arising out of bizarre behaviour induced by the drug have been reported. Repeated use by an addict can lead to permanent psychosis

ML significance
Addiction leads to violent tendency, psychosis, and suicidal as well as homicidal behaviour

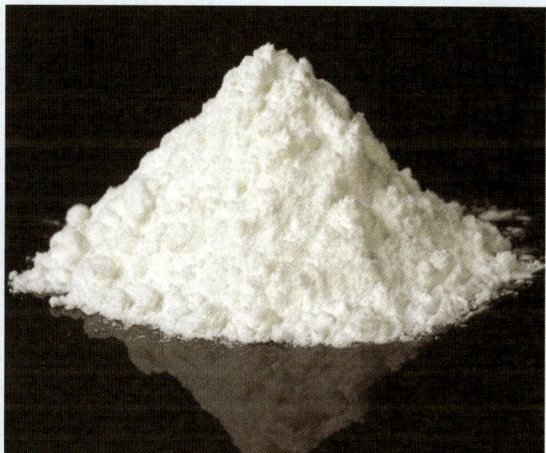

Fig. 15.1: LSD powder

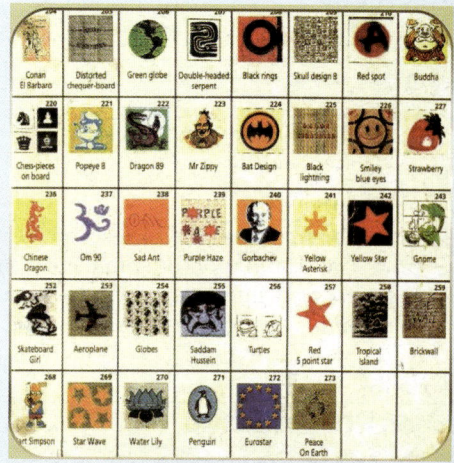

Fig. 15.2: LSD blotter

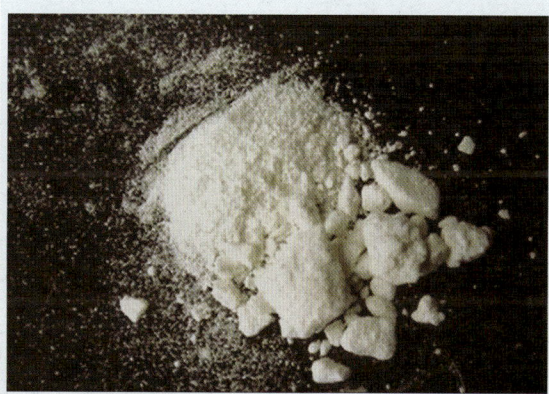

Fig. 15.3: Phencyclidine

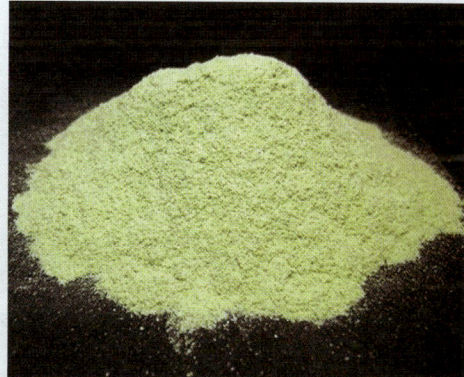

Fig. 15.4: Mescaline

16

Spinal Poisons

Spinal poisons are the poisons which act on the spinal cord. It may either cause stimulation or depression of spinal cord. The stimulation of spinal cord results in spasm and convulsion while depression causes paralysis and loss of sensation. It includes Nux vomica and Gelsemium. Nux vomica is a spinal stimulant and Gelsemium is spinal depression.

STRYCHNINE

Common Name: Kuchila

Plant: Strychnos nux vomica

Toxic part: All part of the plant (maximum concentration in seeds)

Three varieties: Colubrina, Ignati, Tiute.

The fruit is globular yellowish brown with hard covering containing seeds.

Seeds: Biconvex button shaped seeds, 2–2.5 cm in diameter and 0.5 cm thick, bitter to taste, yellowish brown, shiny, hard pericarp with fine hairs over surface (Fig. 16.1).

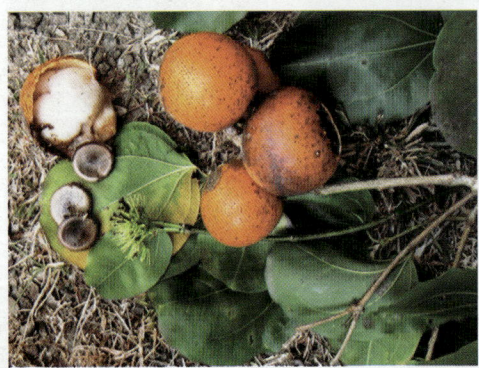

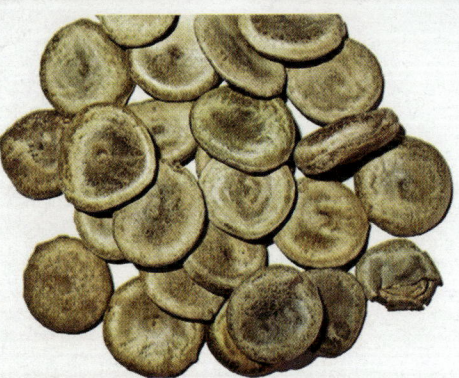

Fig. 16.1: Nux vomica plant, fruit, and seeds

Active principle: Strychnine, brucine, loganine.

Uses

1. Medicinal: As CNS stimulant.
2. Used in popular homeopathic remedy 'Nux Vomica'.
3. Also used in herbal medicine to elevate BP.
4. Used as vermin paste.
5. Rodenticidal agent.

Route of administration: Usually oral

Action

It is a spinal poison acts particularly on the anterior horn cell of spinal cord.

It is a CNS stimulant—produces excitation of all portion of nervous system by increasing the ongoing neuronal activity, through **blocking of post-synaptic inhibitory influence causes convulsion**.

Fatal dose: 1–2 seeds, 30–60 mg strychnine.

Fatal period: 30 mins to 2 hrs.

Clinical Features

1. When swallowed/crushed: Bitter taste with choking sensation in throat. The patient is restless, sensitive, and apprehensive and has anxious look.
2. Twitching/tremor of muscle: First clonic followed by tonic type.
3. Due to extreme degree of contraction of muscle, the **body may assume one of the following positions** (Fig. 16.2) along with the contraction of the muscle of the face leading to widening of angle of mouth with creases appearing in and around the eyelids, (a state known as **'risus sardonicus'**—monkey-like face):

   i. Opisthotonus: Bend backward with convexity facing forward with head—heel touches the ground surface.

   ii. Emphrosthotonus: Bend forward

   iii. Pleurosthotonus: Bend sidewise

4. In between the contraction: Muscles are relaxed. The intercostal muscles fixed leading to difficulty in breathing and cyanosis.

5. The mind is not affected nor is the consciousness.

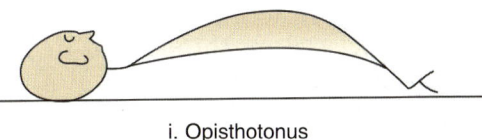
i. Opisthotonus

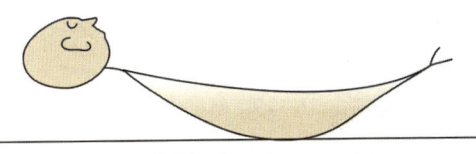
ii. Emphrosthotonus

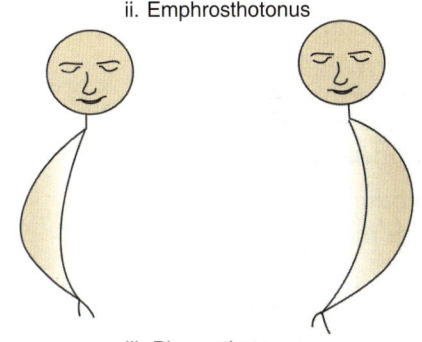
iii. Pleurosthotonus

Fig. 16.2: Different body positions

Differences	Strychnine poisoning	Tetanus
1. Onset:	Sudden	Gradual
2. History of:	Ingestion of some bitter white powder followed by convulsion	Injury
3. Muscle involvement:	All muscles are involved at a time	Muscles are gradually involved
4. Muscle during interval:	Muscles are relaxed	Muscles are rigid
5. Chemical analysis:	Strychnine is detected	Nil
6. Microbiological exam:	Nil	Clostridium tetani present

Death

Due to

1. Respiratory failure due to asphyxia.
2. Medullary paralysis.

Treatment

1. Keep the patient in a dark, noiseless room (because they are easily stimulated).
2. Antidote: Sedation by
   i. Ultrashort acting barbiturates—30–60 mg sodium thiopenton in 10 ml distilled water by slow IV.
   ii. Paraldehyde—45 ml IV.
3. Stomach wash with mixture of 0.1% $KMnO_4$, 2% tannic acid, and activated charcoal.
4. Muscle relaxant:
   i. Mephenesin—30 mg/kg slow IV drip.
   ii. d-tubocurarine—4–5 ml.
5. Artificial respiration: By tracheostomy and O_2 supply.
6. Supportive.

Postmortem Findings

- Nothing specific.
- Rigor mortis—stays longer.
- Signs of asphyxia present.
- Rupture of stretched muscle.

Preservation of Viscera

- Routine viscera
- Blood
- Spinal cord.
  It is present in the tissue for days extending to years.

ML Aspects

1. **Suicidal:** Not common due to painful death.
2. **Homicidal:** Not common, but a few cases have been reported.
3. **Accidental**
   i. By children
   ii. By mistake
   iii. Overdose
   iv. Rat poison
4. **Abortifacient**
5. **Arrow poison**
6. **Cattle poison.**

Peripheral Nerve Poisons

17

Peripheral nerve poisons are the poisons which blocks the action of acetylcholine at nerve ends. It includes Curare and Conium. They cause skeletal muscle relaxant.

Conium	*Curare*
Common name Poison hemlock, Socrates poison	**Common name** Vine
Plant: *Conium maculatum* **Toxic part:** All parts of plant. It belongs to carrot family, grows between 5 and 8 feet tall with smooth green hollow stem. Flowers are small white, clustered in umbels up to 4–6 inch across. When crushed, leaves and root emit a rank, unpleasant odour	**Plant:** *Chondrodendron tomentosum* **Toxic part:** All parts of plant (maximum concentration in bark and stem) It is a long poisonous vine that can stretch up to the canopy. Leaves are large, heart shaped, covered with tiny hairs. Flowers are small and greenish white. Fruits are fleshy but very tiny

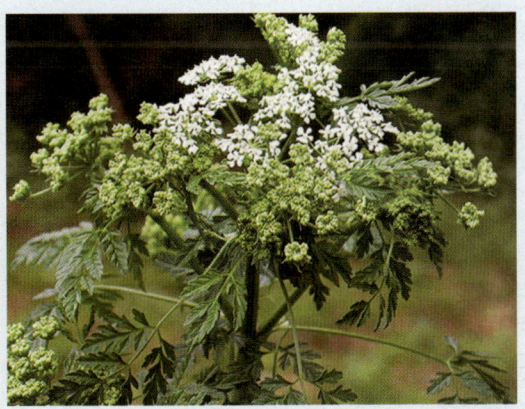 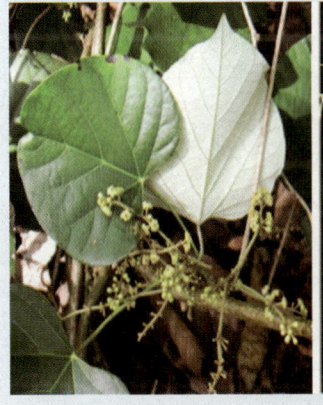 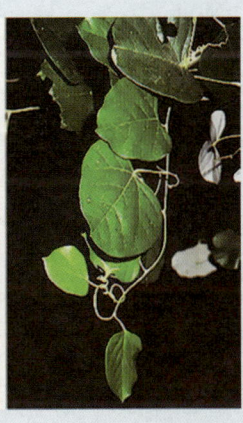

Active principle Coniine, Gamma—Coniceine	**Active principle** Curare, Curariform, Curarine, d-Tubocurarine, Syncurine, Succinylcholine chloride
Uses 1. Medicinal: As muscle relaxant 2. Execution of capital punishment	**Uses** 1. Medicinal: As muscle relaxant during anesthesia 2. As anticonvulsant 3. Used to treat bruise and kidney stones
Route of administration: Usually oral	**Route of administration:** Injectables only

Action

1. It acts at neuromuscular junction as non-depolarizing blockers and causes flaccid paralysis (similar to curare)
2. It also acts on autonomic ganglia producing nicotinic effects

Action

1. It **blocks the action of acetylcholine** at nerve ends
2. It is a skeletal muscle relaxant

Fatal dose: 1 cm of any part of plant
Fatal period: A few hours

Fatal dose: 30–60 mg curarine
Fatal period: 1–2 hrs

Clinical features

1. Nausea, vomiting, abdominal pain
2. Sweating, salivation
3. Mydriasis, tachycardia followed by bradycardia, fall of BP
4. Muscle weakness, paralysis
5. Tremor, convulsion, coma, respiratory failure by paralysis

Clinical features

1. When swallowed: No action.
2. When injected: Inability to move due to flaccidity of muscle which gets paralyzed leading to respiratory failure (due to involvement of muscles of diaphragm and intercostal muscles)
3. Muscle relaxed/flaccid all the time
4. There may be altered consciousness
5. There is also headache, confusion, vertigo, mydriasis, blurring of vision, hyperthermia

Death due to
Respiratory failure: Due to asphyxia

Death due to
Respiratory failure: Due to asphyxia

Treatment

1. Artificial respiration and O_2 supply
2. Antidote:
   Not specific
3. Stomach wash: With activated charcoal
4. Stimulant
5. Supportive

Treatment

1. Artificial respiration and O_2 supply
2. Antidote:
   i. Neostigmine: 0.5–1 mg SC
   ii. Physostigmine: 1–2 mg SC
3. 100 mg of Congo Red in 10 ml of 5% glucose by slow IV drip
4. Stimulant
5. Supportive

PM findings
- Nothing specific
- Stomach—peculiar (mousy) odour
- Suggestive of asphyxia
- Organs—congested

PM findings
- Nothing specific
- Evidence of injection mark
- Suggestive asphyxia

Preservation of viscera
Routine viscera
Blood

Preservation of viscera
Routine viscera
Blood
Skin and underlying muscle at the site of injection

ML aspects

1. Suicidal: Rare
2. Homicidal: In ancient period, it was used for execution of punishments. Socrates was executed by poison hemlock
3. Accidental: Rarely occur

ML aspects

1. Suicidal: Administered usually by person in medical profession—to impart painless death
2. Homicidal: Administered usually by person in medical profession—in dyadic death
3. Accidental:
   i. By mistake
   ii. Overdose during anesthesia
4. Abortifacient
5. Arrow poison

18

Cardiac Poisons

Cardiac poisons are the systemic poison which acts on the heart. Hydrogen cyanide is the most potent cardiac poison. Other examples are aconite, *Cerbera thevetia*, *Nerium odorum*, Tobacco, Quinine, and Digitalis.

Hydrocyanic acid	*Aconitum ferox/napellus*
Synonyms: Cyanogen, prussiac acid	**Synonyms:** Aconite, *Mitha jaher*, (sweet poison), monk hood
Properties Also known as 'Vegetable acid' since it is present in certain fruits kernels. It is very potent, extremely lethal and most rapidly fatal **Chemically:** HCN—colorless gas with bitter almond smell. But can be kept in liquid form in cold temperature and underpressure **Salts:** K/Na cyanide—are dirty white powder **Sources:** Laboratories, industries and kernels of **almonds**, apple, apricot, cherry, plumb, peach, etc.	**Properties** Grows in Himalayan altitude **Toxic part:** All parts of plant is toxic (maximum concentration in dried root). The root is brownish yellow, conical and long shrivelled, sweet taste When fresh root is cut—white surface turns red When fresh horse radish root is cut, it remains white **Active principles:** Aconitine, pseudo-aconitine, aconine, picraconitine
Uses 1. For hardening of metal, metal/gold plating 2. For purifying metallic ores 3. In synthetic rubber and plastic industries 4. In photography and for fumigation	**Uses** 1. Aconite is a pharmacological product marketed as tincture aconitum, has **anodyne properties** (able to relieve pain/mentally soothing) 2. Used in ayurvedic/homoepathic medicines
Action It is a protoplasmic poison that acts by **inhibiting the enzymes cytochrome oxidase** by chelating the metallic moiety of enzyme, thus reducing oxygen utilization in the tissue resulting in histotoxic hypoxia. Thus, it kills person by bulbar paralysis (Cyanogen + cytochrome oxidase = cyanogen-cytochrome complex)	**Action** Stimulates and then depresses myocardium, smooth/skeletal muscle, CNS and peripheral nerves.
Absorption, fate, and excretion Cyanide is absorbed through MM, skin, RT (in gases form). It is metabolized to thiocyanate (nontoxic) and is excreted through urine and expired air	**Absorption, fate, and excretion** Aconite is absorbed through MM of GIT It is metabolized in liver Excreted through urine

Fatal dose/fateal period
HCN gas: 100–200 ppm—immediate
Liquid: 50 ml—2–5 min. Salts: 200 mg—30 mins

Fatal dose: Root—1 gm, aconitine-2–6 mg
Fatal period: 1–6 hrs

Clinical manifestation

The action depends on (i) form of poison (acid/salt), (ii) absence of gastric HCl, (iii) presence of food, (iv) concentration, and (v) route of absorption

In gaseous form and in higher concentration: There is sudden unconsciousness followed by violent breathing, convulsion, and death

When ingested in low dose: Bitter burning sensation in mouth and feeling of constriction in chest, increase salivation, nausea, vomiting, and abdominal pain

With fine froth at mouth and nostrils and strong bitter almond smell in expired air

This is followed by headache, confusion, vertigo, dizziness, dyspnea, delirium, convulsion, collapse, coma

There may be low BP, pulse, respiration with absence of reflex

With cyanosis, pink coloration of skin, which does not improved with oxygen therapy

Clinical manifestation

Tingling/numbness/burning sensation in mouth/tongue/throat with bitter sweet taste and feeling of constriction in chest, increase salivation, nausea, vomiting, and abdominal pain

Tingling/numbness/weakness of muscle and limbs, ringing in ear, impairment of hearing/vision/speech

This is followed by headache, confusion, vertigo, dizziness, dyspnea, delirium, convulsion, collapse, and coma

There may be low BP, pulse, respiration and ventricular fibrillation

Pupils show **hippus reaction** (alternate constriction and dilatation)

Treatment: Hardly any time for treatment
1. 0.2 ml amyl nitrite (3–6 amp), to be stopped if BP <80
2. 3% Na nitrite (10 ml IV) or (IV methylene blue or cobalt acetate/EDTA). The Hb is converted into MetHb, which combines with cyanogen—cytochrome complex to form cyan-MetHb and frees cytochrome oxidase for tissue oxygenation. (Cyanogen cytochrome + MetHb → Cyan-metHb + cytochrome oxidase)
3. 25% Na thiosulfate (50 ml IV).
   Cyanogen → Na thiocyanate
4. Artificial respiration and O_2 supply
5. Stomach wash with mixture of 6% $NaCO_3$ + 15.3% Ferrous sulfate and 3% citric acid in water or with 0.1% $KMnO_4$ or 5–10% sodium thiosulfate solution

Treatment
1. Emesis
2. Stomach wash: $KMnO_4$/tannic acid/charcoal
3. Demulcent
4. Artificial respiration and O_2 inhalation
5. Symptomatic:
   Atropin-1 mg SC-to avoid vagal inhibition
   Lignocaine-0.1% of 50 ml slow IV drip-to relieve tachycardia

PM findings
- Cyanosis
- Suggestive of asphyxia
- Pinkish lividity
- Froth from mouth/nostril with bitter almond smell, corrosion of stomach mucosa

PM findings
- Nothing specific
- Pallor of mucous membrane of mouth
- Stomach: Root remains present

Principles of treatment of cyanide
1. To avoid cyanogen-cytochrome combination
2. To convert Hb to MetHb (by means of nitrite, methylene blue, cobalt acetate). This metHb combines with cyanogen of cyanogen-cytochrome combination to form cyan-metHb and frees cytochrome oxidase for tissue oxygenation
3. To convert free cyanides to harmless complexes (by Na thiosulfate, vitamin B_{12}, dicobalt EDTA)

Hydrocyanic acid	*Aconitum napellus*
Viscera preservation Routine viscera Lungs Brain Preserved in saturated solution of NaCl	**Viscera preservation** Routine viscera Heart Preserved in saturated solution of NaCl or rectified spirit acidified with acetic acid

Medicolegal aspects
1. Suicide: Quite common by goldsmith. Anti-state activities/terrorist usually carry cyanide capsule. They prefer to commit suicide rather than to be caught and to be subjected torture/confession
2. Homicidal: Rare
3. Accidental: From laboratory/industries. (Bhopal gas tragedy, i.e. MIC)
4. Cattle poison: Rare
	Medicolegal aspects
	1. Suicide: Not common, but is painful
	2. Homicidal: Ideal homicidal poison given by oral route, mixed with paan and drinks
	3. Accidental: Mostly due to:
	  i. Mistaken with horse radish route
	  ii. Mixed with country liquor for kicking effect
	  iii. Quackery medicine
	4. Abortifacient
	5. Arrow poison: By parentral route by tribal people of Himalayas
	6. Cattle poison: By parenteral route by tribal people of Himalayas

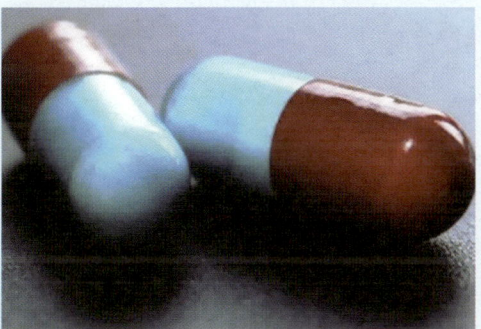

Fig. 18.1: Cyanide capsules (powder)

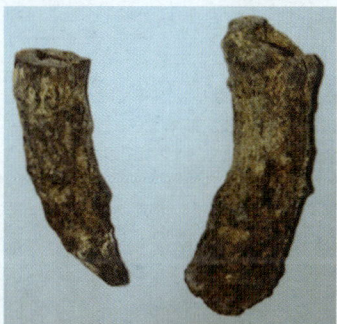

Fig. 18.2: Root of aconite

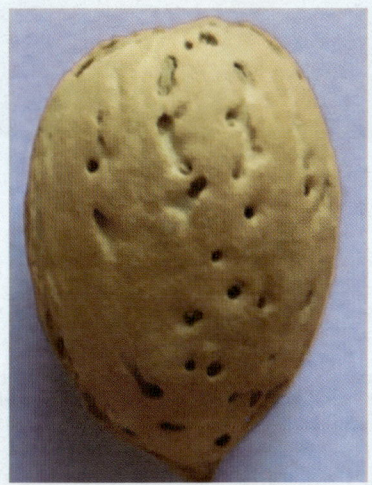

Fig. 18.3: Bitter almond

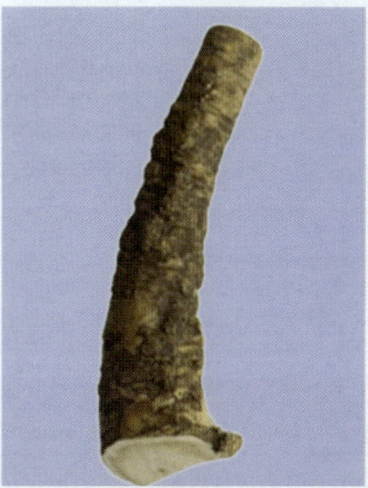

Fig. 18.4: Root of horse radish

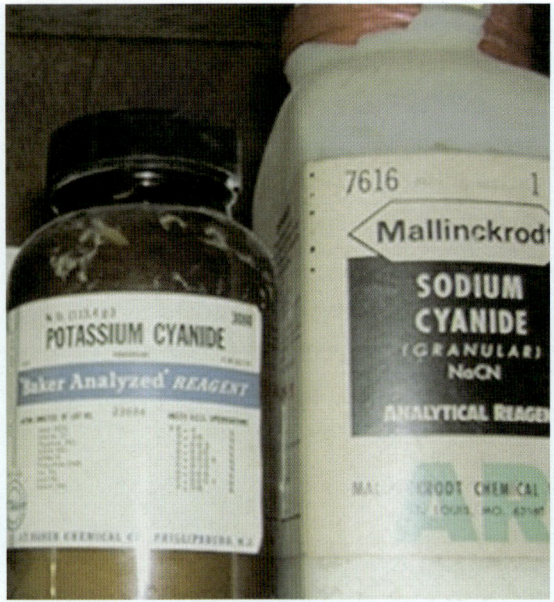

Fig. 18.5: Potassium and sodium cyanide

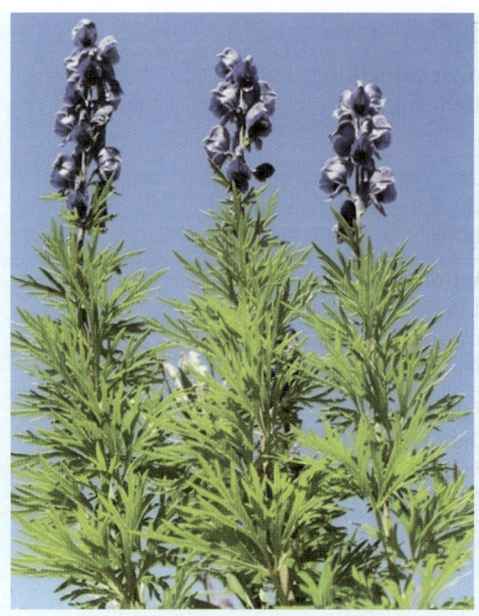

Fig. 18.6: *Aconitum napellus*

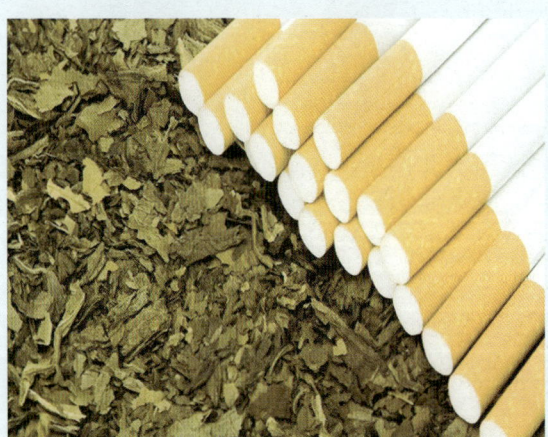

Fig. 18.7: Nicotine dry leaves (tobacco) and cigarette

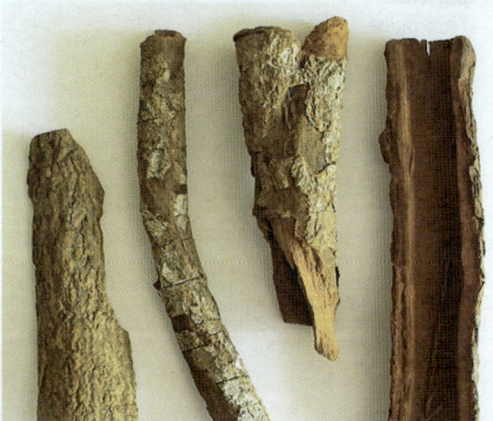

Fig. 18.8: Cinchona bark

Digitalis purpura/lanata	Nicotiana tabacum/lobelia inflata	Cinchona pubescens
Synonyms: Digitalis/fox glove	**Synonyms:** Tobacco (*tambakhu*)	**Synonyms:** Quinine, quina
Grows in: All over world	**Grows in:** All over world	**Grows in:** All over world
Toxic part: All parts of plant (maximum concentration leaves)	**Toxic part:** All parts of plant (maximum concentration leaves)	**Toxic part:** All parts of plant (maximum concentration leaves)

Digitalis	*Nicotine*	*Qninine*
Toxic principles: Digitalin, digitoxin, digitonin, digoxin	**Toxic principles:** Nicotine, nicotianine, lobeline	**Toxic principles** Quinine, quinidine, cinchonine, cinchonidine
Use Medicine: Treatment of cardiac failure	**Use** Dried leaves used as article of luxury (cigarette smoking)	**Use** Medicine: Treatment of malaria and arrhythmia
Action: Prolong diastolic period It increases excitability and improves the function of failing heart	**Action:** Stimulates and depresses heart	**Action:** Stimulates and depresses heart
Fatal dose: Dried leaves: 1–2 gm, Digitoxin: 2–3 mg **Fatal period:** 1–24 hrs	**Fatal dose:** Dried leaves: 20–40 gm, nicotine: 1–2 drops **Fatal period:** 1–5 hrs	**Fatal dose:** Bark: 2–8 gm **Fatal period:** 1–5 hrs

Clinical features
 • Burning sensation in mouth/ tongue/throat with nausea, vomiting, abdominal pain, and diarrhea
  – Slow pulse/heart/respiration rate, with extrasystole, ventricular fibrillation, pericardial distress
  – Headache, confusion, dyspnea, dizziness, delirium, dilated pupil, convulsion, collapse, coma
  – Flat/inverted T wave, prolonged PR and shorten QT interval
	Clinical features
	 • Burning sensation in mouth/ tongue/throat with nausea, vomiting, abdominal pain
	  – Cardiovascular collapse, cardiac irregularities, increased heart rate, extrasystole, ventricular fibrillation, pericardial distress
	  – Headache, confusion, dyspnea, dizziness, delirium, dilated pupil, convulsion, collapse, coma
	 • **Chronic:** Cough, bronchitis, tingling, numbness, tremor, weakness, loss of memory, cardiac systole, anorexia
		Clinical features
		 • Nausea, vomiting, abdominal pain
		  – Slow pulse/heart/respiration rate, with extrasystole, ventricular fibrillation, pericardial distress
		  – Headache, confusion, dyspnea, dizziness, delirium, dilated pupil, convulsion, collapse, coma
		  – Dimness of vision, ringing of ear, loss of vision/hearing
		 • **Kidney:** Oliguria, hematuria

Treatment
 • Emesis
 • Stomach wash
 • Demulcent
 • Artificial respiration and O_2 inhalation
 • Supportive:
  – Atropine
  – IV lignocaine
	Treatment
	 • Emesis
	 • Stomach wash: $KMnO_4$/TA
	 • Demulcent/purgatives
	 • Artificial respiration and O_2 inhalation
	 • Supportive:
	  – Atropine
	  – Adrenaline
		Treatment
		 • Emesis
		 • Stomach wash: $KMnO_4$
		 • Demulcent/purgatives
		 • Artificial respiration and O_2 inhalation
		 • Supportive:
		  – Procainamide
		  – Protect kidney/vision by giving nitrate

PM finding Nothing specific	**PM findings** • Nothing specific, suggestive of asphyxia • Stomach: Inflammation, smell present with leaves ingredient	**PM finding** Nothing specific
ML aspects • Suicidal: Not known • Homicidal: Occasionally used • Accidental: Overdose	**ML aspects** • Suicidal: Unusual • Homicidal: Unusual • Accidental: In chronic case	**ML aspects** • Suicidal: Rare • Homicidal: Rare • Accidental: Overdose • Abortifacient

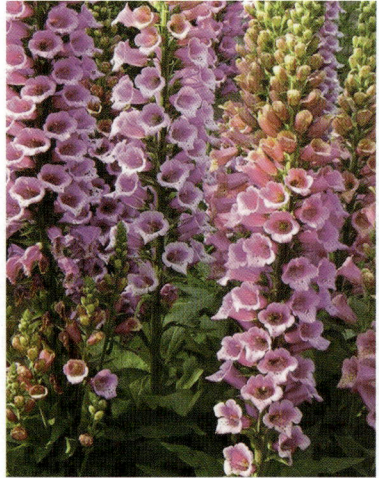

Fig. 18.9: *Digitalis purpurae* plant

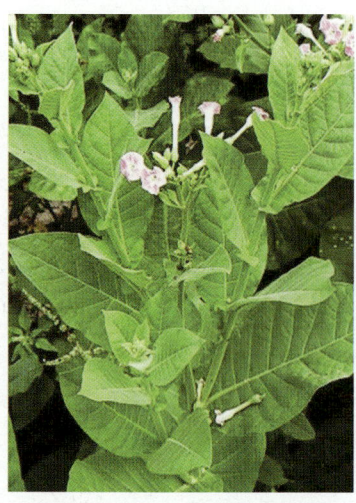

Fig. 18.10: *Nicotiana tabacum* plant

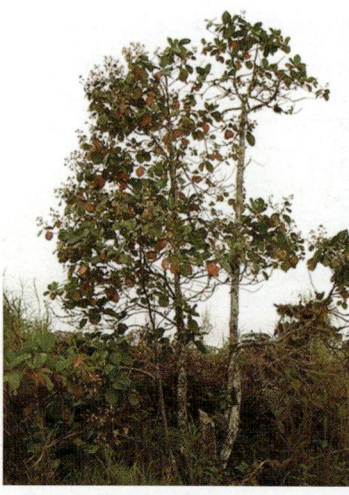

Fig. 18.11: *Cinchona pubescens* plant

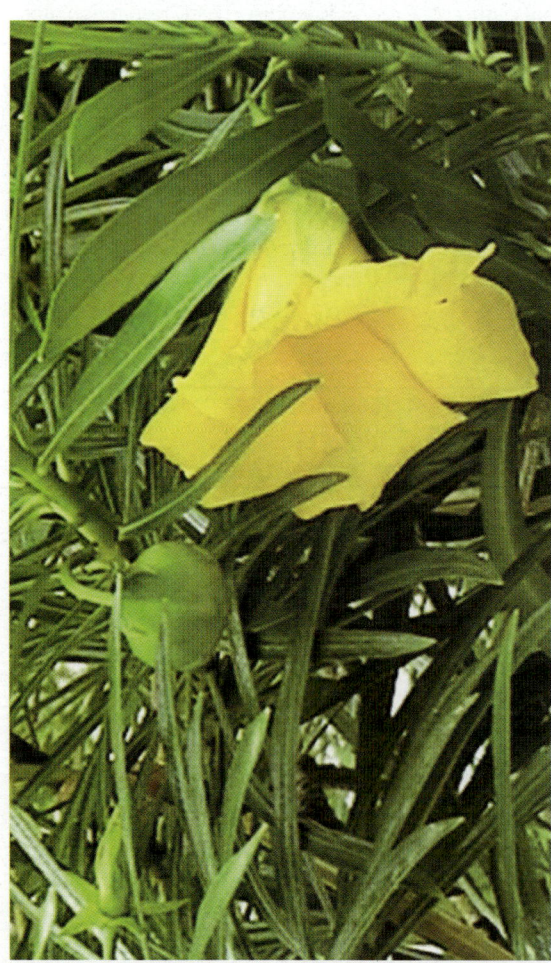

Fig. 18.12: *Cerbera thevetia* with yellow flower and fruit

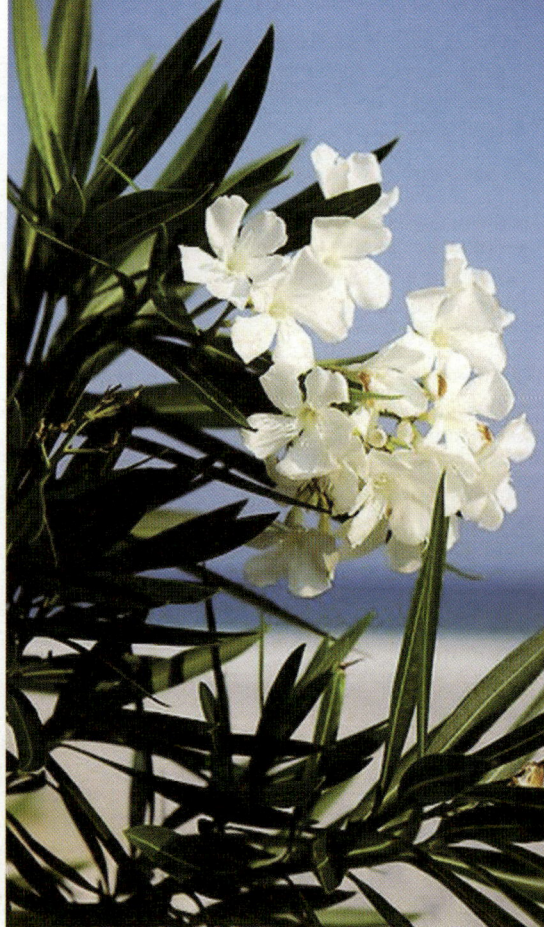

Fig. 18.13: *Nerium odorum* with white flower

Cerbera thevetia	*Nerium odorum*
Synonyms: Pila Kanher Yellow oleander, bitta-green globular fruit	**Synonyms:** Safed Kanher, white oleander
Grows in: All over India	All over India
Toxic parts: All parts of plant (maximum concentration—roots, seeds)	**Toxic parts:** All parts of plant (maximum concentration—roots)
Toxic principles: Cerberin, Thevetin, Thevotoxin	**Toxic principles:** Nerin
Use: Seeds used for playing	**Use:** Medicinal use on ulcer
Action: Cardiac depressant	**Action:** Cardiac depressant
Fatal dose Roots: 15 gm Seeds: 8–10 seeds Fatal period: 2–3 hrs	**Fatal dose** Roots: 15 gm Fatal period: 24–36 hrs

Clinical features
• Tingling, numbness and burning sensation in mouth/tongue/throat with bitter taste, increase salivation, nausea, vomiting, abdominal pain, and diarrhea
  – Cardiovascular collapse, cardiac irregularities, increase pulse and respiration, fall of BP
  – Headache, confusion, dyspnea, dizziness, delirium, dilated pupil, convulsion, collapse, and coma
	Clinical features
	• Difficulty in speech/swallowing, increase salivation with nausea, vomiting, abdominal pain, and diarrhea.
	  – Cardiovascular collapse, increase in pulse and respiration, fall of BP.
	  – Headache, confusion, dyspnea, dizziness, delirium, dilated pupil, convulsion, collapse, coma
	  – Muscle weakness, twitching, tremor, tetany, lock jaw

Treatment
• Emesis
• Stomach wash: $KMnO_4$
• Demulcent
• Artificial respiration and O_2 inhalation
• Supportive:
  – Atropine
  – Infusion of sodium, molar lactate with glucose
	Treatment
	• Emesis
	• Stomach wash
	• Demulcent/purgatives
	• Artificial respiration and O_2 inhalation
	• Supportive

PM findings • Nothing specific • Stomach: Inflammation, seeds/root ingredient • Heart: Subendocardial hemorrhage	**PM findings** • Nothing specific • Stomach: Inflammation, root ingredient • Heart: Subendocardial hemorrhage
ML aspects • Suicidal: Usually in rural areas of West Bengal • Homicidal: Rare • Accidental: Usually to children (by seeds/flower) • Abortifacient • Cattle: Used as cattle poison	**ML aspects** • Suicidal: Rare • Homicidal: Rare • Accidental: Quack medicine • Abortifacient • Cattle: Used as cattle poison

Asphyxiant and Irrespirable Poisons

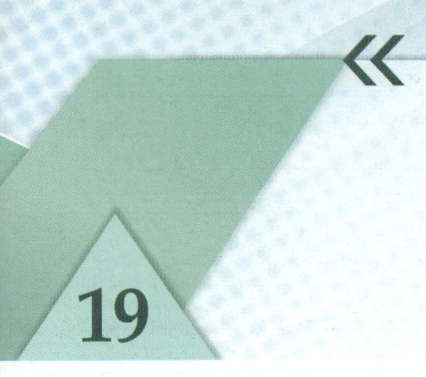

19

Asphyxiant poisons are the gases which causes asphyxia due to one of the following causes.

Causes of asphyxia due to poisons

1. Lack of sufficient oxygen in inspired air: Vitiated air
2. Spasm of RT/larynx: SO_2, mineral acid fumes.
3. Agent which prevents diffusion of gases at alveolar membrane: Phosgene (choking gas)
4. Failure of RBC to pick up oxygen in the lungs: CO
5. Poisons which interferes with the transport of oxygenated blood to tissue: Circulatory depressant.
6. Poisons which prevent the use of oxygen at tissue level: Cyanides, HCN
7. Agent which causes paralysis of respiratory muscle used for respiration: Curare
8. Agents which causes failure of respiratory center: CO_2, H_2S.

Carbon dioxide (CO_2)	Carbon monoxide (CO)
Properties Colorless, odorless, tasteless, heavier than air	**Properties** Colorless, odorless, tasteless, lighter than air
Source: Product of complete combustion • Present in expiration • Decomposition • Fermentation • Explosion of mines	**Source:** Product of incomplete combustion • In Automobiles—5% CO • Coal gas—5–15% • Fuel gas—30% • Explosion gas—60% CO
Uses 1. As respiratory stimulant 2. Fire extinguisher 3. Refrigerant	**Uses** 1. Cheap source of fuel 2. It is used as safety measure where it is mixed with other gas to detect the leakage easily
Action: Respiratory depressant	**Action:** Greater affinity for Hb than O_2, affects carrying capacity of O_2 leading to anemic anoxia
Fatal dose: 2000 ppm **Fatal period:** Min to hrs	**Fatal dose:** 1500 ppm **Fatal period:** Min to hrs
Clinical features • Depends on percentage (%) of CO_2 in air: • 0.04% : Normal in air • 2% : Respiratory stimulants • 5% : Difficulty in breathing • 10% : Vasoconstriction → increase HR, pulse, BP	**Clinical features** • Depends on saturation of CO in blood: • Normally, CO is not found in blood • 0–10% : No signs • 10–20% : Headache, dyspnea • 20–30% : Throbbing headache, dyspnea, weakness

- 20–30% : Respiratory discomfort with sudden fall of respiration
- 40% : Headache, dyspnea, dizziness, confusion, giddiness, tightness in chest, ringing in ears, dimness of vision
- 50% : Paralysis of respiratory centers
- 50–60% : Cardiac irregularities, collapse
- >60% : Unconsciousness, rapid death

- 30–40% : Headache, dyspnea, dizziness, confusion, giddiness, tightness in chest, ringing in ears, dimness of vision, with increase pulse and BP
- 40–50% : In addition to above features, there is pinkish discoloration of skin
- 50–60% : Convulsion, collapse, coma, paralysis of respiratory centers
- >60% : Respiratory arrest

Treatment
- Quick removal from source
- Artificial respiration and oxygen inhalation

Treatment
- Quick removal from source
- Artificial respiration and oxygen inhalation
- Carbogen inhalation (95% O_2 + 5% CO_2)
- Supportive: 5% dextrose, antibiotic cover, mannitol

PM findings
- PM staining: Prominent bluish color
- Organs: Congested, bluish, petechial hemorrhages
- Blood: Dark red fluid blood
- Marked cyanosis

PM findings
- PM staining: Cherry red color
- Organs: Congested, bright red, petechial hemorrhages
- Blood: Bright red fluid blood
- Froth present at mouth and nostrils

ML aspects
- Suicidal: Rare
- Homicidal: Rare
- Accidental: In vulnerable circumstances like inside mines, wells, leakage of fire extinguisher and outbreak of fire, etc.

ML aspects
- Suicidal: Common in male
- Homicidal: Rare by placing a gas tube inside the room of victim when he is sleeping at night
- Accidental: In vulnerable circumstances like outbreak of fire, by cooking gas, exhaust of vehicles, generator, and air conditioner

Autopsy photo: Marked PML lividity and cyanosis

Autopsy photo: PML : Cherry red; Blood/organs—bright red

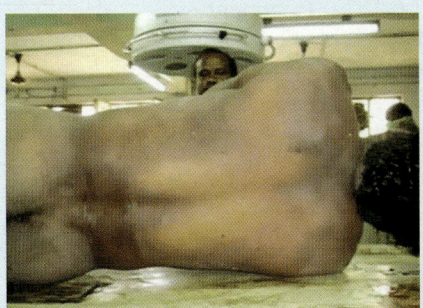

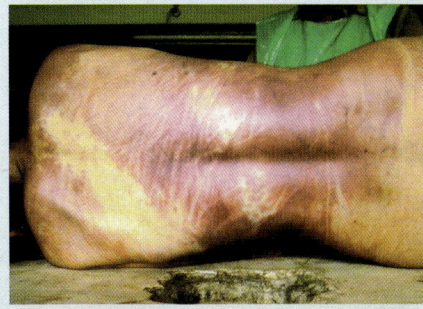

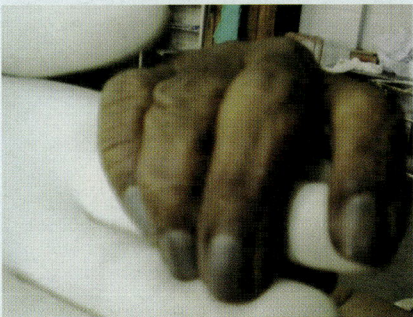

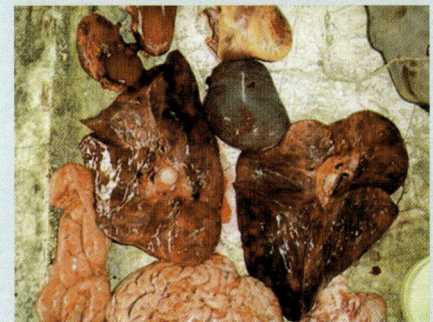

Hydrogen sulfide (H₂S)	Sulfur dioxide (SO₂)	Phosgene (COCl₂)
Metal sulfide + sulfuric acid → salt + H_2S. It is the product of decomposition of organic material containing sulfur	It is prepared by burning sulfur in oxygen/air	The **choking gas** is prepared if CCl_4 is exposed to hot air (i.e. oxidation) or by mixing chlorine gas with carbon monoxide
Properties Colorless, rotten egg smell, burns with blue flame	**Properties** Colorless, pungent	**Properties** Colorless, phosgene smell
Source: Sewer, cess pool, well decomposed body	**Source:** Laboratory, industrial, pollution	**Source:** Laboratory, industrial
Uses: Production of sulfuric acid, manufacture of pesticides, and in laboratories for analytical chemistry	**Uses:** Refrigerant and bleaching agent	**Uses:** Production of isocyanates, used in refrigeration, as a chemical weapon
Action: Respiratory depressant	**Action:** Respiratory irritant	**Action:** Prevent diffusion of gas at alveolar membrane
Fatal dose: 1000 ppm **Fatal period:** Min to hrs	**Fatal dose:** 1000 ppm **Fatal period:** Min to hrs	**Fatal dose:** 1000 ppm **Fatal period:** Min to hrs
Clinical features • Eyes: Lacrimation, photophobia headache, dyspnea, dizziness, confusion, giddiness, weakness, and cramps • This is followed by: – Convulsion, collapse, and coma	**Clinical features** • Eyes: Lacrimation, photophobia + sneezing, coughing, dyspnea, suffocation, constriction in chest • This is followed by: – Laryngeal spasm and convulsion, collapse, and coma	**Clinical features** • Eyes: Lacrimation, photophobia + sneezing, coughing, dyspnea, suffocation, constriction in chest. • This is followed by: – Marked restlessness, rapid respiration, cyanosis, convulsion, collapse, and coma
Treatment • Quick removal from source. • Artificial respiration and oxygen inhalation • Supportive: Respiratory stimulant, antibiotic cover	**Treatment** • Quick removal from source. • Artificial respiration and oxygen inhalation • Supportive: Bronchodilators, antibiotic cover	**Treatment** • Quick removal from source. • Artificial respiration and oxygen inhalation • Supportive: Antibiotic cover
PM findings • Suggestive of asphyxia present • PM staining: Greenish color • Organs: Congested, petechial hemorrhage present • Blood: Dark brown fluid blood • Body decomposes early	**PM findings** • Suggestive of asphyxia present • PM staining: Bluish color • Organs: Congested, petechial hemorrhage present • Blood: Dark red fluid blood	**PM findings** • Suggestive of asphyxia present • PM staining: Bluish color • Organs: Congested, petechial hemorrhage present • Blood: Dark red fluid blood
ML aspects • Suicidal: Not known • Homicidal: Not known • Accidental: Due to chronic exposure/fall in unused wells, and while cleaning of underground sewerage	**ML aspects** • Suicidal: Rare • Homicidal: Rare • Accidental: Rare	**ML aspects** • Suicidal: Unknown • Homicidal: Unknown • Accidental: Leakage of gas

METHYL ISOCYANATE (MIC)

Prorerties: Colorless liquid with a sharp odor, which becomes gaseous at 39°C.

It is an extremely reactive chemically and needs to be stored carefully.

Uses

1. In the manufacture of pesticide carbaryl carbamate.
2. Manufacture of polyurethane articles (plastics, foam, adhesives, etc.).

Action

Powerful respiratory irritant.

Clinical Features

1. Inhalation of gas produces immediate lacrimation, photophobia, cough, dyspnea, chest pain, hemoptysis, pulmonary edema, vomiting, convulsion, and coma.
2. Dermal exposure results in erythema and vesiculation.

Treatment

1. Washing of skin and eyes with saline.
2. Oxygen inhalation.
3. Bronchodilators and corticosteroids.
4. Antidote: Sodium thiosulfate.
5. Supportive.

PM Findings

Suggestive of asphyxia

- **Lungs/brain:** Congested, edematous.
- **Visceral organs:** Congested.

ML Aspect

MIC was involved in one of the most terrible gas disaster which occurred in Bhopal, Madhya Pradesh **(Bhopal Gas Tragedy, 1984)**. There was a leakage of methyl isocyanate from union carbide plant. MIC is required in the manufacture of carbaryl (carbamate). This deadly chemical was stored in huge, double walled stainless steel tanks, one of which burst on the night of Dec 2, 1984, releasing more than 24,000 kg of MIC gas into the atmosphere killing thousands in their sleep and incapacitating several thousands more.

Phosphine (Water + Calcium Carbide)

It is a war gas, being prepared by boiling white phosphorus with a solution of KOH or NaOH. It can be easily prepared by moistening calcium phosphide.

- It is a respiratory track irritant and has acetylene like odor.
- **Fatal dose:** 20 ppm.
- It is released from zinc phosphide and metal phosphide.
- It is used as a fumigant to control insects and rodents in food grains and fields.

20   Drug Dependence and Abuse

Since time immemorial drugs and its abuse is known to mankind. When drug is consumed for non-medical purpose, it is said to have been abused. The abuse of drugs is an international problem, which affects almost every country in the world; India is no exception. Drug abuse is now a major problem faced by our society and it has medical, legal, social, moral, ethical and political ramifications. In 1991, as per survey conduct by UN Narcotics Control Strategy Report, there are over one million opium abusers in India alone.

Drugs are the substance having physiological and psychological effects on human beings and other animals. It is used to sustain/prolong life or to get relief, which should have ideally been the sole use of drugs. But as actions and powers are misused in all fields, the drugs are not spared. This misuse is not limited to therapeutic purpose as follows:

1. To terminate their unsuccessful life.
2. To get relief from tension.
3. To pass undisturbed peaceful time.

Drug abuse: It is an improper and excessive use of therapeutic medicine even in the absence of addiction

Drug addiction (WHO 1950): Addiction is state of periodic or chronic intoxication produced by the repeated consumption of a drug	**Drug Habit:** It is a condition resulting from repeated consumptions of drug, which does not cause much harm to the society
It is characterized by a. Tendency to increase the dose b. Harmful effects to the individual and to the society c. It causes both **psychological and physical dependence** d. An overpowering desire to continue the drug or to obtain it by any means	*It is characterized by* a. Tendency to take the drugs and repeat it as and when convenient b. Harmful effect mainly to the individual c. **Psychological dependence** and not physical dependence

Drug dependence: WHO has coined the term drug dependence to **replace the terms** "Drug addiction and drug habit". It has been defined as a state, psychological or physical, in which a person has the compulsion to take a drug on a continuous or periodic basis either to experience its pleasurable effects or to avoid the discomfort

Physical dependence: It is a biological phenomenon, which depends on the type, dose, and duration of used irrespective of personality factor. If the drug is abruptly stopped withdrawal syndrome will occur.	**Psychological dependence:** Is a compulsive need for a drug in order to maintain state of well-being

CLASSIFICATION OF DRUGS USED FOR ABUSE

I. Depending upon physical or psychological dependence
  a. **Drug of addiction:** Drugs that causes both psychological and physical dependence:
* Alcohols
* Narcotic analgesic: Opium, methadon, morphine, heroin, codeine, pethidine
* Depressant (downers):
    Tranquilizers: Diazepam, chlordiazepoxide
    Hypnotics: Barbiturate, paraldehyde, chloral hydrocarbon, meprobamate
* Methaqualone:

  b. **Drug habit:** Drugs which causes only psychological dependence:
* Tobacco
* Cannabis preparations: Ganja, charas, majun, bhang.
* Stimulants (uppers): Amphetamine, caffeine, ephedrine, methyl phenidate (ritalin)
* Volatile anesthetic solvents: Toluene, known as 'glue sniffing'
* Hallucinogens: Lysergic acid diethylamide (LSD), phencyclidine, mescaline

II. Depending upon their effects:
  a. **Hard drugs**—narcotics
  b. **Soft drugs**—Barbiturates, diazepam, amphetamine, LSD, pentazocaine, alcohol

4. To be out of touch from practical problems.
5. To be in an imaginary state of mental happiness and well being.

The drugs made its path from the doctor's or chemist room to these vulnerable people of the society. Thus, the drugs user may be:

a. **Occasional users:** Depending on the custom and cultural background of the society who accepted the use of alcohol and some preparation of cannabis. However, use of tobacco is almost accepted in all societies.

b. **Heavy users:** They are addicted or dependent on some drugs and cannot do anything without the same.

BRIEF DESCRIPTION OF DRUGS OF ABUSE

I. Opium: It is extracted from unripe fruit of the plant *Papaver somniferum*. Incisions on the unripe fruit produce milky exude which on exposure to air becomes dark brown opium.

Opium is also called 'Black Gold' because of its color and price in international market.

Opioid drugs can be divided into three groups

Natural	Morphine, codeine, thebaine
Semisynthetic	Heroin, oxymorphone, nalorphine
Synthetic	Pethidine, methadon, propoxy-phene, fentanyl

Opioid drugs are known by many names:
* Heroin—smack, dope, Lady Jane, brown sugar.
* Fentanyl—China white.

II. Cocaine: Cocaine is extracted from the leaves of a plant *Erythroxylum coca*, which grows in the mountains of South America and tropical Asia. It is then purified to the hydrochloride salt, which is white crystalline in nature.

Street names of cocaine are: Coke, snow, cadillac, white lady, etc.
* Cocaine + ethanol—it is called liquid lady.
* Cocaine + heroin—it is called speedball or crank.
* Newer type of cocaine is known as crack.

III. Cannabis: *Cannabis sativa/indica* grows all over India, but its cultivation growth and marketing is controlled by legislation.

Active principle: Tetrahydrocannabinol

Preparation of cannabis

Bhang (siddi)	Consist of dried leaves or stem
Ganja	Consist of flowering tops of female plant
Charas 'Hashish'	Concentrated resin extracted from leaves/stem and flower
Majun	Sweet preparation from bhang after **treating with sugar, flour, milk**
Marihuana	It is the extract from American hemp plant
Reefers	Cigarettes preparation of ganja/marijuana

Street names: Marijuana, Mary Jane, pot, weed, grass.

IV. Alcohol

Arrack: Refer to country made liquor usually distilled from palm, cereal or jaggery. In India, adulterant like chloral hydrate (knockout drops) or methanol may be deliberate added to arrack in order to further enhance its effect.

Street names of country liquor: Khopdi, lattha, sura, etc.

V. Tobacco: Is obtained from nicotiana tabacum/rustica.

Active principle: Nicotine—toxic part is leaf.

The dried leaves of tobacco are used in India in the form of smoke/snuff or chewing with lime or alone. Individual begins with tobacco and alcohol, progress later to cannabis and may eventually graduate to opium/heroin. Hence, it is considered as **"Gateway" to drug abuse.**

VI. Sedatives

Barbiturates	Drug of choice for sedation, e.g. gardenal, luminal, veronal
Benzodiazepines	Drug for seizure/anxiolytics, e.g. calmpose, valium, restyl, libruim
Chloral hydrate	Knock out drops, mixed in alcohol for a greater kick

VII. Hallucinogens

Hallucinogens	Street names
Lysergic acid diethylamide	The drug is popular among its uses as 'blue pill'. Acid, microdot, purple haze, white lightnening, etc.
Phencyclidine	It is phenyl-cyclohexyl-piperidine (PCP). Angel dust, Angel's mist, dust killer weed
Mescaline	Extracted from the dried tops of a cactus plant *Lophophora williamsii*

VIII. Designer drugs: These are used to describe the synthesis of drugs by clandestine laboratories; which **are synthetic variations of well-known controlled drugs** with similar pharmacological effects but different molecular structures. This had rendered them immune from the control of the drug enforcement agency.

The most commonly known types of synthetic analog drugs available in the illicit drug market includes:

Derivatives	Street name of designer drug
Amphetamine	Ecstasy/adams/XTC. Love drugs; speed/ice; eve
Fentanyl derivatives	China white. Alpha-methyl fentanyl—3000 times as potent as morphine (detected by RI assay)
Phencyclidine (PCP)	**Angel dust:** Smoking PCP + marijuana **Wack:** PCP + formaldehyde + roach repellent **Spacebar:** PCP + crack (never cocaine)
Flunitrazepam	**Rohypnol 'Roofies':** Reported as being one of the commonest drugs in school and college campuses. It is often combined with alcohol, marijuana or cocaine. It is commonly used for **'Date rape'**

IX. Inhalants: These groups of drug are being used recently. The abuse of these drugs is called 'solvent abuse' because most of these are used as solvents.

Commonly used are hydrocarbons, which are classified as:

Aliphatic	Diesel oil, gasoline, kerosene
Aromatic	Benzene, toluene, xylene
Halogenated	Carbontetrachloride (CCl_4), tetrachloroethane

X. Others

Mandrax	(Methaqualone + diphenhydramine): It is very popular in India. Many factories manufacturing 'Mandrax' were recently unearthed by Gujarat and Maharashtra Police and shut down
Cough syrup	It is a newer type of addiction, common in those who have given up alcohol

INVESTIGATION OF DRUG RELATED OR DRUG ABUSE DEATHS

As a rule, toxicology test results taken alone cannot used to determine the COD. In order to make accurate diagnosis, consideration must

Etiology of drug abuse: Factors related to drug dependence are as follows:	
Factor	*Cause*
1. Personal factor	• Psychological status of a person • Period of stress, strain, curiosity, adventure and experimentation in young age; and is common in males • Tolerance and threshold to different odds of life
2. Social/economic and environmental factors	• Family status/environment/liability/responsibility/attachment/happenings and stress events in family • Neglected childhood, separated parents • Failure in love/exams/achievement/career • Social and mental status of friends/associates • Environment in school, college, hostel, surrounding • Residential and working environment • Emotional trends, habits, likeliness and mental makeup
3. Drug factor	• Self-medication, over medication, wrong medication • Easy availability of drug • Prescription abuse • Tolerance to drug

Routes of administration of drugs for abuse	
Routes	*Examples*
1. Oral	Alcohol, cannabis preparation (bhang, ganja, majun), mandrax, LSD, amphetamine (ecstasy), barbiturates, diazepam, cough syrup
Usually they are mixed with something (alcohol) or sometimes one or two drugs may be combined together for a greater kick	
2. Parental	Accessible sites are preferred
a. Subcutaneous (SC)	Opium, heroin—over thigh/forearm
Drug using SC route is known as 'skin popping' and a person who uses this route is called a 'skin popper'.	
b. Intravenous (IV)	Opium drugs
Drug using IV route is known as 'mainlining' and a person who uses this route is called a 'mainliner'	
c. Intra-arterial	Opium drugs in radial/femoral artery, cocaine injection in venous plexuses
Drug using intra-arterial route is known as 'pinkie'	
3. Inhalation	
Snorting/sniffing	Cocaine—when a powder is inhaled (snuff)
Glue sniffing	Toluene, xylene, benzene—when volatile solvent is inhaled
Chasers	Heroin—when foils containing heroin are burnt and the fumes are inhaled
4. Smoking	Ganja, marijuana, tobacco and crack

also be given to scene investigation, autopsy findings and the circumstances leading to the death (i.e. history). Thus, investigation of drug abuse death involves four steps.

I. Crime Scene Investigation

1. Usually the drugs are taken by addicts at isolated places where the death occurred or may be shifted to any other place.

2. Place/spot should also be searched for presence of drugs, needles, syringes, container of drugs, a cooker and a source of heat. Tubes of plastic glue or plastic bags, aerosol cans, etc. may indicate 'solvent abuse' related death along with soiled clothes with solvent.

3. Clothes of the deceased should be searched for drugs and apparatus. Sometimes drugs may be taped to the body between buttocks, toes, under the breasts or attached to string around tooth.

4. Surrounding area should also be searched for home made local remedies used in an attempt to revive, e.g. injecting saliva, milk or water into the arm, back of hands or buttock.

5. Photograph should be taken.

II. History

The history includes past history of drug abuse, police record, and information from friends, relatives and witness as to past and present behaviour. The drug users may have negative thought—'love is hate, born to lose, loner, die young'.

III. Autopsy Findings

The autopsy in case of death due to drug abuse should concentrate on the external examination and collection of adequate samples for toxicological analysis.

a. External Examination

1. **In most of the cases, there is no specific autopsy finding:** There may be wasting or signs of self neglect may be seen, i.e. unhygienic condition of abuser.

2. **Burns/stain around mouth:** Or on the tips of finger and long fingernails may be seen in cocaine abusers. **Blood tinged froth** oozing from mouth/nostril **with characteristics odor.**

3. **In IV addicts (mainliner), typical linear needle track scars appear as:** 'Railroad tracks' are seen in cubital fossa, forearm and dorsal aspect of hands. They are also seen in area of scalp, neck, sublingual areas, shoulder, inguinal region, penis, vagina, popliteal area, ankle or foot.

In intradermal or subcutaneous drug users—skin popper revealed **typical depressed circular and geographical atrophic scar,** ulceration, infected abscess, etc. Healing by fibrosis may produce hyperpigmented macules, circumscribed scars like that of smallpox vaccination scars.

In nasal inhalation (snorting/sniffing)—there may be irritation, congestion and atrophy of nasal mucosa; and in some cases perforation of nasal septum, especially in cocaine and heroin abusers.

In solvent abusers (glue sniffing)—the face may be red, erythematous pimples or actual excoriations from the irritant action of the solvent. The lesions may become infected, scratched or crusted.

4. **Recent injection sites:** May show zones of inflammation surrounding the puncture site. Incision through skin may reveal a prominent perivenous hemorrhage.

5. **'Soot tattooing':** These are the punctate areas of black discoloration seen along the track of needle due to the deposition of carbonaceous material, as the needle being sterilized over flame. Such tattooing is also called 'turkey skin'.

6. **Tattoos:** May be seen over the areas of needle marks, which are used **to conceal the injection marks.**

b. Internal Examination

Internal findings are not prominent at autopsy:

1. Examination of needle scars reveals **perivenous fibrosis in IV** addicts, and subcutaneous scarring and acute/chronic abscess in the skin popper.

2. Streaks of carbon may be seen in subcutaneous tissue, which are deposited by heated needle tips.

3. Foreign material such as cotton, piece of cloth, talc, starch, etc. are seen in subcutaneous tissues with surrounding foreign body giant cell reaction on microscopy.

4. Peripheral veins may show old or recent thrombosis, phlebitis in mainliners.

5. Lungs are heavy, congested and edematous, especially in heroin addicts called **'Heroin Lung'**. In mainliners, crystals lodge in pulmonary capillaries and lungs show large quantities of talc, starch and cellulose in the foreign body granulomatous reaction. The bronchi and trachea are filled with abundant grey froth. Pleura may show petechial hemorrhage.

6. **Stomach** may show undissolved **tablets/pills**. The entire length of GIT should be searched for evidence of an attempt to hide/smuggled drugs.

7. There may be enlarged lymph nodes near porta hepatis. Liver may be slightly enlarged and may show evidence of cirrhosis. This is especially seen in opioid abusers.

8. Pericardial, pleural and peritoneal effusion may be seen; and heart may show valvular disease.

9. Brain may show edema and focal necrosis of globus pallidus and hippocampus due to hypoxia.

10. Acute muscle neurosis may be present.

IV. Toxicological Analysis

Following samples are preserved for toxicological analysis in drugs related deaths:

1. Routine viscera (V1 + V2) along with gallbladder.

2. **Blood:** Usually venous blood from peripheral sites (femoral vein), kept in fluoride preservative.

3. **Tissue from injection site:** In cases of parenteral users.

4. **Urine:** Usually in opium, datura, cannabis, alcohol, amphetamine, cocaine. Addicts are known as **'Liquid Gold'**.

5. **Nasal swabs:** In cases of nasal inhalation of drugs.

6. **Hepatic lymph nodes:** In opiates.

7. Any soiling with adhesives or solvent stain.

8. In cases of death due to volatile substances:

i. **Blood in a glass tube** filled to the top with an aluminium foil lined cap.

ii. **Whole lungs** with main bronchus and pulmonary vessels, which are to be ligated, should be kept **in a nylon bag** (and not in polythene bags which are permeable to volatiles) and securely tied.

iii. Brain half in opium, barbiturate, diazepam, solvent abuse, cocaine, etc.

CAUSES OF DEATH

I. Mostly due to Drug Overdose/Toxicity

Drug toxicity	Effects
Ethyl alcohol	Alcoholic intoxication
Methyl alcohol	Metabolic acidosis, renal failure
Heroin	Due to combination with alcohol or cocaine
Cocaine Phencyclidine	Cardiac arrhythmia, convulsion. Hypothermia, intracranial hemorrhage, cardiac failure
LSD	Traumatic death due to fall from height because the person under influence of LSD think that he can fly and thus project himself out of window
Body packer syndrome	It is due to rupture of packet containing smuggled drugs in the body used as body packer

II. Due to the Complication, Secondary to Unsterile Injection or Adulteration

i. Infection-bronchopneumonia, bronchitis, viral hepatitis, AIDS, infective endocarditis, tetanus, acute myopathy, meningitis, and brain/lung abscess.

ii. Malnutrition, anemia and cachexia.

iii. Acute muscle neurosis with myoglobinuria and renal failure, malaria, syphilis.

MEDICOLEGAL ASPECT

The drugs are sold to people under many funny names at the rate of ₹ 10/– for 10 gm for charas to very costlier drugs like opium (Black Gold). In spite of stringent legislation, the drug trade is increasing day by day and often lead to varieties of criminal offences.

1. Body packing: For smuggling drugs, person swallows a small packet containing drugs.

2. Drug abuse and crime

Drug	Crime
Cannabis	Rum amok
Heroin	Assault, mugging to extort money for purchase of drug.
Alcohol	Sexual assaults/rape, etc.
Exchange of drugs for weapons	Narco terrorism
Drug addicts parent	Battered baby syndrome
Morphine	Infanticide

3. Drugs abuse and suicide: Barbiturate/diazepam are commonly used for suicide.

4. Drugs abuse and accidents

Drug	Accidents
Alcohol	Vehicular accident if under influence
Alcohol	Industrial hazards
Aphrodisiacs drugs—viagra, cocaine	Accidental death due to excessive dose
Barbiturates	Automatism

5. Drugs abuse and insanity

Drug	Insanity
LSD	Hallucinogens
Datura	Deliriant, stupefying
Cocaine, morphine	Maniacs
Alcohol withdrawal	Delirium tremens

EFFECTIVE DEALING OF THE PROBLEM OF DRUG ABUSE

The association of drugs with AIDS on one side and terrorism on the other makes it the most dreaded and burning menace the world has ever faced. Following measures are important while dealing with the problem of drug abuse:

1. **Mass education:** Only mass education will not solve problem.

2. Running of de-addiction **centers and counselling**.

3. **Stringent legislation** and strict implementation of the provisions in the law regarding drug trafficking or peddling.

4. **Encouragement for de-addiction:** Effort should be taken to identify the abusers and potential abusers, the factor influencing the abuse and **effective methods to stop drug trafficking/peddling.**

5. There should be adequate numbers of **laboratories for drug testing** and treatment centers for the drug dependents.

6. There should be meaningful **rehabilitation** programmes for de-addicted persons.

It must be remembered by all that drugs are blessed discoveries for the safety and well-being of members of the society and not to cause any harm to any of its members.

21

Food Poisoning

Definition: These are the illnesses resulting from ingestion of food containing bacterial or non-bacterial products. However, the term is restricted for the acute gastroenteritis due to bacterial infection of food or drink. Food poisoning is due to following causes:

1. Food contaminated with bacteria (bacterial food poisoning)
2. Poisonous food of vegetable origin
3. Poisonous food of animal origin
4. Food contaminated with chemicals

BACTERIAL FOOD POISONING

It is commonly seen in summer season or rainy season and usually occurs in isolated/small outbreaks. The poisoning spreads by consumption of infected food. It is of two types:

a. Infection type
b. Toxin type

a. Infection type: It occurs due to ingestion of viable microorganism that multiplies in the gastrointestinal tract producing gastroenteritis. It is mainly due to Salmonella group of organism and *E. coli*.

Treatment

1. Fluid replacement therapy
2. Antibiotics

b. Toxin type: In this type, toxin is either produced/present in the contaminated food (exotoxin) or produce after ingestion of contaminated food (enterotoxin).

Infection type	Source	Incubation period	Clinical features	Diagnosis
Salmonella infection	Beef, poultry products, eggs, dairy products	12 to 48 hours	Main feature is watery diarrhea (foul smelling mixed with blood or mucus), fever and muscle weakness	Widal test, stool culture, isolation of bacteria in suspected food
Escherichia coli (normal flora of intestinal tract of human)	Contaminated food like salad, cheese, meat, water, raw vegetables, apple juice, etc.	1–3 days	(Copious outpouring of fluids from gastrointestinal tract) severe vomiting and diarrhea resulting in dehydration, abdominal cramps, fever and bloody diarrhea	Stool culture, clinical features
Campylobacter jejuni	Water, milk and meat	2–10 days	Watery or bloody diarrhea along with fever, abdominal pain and headache	Stool/blood culture with special media at 43°C, dark field microscopy

1. Exotoxin Variety (Botulism)

Botulism: It results from consumption of preformed botulinum toxin (exotoxin) in the preserved food due to infection by *Cl. botulinum*. The toxins bind to the presynaptic nerve terminal at the neuromuscular junction and cholinergic autonomic sites. This prevents the release of acetylcholine and blocks neuro-transmission.

Treatment: It involves clearing of airways, ventilation and intravenous trivalent antitoxin.

2. Enterotoxin Variety

In this food poisoning, the toxins are produced after consumption of the contaminated canned or tinned foods by bacteria. It is due to con-tamination with Staphylococcus, *Bacillus cereus, Clostridium perfringens*, Shigella and cholera. It acts by producing enterotoxin after consumption of food.

Treatment of enterotoxin variety of food poisoning:

1. Replacement of fluids and electrolyte losses.
2. Antibiotics.
3. Supportive care is the mainstay of treatment. Close attention to oxygenation and hydration is important.

FOOD POISONING FROM VEGETABLE ORIGIN

It occurs due to direct toxin effect of the plant or due to the decomposition/contamination.

Toxin type	Source	Incubation period	Clinical features	Diagnosis
Cl. botulinum	Under processed sausages, potted meat, tinned fish, canned acidic vegetables and fruits, etc.	A few hrs to 36 hours	Initial signs and symptoms include blurred vision, mydriasis, ptosis, dysphagia, and dysarthria, dysphonia, and muscle weakness. After 24–48 hours, neuromuscular manifestations progress to symmetric descending paralysis and respiratory failure	Stool culture, isolation of bacteria in suspected food
Staphylococcus	Contaminated meat, milk, dairy products, potato, eggs, salad, etc.	2–12 hours	SEB produces nonspecific systemic illness that is characterized by fever, chills, headache, nausea, vomiting, dyspnea, chest pain, myalgia, and a nonproductive cough	Stool culture
Bacillus cereus	Consumption of fried rice, dried fruits, powdered milk, etc. produce toxicity	Two types of toxin 1. 8–16 hours 2. 3–6 hours	Two types of toxins: 1. One is heat labile large molecular protein which produces diarrhea as the main symptom 2. Other toxin is heat stable, low molecular weight peptide which produces severe vomiting	Stool culture, culture of contaminated food
Clostridium perfringens	Consumption of contaminated food particularly canned food, meat, etc.	8–16 hours	Poisoning is characterized by sudden onset of profuse diarrhea and occasionally vomiting	Stool culture
Shigella	Potato, raw milk, eggs, vegetables, lettuce, salad, fruits, etc.	12–96 hours	Patient presents with sudden onset of diarrhea, often with blood and pus in stool, cramps, tenesmus, and lethargy	Stool culture
Cholera	Contaminated water	12–72 hours.	The syndrome is characterized by sudden onset of nausea and vomiting and profuse diarrhea with classic rice water appearance	Hanging drop preparation of stool-motile bacteria. Stool culture

Food poisoning from vegetable origin occurs due to:

a. *Lathyrus sativus*	Due to neurotoxin BOAA
b. Food substance	
Argemone oil	It is mixed with mustard oil
Badly stored groundnut seeds	Contaminated with *Aspergillous flavus* produce aflatoxin causing hepatic damage
Badly stored wheat, rye, oat, barley, etc.	Allows growth of fungus *Claviceps purpurae* leads to ergot poisoning
Potato	Produces solanin
Cotton seeds	It has gossypol which makes lysine unavailable to the body
Cabbage	It has sulfur containing compound which inhibits thyroxine secretion
Soya bean	It has trypsin inhibitor which makes protein unavailable to the body
Poisonous berries, e.g.	Atropa belladonna
c. Food allergy	Particularly with tomato, bean (gavar), milk
d. Mushroom	*Amanita muscaria/phalloides*

Lathyrus sativus

Common name: Kesari, lakhori/tiwra daal.

The seed of this plant is a staple food for low income groups in some areas of central India. The plant is not poisonous and the leaves are used as green vegetables. They have 4–6 cm long beans containing seeds similar to tur daal. The toxic principle is present in the seeds. However, the seeds are used in making different food preparations (Figs 21.1 and 21.2). Consumption of *Lathyrus sativus* seeds in quantities more than 30% of the total diet for more than six months have been known to cause paralysis (neurolathyrism).

Toxic principle: It contains a neurotoxin known as BOAA (beta oxalyl amino alanine) as a free amino acid in seeds cotyledon which has an affinity for pyramidal systems.

Clinical features: The onset of symptoms due to the BOAA is acute, subacute or gradual. There is an agonizing pain in calf muscles with paralysis of limbs. While working in the field, there may be weakness in the leg with difficulty in sitting. Soon the patient become unable to walk without help of a stick; the legs tremble and drag along with difficulty. Later, the patient has spastic gait characterized by a walk on tiptoes with scissor-like crossing of legs. This is followed by paraplegia but there is no atrophy/degeneration or loss of tone of muscle.

Treatment

1. No specific treatment.
2. Exclude pulses from diet.

Argemone mexicana

Common name: Sial Kanta (Bengal), Pila Datura/Bharam Dandi (Maharashtra) and Darvdi (Gujarat).

Mustard oil is widely used for cooking purpose in certain parts of India which is more often adulterated with oil of *Argemone mexicana*. This plant grows all over the India.

All parts of the plant are poisonous but maximum concentration is in the seeds. It has sessile, spiny, thistle-like leaves. The flowers are yellow with prickly oblong/elliptic capsular fruit of size 2–4 cm long containing seeds (Fig. 21.3). The seeds are dark brown in color and granular in shape but smaller in size in than mustard seeds.

Active principle: It contains alkaloids—*berberine and protopine* and sanguinarine and dihydro-sanguinarine in seeds. The oil of Argemone seeds causes **epidemic dropsy**. This oil is used as an adulterant of mustard oil or other edible oil.

Clinical features: The symptoms appear slowly with loss of appetite, nausea, dyspepsia, diarrhea, edema of legs or even generalized anasarca. There is enlargement of liver with breathlessness on slight exertion.

Treatment: It includes supportive treatment, diuretics and prednisolone. Good nutritious diet, vitamins B_1 and B_{12} and mineral in adequate dose will help in early recovery. Avoid consumption of contaminated oil.

Chemical test: 5 ml adulterated mustard oil + 5 ml nitric acid → shake the test tube.

Orange yellow color develops, if argemone is present.

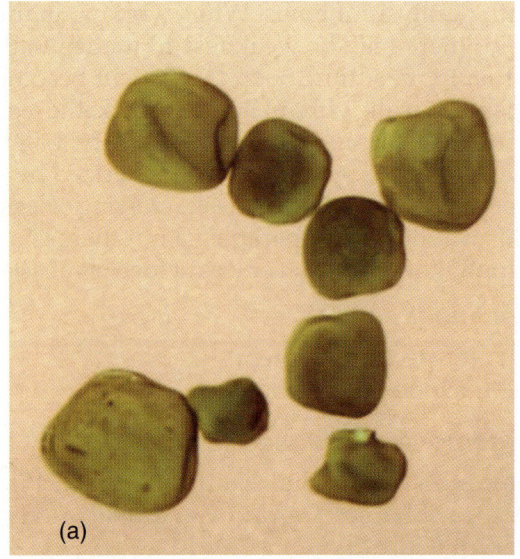
(a)

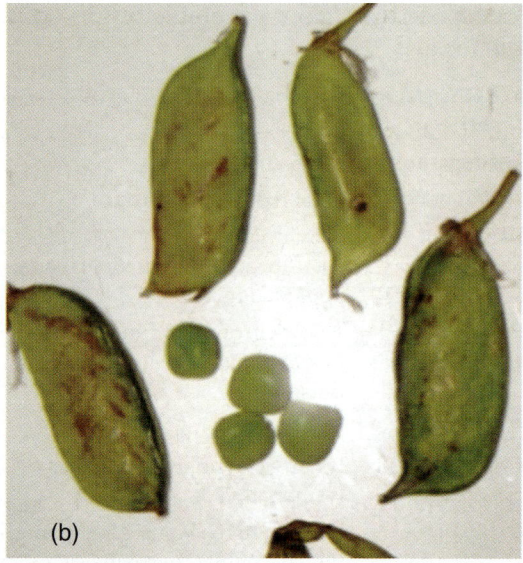
(b)

Figs 21.1a and b: Beans and seeds of *Lathyrius sativus*

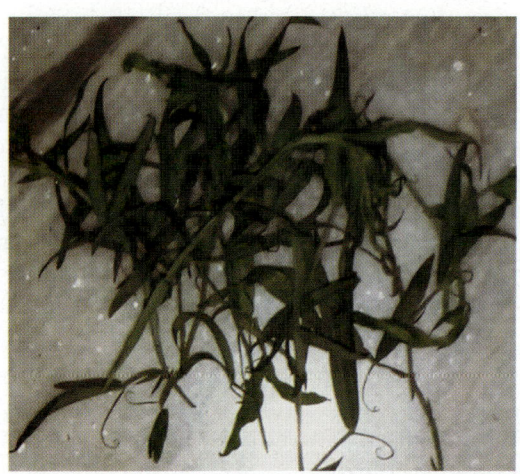

Fig. 21.2: *Lathyrius sativus*

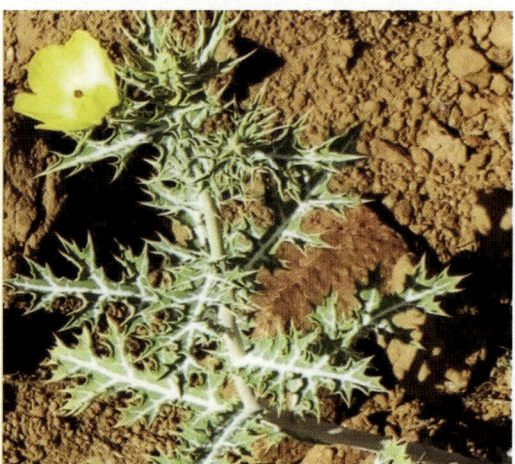

Fig. 21.3: *Argemone mexicana*

Food Allergy

It occurs in people who are sensitive to particular food product (usually proteinaceous substance) and may show allergic manifestations like rashes, vomiting, diarrhea, asthmatic attack, and circulatory collapse.

Treatment

1. Anti-allergic/anti-histaminic.
2. Symptomatic.
3. Avoid food responsible for allergy.

POISONOUS MUSHROOMS

These are actually the **reproductive portion of the fungus** which grows from an underground mycelium or hyphae constituting the vegetative portion of the fungus. *Some species of the mushrooms are non-poisonous and are used as food. Amanita phalloides/muscaria are the common* varieties of poisonous fungi.

Poisonous mushrooms usually have a bitter, astringent, acid or salt taste. On cut section, brown/green/blue color may be seen on exposure of cut surface. However, it is very difficult to differentiate poisonous mushrooms.

Amanita muscaria: It grows singly in sandy soil. It has a hollow stalk which is solid and bulbous at the base, and has gills which are white. The pileous (top flower-like) varies in color from yellow to orange or red and is covered by warty scales (Fig. 21.4). It contains toxic alkaloids—muscarine, the action of which resembles stimulation of parasympathetic postganglionic nerves.

Amanita phalloides: It is white in color and grows in woody places to a height of 15–20 cm. It has a hollow stalk with a permanent bulb at the base. The pileus is usually white, pale yellow or olive; and has gills covered with white spores on its undersurface. It contains polypeptides which are powerful inhibitors of cellular protein synthesis.

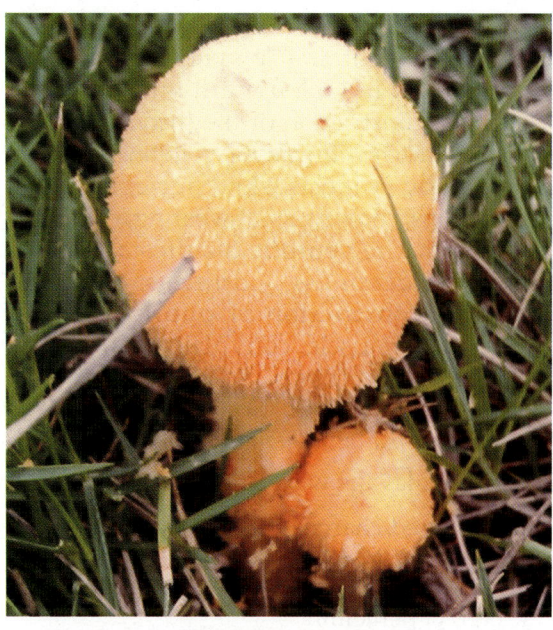

Fig. 21.4: Mushroom: *Amanita muscaria*

Species of mushrooms	Common name	Toxin
Amanita muscaria	Fly Agaric	Amatoxin, phallotoxin, virotoxin
Amanita phalloides	Death Cap	Amatoxin, phallotoxin, virotoxin
Amanita pantherina	Panther Cap, False Blusher	Amatoxin, phallotoxin, virotoxin
Amanita virosa	Destroying Angel	Amatoxin, phallotoxin, virotoxin
Clitocybae dealbata	Sweater	Muscarine
Coprinus atramentarius	Inky Cap	Coprine
Galerina autumnalis	Deadly Galerina	Gyrometrin
Gyrometra esculenta	False Morel	Gyrometrin
Psilocybe caerulipes	Blue Foot	Psilocybin, psilocin
Psilocybe semilenceta	Liberty cap, Magic Mushroom	Psilocybin, psilocin
Lycoperdon	Puffball Mushrooms	Amatoxin

S. no.	Classification of mushrooms into 8 groups	Species name
1.	Cyclopeptide containing mushrooms	Amenita, Galerina, Lepiota
2.	Monomethylhydrazine containing mushrooms	Gyrometra, and Lycoperdon
3.	Muscarine containing mushrooms	Clitocybae, and Inocybe
4.	Coprine containing mushrooms	*Coprinus atramentarius*
5.	Ibotenic acid containing mushrooms	*Amanita muscaria, Amanita pantherina*
6.	Psilocybin containing mushrooms	*Psilocybe caerulescens, Conocybe cyanopus*
7.	Gastroenteritis containing mushrooms	*Agaricus augustus, Boletus sensibilis*
8.	Orelline and orellanine containing mushrooms	Cortinarius

Clinical features: Mushroom poisoning is usually accidental. The symptoms are the combination of GIT irritant and neurotic. There is a constriction of the throat, burning pain in stomach with nausea, vomiting, diarrhea followed by cyanosis, slow pulse, laboured respirations, convulsions, sweating, collapsed and death. The neurotic manifestations are headache, dizziness, giddiness, delirium, diplopia, constriction of pupils, cramps, twitching of muscle, convulsion, salivation, bradycardia and coma.

Treatment of poisoning with mushrooms

1. Gastric lavage with $KMnO_4$.
2. Activated charcoal.
3. Forced diuresis/hemodialysis.
4. Benzyl penicillin
5. Atropine sulfate
6. Symptomatic

FOOD POISONING FROM ANIMAL ORIGIN

It is due to the following reasons

a. **Decomposed flesh**—forms ptomaine which produce manifestation like that of atropine.
b. **Venomous fish.**
c. Poisonous aquatic animal.
d. **Food allergy** to fish, prawn, etc.

Ptomaine Poisoning

Ptomaine is produced by the action of saprophytic microorganism upon nitrogenous material during the decomposition. They also known as **cadaveric alkaloid** when found in dead tissues. And alkaloids secreted during metabolism by **living cells** are called **leucomaines.**

Ptomaine resembles vegetable alkaloids like morphine, codeine, veratrine; mostly non-poisonous except neurine and mydaleine, which are actively poisonous and **produce symptoms resembling those of poisoning by atropine, muscarine and aconite.** But, by the time ptomaine is formed, the food becomes so unpalatable that it is not likely to be eaten.

Poisonous Fish

Poisoning resulting from fish and other marine creature is known as **ichthyism.** Poisonous fish is divided into three subgroups:

a. Ichthyo-sarcotoxic fish: Contain toxin within their flesh
b. Ichthyo-hemotoxic fish: Contain poisonous blood
c. Ichthyo-otoxic fish: Contain toxin mainly in gonads

Based on nature of toxin, there are six types of sea fish poisoning (Table 21.1).

Table 21.1: Types of sea fish poisoning based on the nature of toxin

Type of sea fish	Toxin	Source
Scombroid	Histamine and saurine	Tuna, needle fish, king fish, blue fish
Ciguatera	Ciguatera, maitotoxin, scaritoxin, okadaic toxin, polytoxin	Parrot fish, barracuda, sea bass, red snapper, grouper, king fish
Tetradotoxic	Tetradotoxin	Puffer fish, newts, salamander, blue ring octopus, Ballon fish, Globe fish, toad fish, horseshoe crab eggs
Paralytic shellfish	Saxitoxin, neosaxitoxin	Shellfish like oysters, clans
Neurotoxic shellfish	Brevitoxin	Dinoflagellate, *Ptychodisus brevis*
Amnesic shellfish	Domoic acid	Diatom Nitzschia pungens

Poisonous Aquatic Animals

1. California mussel (which eats planktons having deadly toxins): May cause sensory and motor disturbances like tingling, numbness, muscular weakness and paralysis.
2. Some shells, shrimps and crabs: May cause chronic arsenic poisoning
3. Puffer fish: Cause tetradotoxin poisoning leading to vomiting, retching, lethargy, muscular weakness, fall of BP and respiratory distress.

Treatment

Symptomatic

POISONING FROM INGESTION OF CONTAMINATED FOOD WITH CHEMICALS

a. Contaminated with chemicals, intentionally added flavouring agents to processed food, mixing of preservatives or coloring agents to the food, use of hydrocarbon to extract fat from the food.

b. Accidentally added or contaminated with pesticides/insecticides.

c. Produced as a result of food processing, e.g. smoking of fleshy food.

d. Radionuclides.

22

War Gases: Chemical and Biological

The term 'War gases' includes **any chemical** (gaseous, liquid or solid) **or biological agents** which is used to cause destruction or damage mostly in times of war but does not includes explosives. **Warfare agents are the agents used to kill, injure or incapacitate the enemies mostly during war**. However, in civil conditions, these gases are used to disperse the unruly mob. When chemical substance is used, it is called 'chemical warfare', and when biological agent is used, it is called 'biological warfare'.

Chemical warfare: It is the warfare in which there is offensive use of chemical substance having toxic properties to kill, injure or incapacitate the enemies. A chemical used in this warfare is called **chemical weapon agent (CWA)**. About 70 different chemicals have been used or stocked piled as CWA during 90th century which may be in liquid gas or solid form, which are classified as weapon of mass destruction by the United Nations, and their production and stock piling was outlawed by the chemical weapon convention of 1993. Some substances are lethal, and some injure or incapacitate people. These agents are dispersed as tiny droplets through chemical shells, spray tanks, bombs and missiles. Harmful effects are caused when the chemical is inhaled, ingested or when it comes in contact with skin or mucous membrane.

There are other chemicals used in military operations that are **not technically considered to be CWA** such as:

1. **Defoliants:** That destroys vegetations. For example: Agent orange contained dioxin is known for its long-term cancer effects and for causing genetic damage leading to birth deformities.

2. **Incendiary/explosive chemicals:** Their destructive effects are primarily due to fire or explosive force and not direct chemical action. For example Napalm and dynamite

Classification of warfare agents

1. Lacrimators: Tear gases
2. Lung irritants: Asphixiant gases
3. Vesicants: Blistering gases
4. Sternutators: Nasal irritant
5. Paralysant: Nerve poison
6. Nerve gases: Acetylcholine like action

Biological warfare: It is the offensive use of living microorganisms to kill, injure or incapacitate the enemies. **Biological weapons (BW)** are defined as microorganisms or their products of metabolism that infect and grow in the target host producing a clinical disease that kills or incapacitates humans or animals. Such microbes may be natural, wild-type strains or may be genetically modified. These include biological toxins and substances that interfere with normal behavior, such as hormones, neuropeptides and cytokines (Table 22.1).

Biological warfare agents: *Bacillus anthracis*, small pox virus, botulinum toxin and ricin are commonly used biological agents followed by bacteria causing plague, cholera, typhus, brucellosis, Salmonella, ebola virus, abrin toxin, etc. Very small amounts of biologica

Table 22.1: Clinical manifestation of different warfare agents

Type	Examples	Signs and symptoms	Treatment
1. Lachrymators or tear gases (These are the tear gases and causes tearing of eyes)	Chloracetophenone (CAP) Bromobenzyl cyanide (BBC) Ethyliodoacetate (KSK) They are fired in artillery shells or pen guns	The vapors cause intense irritation of the eyes with a copious flow of tears, spasm of the eyelids and temporary blindness. They also cause irritation of air-passages. In long-continued exposure there may be nausea, vomiting and blistering of skin. The effects are transitory	1. Removed the patient to the fresh air 2. Eyes washed with warm normal saline or fresh water or boric acid 3. Application of weak solution of soda bicarb to the affected skin 4. IV aminophylline or salbutamol inhalation
2. Lung irritants or asphyxiants (These are the asphyxiant and causes choking of respiratory track)	Chlorine and phosgene chloropicrin and diphosgene Nitrous oxide, sulfur dioxide, ammonia (choking gases). They can be released from tanks, and gas shells. Phosgene is ten times and chloropicrin four times more toxic than chlorine	The signs and symptoms develops within 2–4 hours of inhalation. Lacrimation, conjunctivitis, coughing, dyspnea with intense air hunger with feeling of pain and tightness of chest. There is headache, vomiting, restlessness, stertorous breathing, cyanosis and collapse Death occurs in 24 to 48 hours due to acute pulmonary edema	1. Eye wash with boric acid. 2. Oxygen and adrenaline. 3. Antitussives. 4. Antibiotics. 5. Atropine for pulmonary edema.
3. Vesicant or blistering gases (These are the agents that causes blisters)	Mustard gas, lewisite (arsenic) sulfur, phosgene, oximes. They are discharged in artillery shells so as to saturate the area of attack	**Mustard gas** causes irritation of the eyes, nose, throat and respiratory passages. There is lacrimation, conjunctivitis, photophobia with nausea, vomiting and abdominal pain. There is intense itching, redness, vesication, and ulceration especially of the moist areas as it passes through the clothes into the skin. **Lewisite** causes rapid blister with inflammation of mucosa of larynx, trachea and bronchi. It also causes hemolysis, leucopenia and features similar to arsenic poisoning	1. Shift the patient to fresh air 2. Remove all clothing and wash the body with soap and water 3. Irrigation of eyes/nose with cold water/sodium bicarbonate solution 4. Wash the affected part with soda bicarb solution 5. BAL—in lewisite poisoning

(Contd...)

Table 22.1: Clinical manifestation of different warfare agents (*Contd...*)

Type	Examples	Signs and symptoms	Treatment
4. Sternutators or nasal irritants (These are the agents that are nasal irritant)	Diphenyl-chlorarsine (DA), Diphenylamine chlorarsine (DM), and diphenyl-cyanarsine (DC). DM (sickening gas) is about six times as heavy as air. These are solid, organic compounds of arsenic and are fired in artillery shells	The manifestation is due to inhalation or drinking of contaminated water. The vapors cause intense pain and irritation in the nose and sinuses. There is sneezing, headache, salivation, nausea, vomiting, tightness in the chest and prostration	1. Shift the patient to fresh air 2. Remove all clothing and wash the body with soap and water 3. Irrigation of eyes/nose with cold water/sodium bicarbonate solution
5. Paralysants	Hydrocyanic acid, hydrogen sulfide, carbon monoxide	Already described in respective chapters	Depends on the type of poisons
6. Nerve gases (These are the agents which have acetylcholine-like action. They inhibit the acetylcholinesterase)	GA (Tabun), GB (Sarin), GD (Soman) VE, VM and VX. The vapors are heavier than air, so they tend to sink into valleys, trenches and basements. They are colorless and odorless volatile liquids. They are the most toxic of the known chemical agents	They cause **inhibition of cholinesterase and produce features of acetylcholine poisoning** with constriction of pupil, choking, bronchial constriction and photophobia. Exposure to a large amount of vapor will cause loss of consciousness within seconds, followed by convulsions. Muscles become flaccid and breathing stops	Treatment is similar to organo-phosphates: 1. Decontamination 2. Irrigation of eyes/nose 3. Atropine 4. Oximes 5. Diazepam for convulsion
Chemical crowd control agents used by law-enforcement agencies and the military	Ortho-chlorobenzylidenemalano-nitrile (CS, tear gas), CN (Mace). Oleoresin capsaicin (pepper spray, OC) is an extract of hot peppers consisting of capsaicin. These agents are available in varying concentrations and several vehicles, in aerosols or fumes and vehicles, in particulate form with dispersal device. They are also available in grenades or canisters that can be propelled either by throwing or with a projectile device	**Eyes:** Burning, stinging or pain, conjunctivitis, lacrimation, transient impairment of vision **Nose and mouth:** Burning, stinging or pain, increased secretions **Skin:** Burning, stinging or pain, erythema **Respiratory tract:** Burning and irritation, increase secretions, coughing, tightness in the chest	1. Remove the patient to fresh air 2. Irrigation of eyes/nose with cold water/sodium bicarbonate solution

agents or toxins can cause mass casualties. The agents are odorless, tasteless and invisible to the naked eye. It is spread through aerosol spray, explosives or food or water contamination.

Precaution while handling the body: The body should be cleaned with **0.5%** hypochlorite or phenol disinfectant and transported to mortuary in an impermeable double bag. Certain bio-agents, such as small pox, tularaemia, viral hemorrhagic fever, ganders, Q fever, can be transmitted to persons performing autopsies. Collect blood, CSF and tissue samples or swabs for isolation of bacteria and virus.

Appendix

Table 1: Fatal dose, fatal period and antidote of different poisons

Poisons	Fatal dose	Fatal period	Antidotes
Inorganic strong acids	10–20 ml	12–24 hrs	CaO, MgO
Oxalic acid	10–15 gm	2–12 hrs	Lime, CaO, Ca-carbonate
Carbolic acid	10–20 gm	2–12 hrs	Magnesium sulfate
Alkalies	Hydroxides: 5–10 gm Carbonate: 15–30 gm	12–24 hrs	Weak acid, vinegar, citric acid
Phosphorus	50–100 mg	12 hrs to 1 week	Copper sulfate
Iodine	2 gm	24 hrs	Starch solution sodium thiosulfate
Arsenic	200 mg	24 hrs	Ferric oxide, BAL
Lead	20–30 gm	24 hrs	Mg/Na sulfate, calcium EDTA
Mercury	0.5–1 gm	2–3 days	Egg albumin, Na formaldehyde sulfoxylate, penicillamine, BAL
Copper	15–30 gm	2–3 days	Pot ferrocyanide, penicillamine
Potassium iodate/ $KMnO_4$	12–15 gm	–	Calcium chloride/gluconate
Iron–$FeSO_4$ tablets	10–5 tabs	–	Desferroxamine, deferiprone
Organophosphorus	30 mg to 60 gm	30 min to 3 hrs	Atropine, oximes
Organochlorine	30 mg to 5 gm	Within 24 hrs	–
Carbamates	–	Uncertain	Atropine
Pyrethroids	–	Uncertain	–
Alum/zinc phosphide	3–5 gm	12–24 hrs	–
Abrus precatorius	1–2 seeds	12 hrs to 3 days	Anti-abrin
Castor/croton/ semicarpus	6–8 seeds	12 hrs to 3 days	–
Poisonous snakes	6–12 mg	Cobra: 20 min Viper: 2–4 days	ASV serum
Opium/morphine	2 gm/100–200 mg	6–12 hrs	Naloxone/nalmefene
Ethyl alcohol	150 ml in non-addict	12–24 hrs	–
Methyl alcohol	60–120 ml	24–36 hrs	Ethyl alcohol, fomepizole
Formaldehyde	30–90 ml	12–24 hrs	Sodium bicarbonate
Fuels—kerosene	30 ml	A few hrs	Liquid paraffin
Datura/atropine	75–100 seeds; 60 mg	24 hrs	Physostigmine/pilocarpine
Cannabis	2–10 gm/kg body wt	12 hrs	–
Cocaine	1 gm	2hrs	Amyl nitrite inhalation
Barbiturates	4–5 gm	1–2 days	–
Benzodiazepines	5–10 gm/variable	1–2 days	Flumazenil
Nux vomica/strychnine	1–2 seeds/30–60 mg	30 min to 2 hrs	Barbiturates, d-tubocurarine
Conium plant	1 cm of any part	A few hrs	–
Curare	30–60 mg	1–2 hrs	Neostigmine/physostigmine
Hydrocyanic acid/salts	200 ppm/200 mg	Immediate/30 min	Nitrites/Na thiosulfate
Aconite	1 gm root	6 hrs	–
Oleander	15 gm root	24–36 hrs	–
Paracetamol	10 gm	–	N-acetyl cysteine, methionine

Table 2: Characteristic smell of poison

Typical smell	Poison
Garlicky	Arsenic (Arsine), OP, phosphorus, aluminium/zinc phosphide, selenium, thallium
Phenolic/sweetish	Carbolic acid
Vinegar	Acetic acid
Fruity	Alcohol
Kerosene/petrol	Petroleum products
Bitter almond	Cyanides
Burnt rope-like	Cannabis
Raw flesh	Opium
Kerosene/turpentine	Insecticidal poisons
Burnt coal gas	Carbon monoxide
Rotten egg	Hydrogen sulfide
Shoe polish	Nitrobenzene
Tobacco	Nicotine
Iodine	Iodine
Mothball	Naphthalene
Formalin	Formaldehyde

Table 3: Characteristic taste of poison

Typical taste	Poison
Sweet	Aconite, carbolic
Bitter	Datura, strychnine
Sour	Acids
Metallic	Metallic irritant

Table 4: Poison acting on enzyme system

1. Metallic irritants
2. Phosphorus
3. Organophosphorus
4. Carbamates
5. Cyanides

Table 5: Poison imparting different colors

1. Urine

Green	Phenol
Red	Lead (corpoporphyrin-3), cantharides, phenolphthalein
Orange	Rifampicin, phenothiazines
Blue	Methylene blue
Brown to black	Naphthalene, thymol
Pink	Aniline, eosin, mercury
Yellow	Arsine, dinitrophenol

2. Vomitus

Green	$CuSO_4$, copper arsenite, copper acetoarsenite
Blue	Iodine
Brown	Acid, alkali, zinc phosphide
Red	Lead tetraoxide/monoxide, mercury sulfide
Curdy white	Lead
Dark, luminous	Phosphorus

3. Stool

Dark, luminous	Phosphorus
Black	Lead
Colorless, watery	Arsenic

4. Tears

Red	OP (due to porphyrin)

Table 6: Skin manifestation in poisons

Skin manifestation	Poisoning
Dry skin	Datura
Moist skin/sweating	OP, opium, arsenic, pilocarpine
Flushing	Alcohol, datura, arsenic, cyanide,
Blister/vesicles	Barbiturates, viper bite, CO, semicarpus juice, calotropis, plumbago, croton oil, iodine, arsenic, mustard gas, lewisite gas
Petechiae, purpura, hemorrhagic lesion	Arsenic, phosphorus
Pigmentation	Arsenic
Hair loss	Arsenic
Hypothermia	Opiates, alcohol, barbiturates, CO
Hyperthermia	Datura, cocaine, strychnine

Table 7: Poison causing eye changes

1. Constriction of pupil	Opium/morphine, OP, carbolic, mushroom, cannabis
2. Dilatation of pupil	Datura/atropine, cyanides, cocaine, cannabis, CO, curare, conium
3. Alternate const/dilatation	Aconite, barbiturate
4. Nystagmus	Alcohol
5. Diplopia	Opium, cannabis, alcohol
6. Lacrimation	Irritant gases, OP, carbamates, pyrethroids
7. Ptosis	Snakebite—cobra, botulinism
8. Blindness	Methyl alcohol, chloroquine, arsenic, lead, mercury, tobacco, ergot
9. Photophobia	Irritant gas, iodine, nitric acid fumes

Table 8: Poison causing oral changes

1. Dryness of mouth	Datura, lead, cocaine
2. Excess of salivation	Corrosives, OP, carbamates, pyrethroids, vegetable irritants, aconite, scorpion bite
3. Stomatitis/glossitis	Cyanide, calotropis, iodine
4. Discoloration of gums/teeth	Blue-copper, mercury, lead, iron, thallium, silver; fluoride, tetracycline

Table 9: Poison causing GIT manifestation

1. Vomiting	Almost all poisons, copper sulfate is potent emetic
2. Diarrhea	Organic acids, alkalies, arsenic, food poisoning
3. Constipation	Inorganic acids, lead, opium
4. Gastroenteritis	Almost all local poison; arsenic, oleander, phosphorus
5. Abdominal pain	Corrosives, irritant, cocaine, iron, oleander, formaldehyde, kerosene
6. Thirst	Corrosives, arsenic, lead, phosphorus, atropine
7. Dysphagia/odynophagia	Corrosives, metallic poison

Table 10: Poison causing genitourinary system manifestation

1. Oliguria	Corrosives, arsenic, lead, mercury, copper, phosphorus
2. Polyuria	Alcohol, digitalis, mercury
3. Dysuria	Mushrooms, OP, arsenic
4. Hematuria	Organic corrosives, arsenic, mercury, lead, copper, phosphorus
5. Albuminuria	Organic corrosives, arsenic, mercury, lead, copper, phosphorus
6. Hemoglobinuria	Snake bite, acetic acid, arsenic, copper
7. Glycosuria	Morphine, anesthetic agents
8. Porphyrinuria	Lead, mercury

Table 11: Poison causing CVS manifestation

1. Bradycardia	OP, aconite, digitalis
2. Tachycardia	Datura, conium, cannabis, CO, amphetamine
3. Hypotension	OP, aconite, snake bite, arsenic
4. Hypertension	Amphetamine, zinc phosphide

Table 12: Poison causing RS manifestation

1. Dyspnea	CO, phosphine, irrespirable gases, strychnine, arsine
2. Pulmonary edema	OP, OC, snake bite, opium

Table 13: Poison causing CNS manifestation

1. Coma	Alcohol, CO, opium, organophosphorus
2. Convulsion	Strychnine, cyanides, phosphorus, arsenic, lead, copper, opium, datura, cobra bite, alcohol, OP, aconite, CO
3. Paralysis	Arsenic, lead, curare, conium
4. Paresthesia	Arsenic, lead, conium, alcohol, aconite, cannabis
5. Delirium	Datura, cannabis, cocaine, calotropis
6. Psychosis	Datura, cannabis, cocaine, alcohol

Table 14: Poison causing blood manifestation

1. Anemia	Arsenic, lead, copper
2. Leukocytosis	Snake poisoning
3. Leukopenia	Arsenic, lead, antimony
4. Hemolysis	Sea snakes, viper bite, copper sulfate, lead, arsenic
5. Methemoglobin	Nitrobenzene, mthylene blue, copper
6. Basophilic stippling	Lead, antimony, bismuth

OP	: Organophosphorus	OC	: Organochlorines
CO	: Carbon monoxide	GIT	: Gastrointestinal tract
CVS	: Cardiovascular system	RS	: Respiratory system
CNS	: Central nervous system		

Index